PRAISE FOR *DOCTOR DOGS*

"This is a fascinating book about the amazing ways dogs can, and do, help people with physical and emotional problems. The title isn't stretching the truth: They really are 'Doctor Dogs.' On the other hand—and I mean this as a compliment—they would make terrible lawyers."

—Dave Barry, Pulitzer Prize–winning, *New York Times* bestselling author of *Lessons from Lucy: The Simple Joys of an Old, Happy Dog* and dozens of other books

"Goodavage has done it again, with her fascinating investigation into the world of doctor dogs. Goodavage has expertly synthesized the latest scientific research on how dogs can even save us from invisible dangers lurking in our bodies. A testament to the extraordinary connection between dogs and ourselves, and one more piece of evidence that their love for us truly knows no bounds."

—Brian Hare, *New York Times* bestselling author of *The Genius of Dogs*

"*Doctor Dogs* is fascinating, beautifully researched and written—and deeply moving. Maria Goodavage takes the reader around the globe—from laboratories developing a better e-nose or working to understand what compounds dogs may be alerting to in cancer samples, to homes where service and detection dogs are saving the lives of their owners on a daily and even hourly basis, and to facilities doing sophisticated and nuanced training with dogs that have fine noses and love treats, toys, and praise. The reader will meet seizure-detection dogs, dogs who can detect the dangerous bacterium *C. diff*, and dogs who can calm their humans suffering from PTSD. Goodavage doesn't shy away from the training challenges, the sometimes disappointing study results, and the problems with dishonest organizations taking advantage of desperate families. But the reader comes away feeling hope and profound admiration for the complex new roles that dogs are playing in helping humans—and for the dedicated researchers, trainers, and owners who work tirelessly and lovingly with our best friends."

—Cat Warren, author of the *New York Times* bestseller *What the Dog Knows*

"It's often said that dogs are man's best friend, and *Doctor Dogs* depicts the healing power of canines in a very literal sense. I was completely enthralled by Goodavage's research and stories of dogs in the medical field, and in awe of its dramatic takeaways. This book is equally enlightening as it is heartwarming."

—Craig Grossi, author of *Craig & Fred: A Marine, a Stray Dog, and How They Rescued Each Other*

"Introducing us to a memorable international cast of dogs and their humans, *Doctor Dogs* captures how dogs are putting their natural abilities to work on behalf of human physical, neurological, and psychological health; explains the science behind these feats; opens a window into expanding possibilities for medical service dogs; and most of all honors the extraordinary social intelligence of dogs and the life-enhancing relationships people forge with them."

—Hilary Hinzmann, co-author, with John W. Pilley, of *Chaser: Unlocking the Genius of the Dog Who Knows a Thousand Words*

"Blending painstaking research with journalistic prowess, Maria Goodavage takes the reader into the inspirational world of 'canine clinicians,' highlighting the gifts of an exceptional nose and soulful eyes. Fetch a copy to be enlightened, humbled, and amazed, as Maria never loses sight of the most important intangible of all, the emotional connectivity we recognize and love in every dog."

—Nick Trout, *New York Times* bestselling author of *The Wonder of Lost Causes*

"If you're a dog lover, *Doctor Dogs* is bound to become one of your all-time favorite books. It's a hope-inspiring testament to the power of the human-animal bond—a bond that science is showing to be even more powerful than we ever suspected. You'll fall in love with every dog in this book, and you'll swoon with happiness and relief for all the humans they've helped. *Doctor Dogs* gets four paws up!"

—Laura T. Coffey, author of the national bestseller *My Old Dog: Rescued Pets with Remarkable Second Acts* and a senior writer and editor for *Today*

"If you take an amazing subject and put it in the hands of a wonderful writer, you get . . . SPOILER ALERT . . . a truly fantastic book. Every single page of Maria Goodavage's *Doctor Dogs* is made up of remarkable research and storytelling."

—David Rosenfelt, national bestselling author of *Dogtripping* and thirty-one other books

"*Doctor Dogs* is a captivating, groundbreaking, meticulously researched book about the incredible new ways dogs are sniffing out disease and helping people with physical and mental health issues. Maria Goodavage, who has been writing beloved books about dogs for thirty years, brings readers behind the scenes around the world and immerses them in the fascinating, cutting-edge research dogs are doing, as well as the riveting stories of how doctor dogs are saving the lives of their humans every day. You'll laugh, you'll cry, you'll want to hug the nearest dog! (The life a doctor dog saves may one day be your own.)"

—Dr. Marty Becker, "America's Veterinarian," founder of FearFreeHappyHomes.com

"Maria Goodavage takes the reader on a fascinating journey to uncover the amazing things dogs can do for their human friends. From canines that calm the veteran with PTSD and the child called upon to face her tormentor in court, through dogs that sniff out cancers, malaria, and other diseases, to the dogs' finding unprecedented roles supporting people with autism, schizophrenia, and myriad other ailments. Goodavage shows that there are many people who, when they say, 'My dog saved my life,' mean this, not in some metaphorical sense, but in a completely concrete way: without their dog they would not be alive, or certainly their lives would be greatly constrained. Along the way, Goodavage is a witty and compassionate guide, and supremely well-informed. I learned a lot!"

—Professor Clive Wynne, director of the Canine Science Collaboratory at Arizona State University and author of *Dog Is Love: Why and How Your Dog Loves You*

ALSO BY MARIA GOODAVAGE

Soldier Dogs

Top Dog

Secret Service Dogs

DOCTOR DOGS

✚

HOW OUR BEST FRIENDS
ARE BECOMING
OUR BEST MEDICINE

MARIA GOODAVAGE

DUTTON

DUTTON

An imprint of Penguin Random House LLC
penguinrandomhouse.com

Previously published in a Dutton hardcover edition in October 2019

First Dutton trade paperback edition: November 2020

THE LIBRARY OF CONGRESS HAS CATALOGUED THE HARDCOVER EDITION AS FOLLOWS:
Names: Goodavage, Maria, 1962– author.
Title: Doctor dogs: how our best friends are becoming our best medicine / Maria Goodavage.
Description: New York: Dutton, an imprint of Penguin Random House, LLC, [2019] | Includes bibliographical references and index.
Identifiers: LCCN 2019004511 | ISBN 9781524743048 (hardcover) | ISBN 9781524743055 (ebook)
Subjects: LCSH: Dogs—Therapeutic use. | Service dogs. | Human-animal relationships.
Classification: LCC RM931.D63 G66 2019 | DDC 615.8/5158—dc23
LC record available at https://lccn.loc.gov/2019004511

Dutton trade paperback ISBN: 9781524743062
1 3 5 7 9 10 8 6 4 2

Book design by Nancy Resnick

To Laura Altair,
Keep reaching for the stars, and always remember to look at the world
with twinkling eyes. And to floss.
Love,
Your proud mother,
Mama

CONTENTS

DOCTOR
DOGS

THE DOCTOR'S NOSE

The dog nose arrived at my house in a box that said it contained a Corelle eighteen-ounce soup/cereal bowl. At the time, I had no idea what was actually inside. Gus barked the UPS truck good riddance while I checked the name on the return address. It was definitely not a bowl.

It had been weeks since Matthew Staymates, PhD, a fluid dynamicist and mechanical engineer with the National Institute of Standards and Technology (NIST), had said he would send me something interesting. It felt like Christmas in May as I drew the knife in a shallow track along the tape. The top of the box popped open like double doors to reveal a wad of crinkly brown paper. What could it be?

Gus was curious, too. He stood by me at the kitchen counter, his yellow Lab face smiling, his big brown eyes glancing from me to the package and back to me.

Open it! Open it! What did we get?!

I pulled away one corner of the paper, then the next. Something white and cylindrical peeked out. It looked like a cup. A *cup*? I ripped through the rest of the paper.

In my hands I now held a heavy-duty hard plastic replica of a dog's nose. Not some cheap costume-shop version, but a 3-D-printed model of the exterior of a real dog's snout, life-size. It was all white except for the soft black rhinarium (the cold wet part of a dog's nose), with a perfect rendition of the nostrils, down to the little curvy slits on the side.

The inside of this particular nose was mostly hollow. It wasn't anything like the intricate interior anatomy that makes a real dog's nose such a superb sniffer. When I held it with the nostril end facing down, it looked like a strange Japanese teacup that would never balance on a table. "NIST" was written in it with a Sharpie.

From my interviews with Dr. Staymates, I knew he had created this nose himself on a 3-D printer. He used CAD (computer-aided design) files that had been supplied to him by fellow fluid dynamicist Brent Craven, PhD, who had created models of the complex *inside* of this same dog's nose.*

Compared with Dr. Craven's model, this nose was simplicity itself. And yet even this simple structure has been shown to vastly improve detection of odors when applied to a "sniffing" system. When Dr. Staymates and his colleagues used a similar design on a vapor detection system and had it mimic the way dogs sniff—inhaling and exhaling about five times a second rather than just drawing in air—vapor detection improved sixteen-fold.

This kind of canine biomimicry, when put to use with technology that already exists, could have far-reaching effects for future scent detection. As Dr. Staymates and his colleagues wrote in *Scientific Reports,* "These lessons learned from the dog may benefit the next-generation of vapor samplers for explosives, narcotics, pathogens, or even cancer . . ."

The mere shape of the outside of a dog's sniffer can lead to possibly lifesaving technologies? This was my cup of nose.

---

*Who was this dog whose nose went under the proverbial scientific Xerox machine? She was a Labrador retriever whose head Dr. Craven and Dr. Staymates had received when they were roommates in grad school at Penn State and doing research at the gas dynamics laboratory. They were working on ways to improve detection of explosives and narcotics, and wanted to get a really good computer model of the "amazing chemical detector" that is a dog's nose. They kept the Lab's head in a refrigerator in formaldehyde until they could make an MRI model of the inside and outside of her head and nose.

I've been writing about dogs for thirty years. It's been a joy to be able to focus part of my journalism career on these loyal, fun, intelligent, beautiful creatures. And now is an especially exciting time to be writing and reading about dogs. Never has there been so much interest in the hearts, minds, and noses of dogs as there is today.

As I wrote this book, I kept the nose on an empty corner of my large desk. It stared at me with its soft plastic nostrils, cheering me on and reminding me of a key theme at the core of the book.

Dogs can smell in parts per trillion. Craig Angle, PhD, codirector of Canine Performance Sciences at Auburn University's College of Veterinary Medicine, likens this to being able to sniff out a teaspoon of a chemical in a million gallons of water—or the equivalent of nearly two Olympic swimming pools.

Our own sense of smell is much better than most of us think it is. But we're limited. Dogs have a big advantage by virtue of their olfactory anatomy. We have about six million olfactory receptors in our noses. Dogs have up to three hundred million. They sniff in 3-D, with each nostril sampling air separately, which helps them locate a scent. And the brains of dogs are better equipped to make sense of the scents.

Yet as good as they are, dogs don't rank among the best sniffers in the world, at least when measuring olfactory receptor genes. In a Japanese study of thirteen mammals, African elephants had twice as many functional olfactory receptor genes as dogs. Also ranking above dogs were rats, mice, cows, and horses. Humans placed just barely above other primates, which had the lowest number of genes associated with smell in the study. The researchers didn't include bears, which are known to have a phenomenal sense of smell. Sharks and other nonmammals known for their olfactory abilities also weren't part of the study.

Even if canines aren't the olfactory superstars of our planet, they're top dog when it comes to working alongside us to detect scent. They've long been our faithful assistants for jobs like explosives and narcotics detection, search and rescue, hunting, human tracking, bedbug detection, sniffing for cell phones in prisons, and rooting out certain foods from luggage at airports.

They've recently been helping humans in unprecedented ways. The list of jobs involving a dog's sense of smell continues to expand as training techniques and our knowledge of dogs improve.

Dogs are searching for the feces of several species listed as vulnerable, threatened, or endangered, including orcas, tigers, giant anteaters, jaguars, and certain bears and wolves. This helps conservationists keep track of everything from the populations of these animals to their illnesses and diets. Dog noses are also tracking down water leaks in Western Australia, rhino poachers in Africa, cremated remains,* old bones of interest to archaeologists, elephant tusks, counterfeit money, and ancient artifacts.

And recently dogs have been using their olfactory skills on something that might prove most important of all: our health. Scientists and top-notch trainers are working together around the world to help canines help us with some of our biggest health concerns—everything from early cancer detection to diabetes control to stopping the spread of deadly bacteria. The dogs in this book are on the cutting edge of science.

Some of these coveted "biodetection" dogs work in homes, as service dogs. Others are regular pets whose people bring them into training centers and laboratories (which are truly fun places) to help researchers uncover the scents of disease. Most of the dogs in this book rely on their noses for their jobs, although many of the service dogs use a variety of senses.

Traditional service dog jobs like guiding the blind and helping the hearing impaired will always be in demand. But the world of the new "doctor dogs" is using the talents of dogs in ways we never would have dreamed of at the beginning of this century.

---

*Dogs who sniff cremated remains ("cremains") have unfortunately been extra busy lately because of the wildfires in the West. The dogs are not looking for fire victims, but for the cremated remains of the loved ones of people who lost their homes. These dogs can swiftly find cremains—whether or not the urn survived—under up to several inches of ash.

. . .

Some dogs use their noses for a living.

Gus smells for a living.

There is a difference.

It seems to be Gus's calling to want to *become* certain scents. Or at least to wear them in style. If he really likes something, he'll do his best to get it all over his body. This is usually accomplished by rolling in the scent, or at least sliding into it with his head and shoulders.

Gus is selective about the substances he likes to wear. They're usually one of two categories: poop or dead animals. He will roll in grass, like normal dogs, but only if it has a specimen from one of these categories.

Sometimes he also goes for urine. In Golden Gate Park, we often pass by the police horse stables on our walks. Lately we've been coming across mounds of used straw near the corral. The first time we encountered one, Gus sniffed the air and dived into it, joyfully rolling and scratching his back for a few seconds, standing up, and crashing into it again.

I laughed to myself about him having a literal roll in the hay. But Gus got the last laugh, because as we continued our walk, I noticed a wretched stench—like used diapers festering in a bin. I sniffed and looked around for the source because I couldn't shake it. Then I realized it was emanating from the bouncy, grinning Labrador retriever, and the stink was old horse urine.

Why, Gus, *why?*

I later learned that some wolves like to roll in the poop of carnivores such as cougars or black bears. And gray foxes seek areas frequented by male mountain lions and rub their faces in it. Could it be a form of camouflage? Some researchers think so. Others think it might be a way of carrying the odors of their journey back to the pack—kind of like the canine version of Instagram or Facebook.

Maybe. Or something else? On a sunny mid-February hike along a rugged leashes-optional coastal trail about fifteen minutes south of home, Gus cantered off ahead about twenty feet and threw himself down into something I couldn't see. When I caught up with him a few seconds later, he had just completed a thorough body rub on his left side.

"Gus!"

He stood up and looked at me.

Yeah, I know, can you believe I found this? It's so great, isn't it?!

I looked where he had been rolling and saw what had lured him. It had the familiar shape of feces, but consisted primarily of a former animal, or part of one. It was hairy, twisted, and dark gray.

Coyote poop.

Gus beamed. He held his head high and wagged his tail in the same proud way he does when gets a new bone or ball. It struck me that he felt like he was now part coyote (not that I read into my dog's behaviors or anything).

A little way down the trail, as I was admiring the ocean view, he plowed to the ground again, left shoulder first. This time it was a pile of fresh horse manure. When I stopped him, he stood up and seemed just as thrilled as he had with the coyote-poop incident. Now he was part horse, part coyote, and part Gus.

As we came to other dogs on the trail, he approached them in a different manner than normal—still friendly, but with a *check ME out* vibe. Sure enough, the dogs would run up to him and sniff Gus—this multi-animal wonder. They lingered on his left side, where he apparently smelled of both horse and coyote. (Thankfully, unlike during the horse-urine incident, his odor wasn't obvious to the human nose.)

The older dogs would move along after a good inspection, but the younger dogs followed him around, sniffing more, wagging fast—clearly in admiration of this cool guy. He seemed to revel in the attention, walking slowly by them and standing with his left side for them to ogle again with their noses.

When we got home, the hose came out and washed away his hard-won glory.

. . .

I've often wondered if Gus could be a detection dog of some sort if he had the training. He's only three years old, and he has the nose for it, a high drive for a reward of food or a ball, and he enjoys learning new skills. But what kind of detection would he do?

For personal reasons, it would be handy to me if he could be a cancer-detection dog. Even just a self-trained one.

When it comes to cancer detection, I have a dog in this fight— skin in the game. Or, actually, body parts in the game. In 2001, after a lifetime of radiant health, my amazing mom, Evelyn DeMagistris Goodavage, was diagnosed with stage IIIC ovarian cancer at age sixty-eight, seemingly out of the blue. A large mass was discovered during a routine annual checkup. There had been no sign of anything amiss during her previous exams.

Less than two years later, after two massive surgeries, chemo-therapy, and a cruise through the Panama Canal, Mom was gone.

I would later discover that a few relatives on the Italian side of the family died from this cancer. I did the genetic tests my doctor recommended, and nothing came up as positive. But the geneticists still think I'm at high enough risk for the disease that I should consider preventative surgery. This is not something I want to have to do.

The problem is that, as with several other cancers, there's no good early screening for ovarian cancer. The American College of Obste-tricians and Gynecologists issued a statement saying, "Unfortunately, the existing evidence does not support any test to effectively screen for ovarian cancer. More research is still needed . . . [A]t this time, there is no effective strategy for ovarian cancer screening. Available ovarian cancer screening tests . . . are neither accurate nor reliable to screen asymptomatic women for early ovarian cancer."

Ovarian cancer is known as "the silent killer." Often there are no symptoms, or if there are, they're so common—like bloating, indiges-tion, and lower back pain—it's easy to attribute them to something more benign. As a result, most cases of ovarian cancer are found in later stages, when survival rates are low. It's the fifth-leading cause of cancer deaths in women in the United States.

Living without a cancer safety net can be unnerving. I try not to think about it. But in the beginning of researching this book, I drove up to the In Situ Foudation, in Chico, California, to meet with Dina Zaphiris, a dog trainer who was involved in one of the earliest studies using dogs to detect cancer. And I did something I'm embarrassed to admit.

Dina's star dog, Stewie, an Australian shepherd, has been trained to detect the presence of breast and ovarian cancer in laboratory samples. As you'll see throughout the book, scientists think that dogs who detect cancer and other diseases or conditions may be picking up on volatile organic compounds (VOCs).

In a nutshell, VOCs are chemical substances released into the air. They can be natural or man-made. You may have heard of this term in relation to paints or solvents, but scientists reported in the *Journal of Breath Research* that they detected 1,840 VOCs in healthy humans. (They considered breath, saliva, blood, milk, skin secretions, urine, and feces.) Dogs like Stewie seem to be able to detect disease-specific VOCs.

Stewie is just a regular dog most of the time, enjoying a hearty belly rub or a chase around the pasture as much as any canine. But Dina explained that sometimes Stewie finds it hard to find the "off" switch outside In Situ's research facility—a pleasant farm-style building on the outskirts of town.

Stewie sometimes approaches people on her own, sits down, and paws at them repeatedly—much as she would do with a cancer sample in the laboratory. Dina tries to discourage this and moves Stewie along. But she said it's something Stewie seems compelled to do.

This puts Dina in a tough spot. Could Stewie be smelling cancer? Should she let the person know the possible significance of Stewie's pawing, just in case? She told me she's been hesitant to say anything, but if the situation allows, she will sometimes mention Stewie's line of work. On several occasions, she's learned that the person Stewie sought out does have cancer. Still, Dina doesn't like to assign any status to Stewie's occasional moonlighting.

"It's not at all scientific. There are so many factors at play," she says. "These dogs are trained on samples, not people."

I couldn't wait to meet Stewie, in part because this would be my first in-person encounter with a biodetection dog for this book.

There was another reason for my excitement. But I couldn't tell Dina. She'd never approve. This had to be between Stewie and me.

On a sunny winter afternoon, I pulled into the driveway of In Situ's training center. Dina was busy wrapping up a session, so an assistant came out to greet me. At her heels was a fluffy Australian shepherd. Stewie! I was in luck.

As Stewie trotted closer, I could see that one of her eyes was brown, the other half light blue and half brown, almost right down the middle. She held me in her gaze, her striking eye taking me in, her nostrils doing a little jig. I held my breath and steeled myself, with only one thought.

Please do not give me your paw.

My hope is that one day dogs will lead us to early detection of all kinds of cancers for which there is no "gold standard" test. But for now, just this once, I had an impromptu appointment with a talented early pioneer in this field.

To my relief, Stewie did not paw at me. She rolled over for a belly rub, then sidled close for a snuggle and ran off to greet another visitor. I realize her lack of signaling meant nothing and wasn't based on science in the least. But still, it felt reassuring.

Gus may never be a cancer-detection dog, but he enriches my life in so many ways that I'm sure I'm healthier for it. When I'm having a bad day, I can talk to him and he'll listen. Always. He loves me when I'm on a tight deadline and look like the Creature from the

Black Lagoon as much as he does when I'm my more kempt self. (At least he pretends to.) He makes sure I get out in fresh air for long walks. He's always good for a snuggle. He's by my side when I take sick. And he makes me laugh.

Of course, he's not perfect. He's the reason the plastic nose now sits on a shelf instead of my desk. One afternoon I came home from the gym and he greeted me at the front door with something in his mouth. He always brings people gifts upon their return, so this was no surprise.

"What did you get me, Gus?"

He fast-wagged in joyful circles. I saw a flash of nostrils.

Not his nostrils.

"Drop it."

He stopped prancing and opened his mouth. The hard plastic nose thudded to the floor, landing nostrils up.

I rinsed off the slobber and placed it on a shelf above my desk. Gus can't reach it and doesn't seem to care about it anymore. He's been there, done that.

Most of the doctor dogs in this book go through extensive training to do their jobs—the canine version of medical school, minus student debt. It can take years to get seizure dogs or cancer-detection dogs ready for doing their precision work. But some rare dogs—clever pets—just wing it, somehow figuring out what's amiss at home and telling their people about it as best they can.

While trainers and scientists from around the world spoke different languages and were working toward unique goals, they all had approaches that respected the dogs as collaborators. The training was all carrot, no stick. Rewards of toys and sometimes treats were given with love and enthusiasm. If a dog missed something in training, no biggie. The dog didn't get the reward but was encouraged to try again.

With rare exceptions, the dogs I saw seemed to be crazy about their jobs. Those who work as service dogs were profoundly devoted to their mission and their people. The dogs who go to research centers to find disease in laboratory samples were equally excited about their work. They approached their tasks with the kind of focus and enthusiasm that managers wish their employees would have.

As I traveled, I interviewed dozens of people and watched their dogs at work. Whatever the culture, dogs smoothly, happily fit the needs, emotions, and lives of their humans.

In Japan, mobility-assistance dogs are sometimes trained to open packets of chopsticks and help pry them apart for people with limited hand mobility. Some can unwrap rice balls. Naoto Anzue, paralyzed from the chest down, drove me around Tokyo with his ultra-chill service dog, a yellow Lab named Dante. Dante flanked him as we ascended Tokyo Tower, had no fear of looking down the dizzying heights, navigated packed elevators calmly, and was a perfect gentleman as we later toured Edo Castle—better than some of the tourists.

In Amsterdam, I watched guide dogs learn to navigate the dizzying lanes of bicycle traffic. With more than 880,000 bikes in the city—four times the number of cars—it's easy to stumble into bike territory if you don't know what you're doing. The dogs were brilliant.

In Croatia, I witnessed a beautiful service dog—a happy golden retriever named Freddi—as he balanced the needs of the twin teenage boys in his care, no matter what the weather, the pressures of school, or the boys' condition. Leone and Renato Brašnić have had cerebral palsy since age two. Freddi helps them with some mobility issues and always seems to know when they're sick—even before they know. The night before one of these bright, personable boys shows symptoms, Freddi will snuggle up to that boy and stay near for the duration.

"The medicine Freddi brings our family goes so much beyond the job he's trained to do," said their mother, Zeljka. "He fits our family perfectly and fills our souls with such happiness."*

---

*Freddi is mostly angelic, but he is in cahoots with the family's giant cats, who

This book is divided into three parts. In the first section, you'll meet dogs who are detecting cancer and Parkinson's disease, and dogs who alert their people to seizures, diabetic lows or highs, and other life-threatening physical ailments. The second section features doctor dogs who are stepping into new fields such as sleep disorders, and even protecting us from antibiotic-resistant bugs and potential epidemic catastrophe. In the third part, we'll look at the dogs helping people who are struggling with debilitating mental health problems such as anxiety, depression, schizophrenia, and post-traumatic stress disorder in its many guises.

The service dogs in this book are top dogs. They perform their jobs exquisitely. I don't write about dogs with such poor training that they're little more than glorified pets, and I don't go into the stories of people who have spent a fortune on those dogs. But it happens, and it's heartbreaking. There are well-meaning trainers out there who may not be producing great dogs, and there are some organizations that are considered moneymaking scams. Please do your homework diligently if you're in the market for a service dog.

I also don't get into the minefield that is service dog law and "fake" service dogs. This book is about dogs and what we are learning from them. It's not about law. I'll leave that for others to tackle.

But there will be a few cats. Cats have refined senses of smell. One study showed they might beat dogs in a couple of olfactory traits. As befits the feline stereotype of independence, cats who have alerted their people to health problems weren't trained by anyone. They figured it out for themselves. So far I haven't heard about any cats who have been taught to detect human illness, but cat experts think that with early socialization and training, it could well happen. In which case, my next book will be called *Clinician Cats*.

They'd be joining a growing parade of other animals already

---

fling him treats from the tables when they can get away with it, and once even batted a loaf of bread down to him.

ensconced in the biodetection field. African giant pouched rats (sur-prisingly cute critters, known for their brains and trainability) do an excellent job rapidly sniffing sputum samples for tuberculosis—one of the top ten causes of death worldwide.* Mice have been trained to detect bird flu in duck poop. Genetically modified fruit flies can ac-curately detect breast cancer cells using their olfactory senses.

Even worms seem to be able to detect cancer. While in Japan, I spent some time at Hirotsu Bio Science outside Tokyo. Researchers there are developing a cancer-screening method based on their finding that nematodes can detect the smell of cancerous cells. I watched as several wee worms waggled their way toward a dot of urine from someone with cancer, and away from a dot of urine from someone without cancer. The race to the mini pee pool took place in a petri dish. To the naked eye there wasn't a lot of action. But as I stared through a microscope, it was clear that these were worms with a mission.

I wanted to interview them and ask them just one question: "*Why?*"

It's a question I don't have to ask doctor dogs.

"These working dogs share a tight emotional bond with their han-dler. Consequently, they find working together with a person they love tremendously satisfying," says Clive Wynne, PhD, a behavioral scientist who directs the Canine Science Collaboratory at Arizona State University. "In modern working dogs we see the powerful con-nection that underscores everything about dogs' lives with us."

Could it be love?

The scientific jury is still out on whether dogs truly feel love. Some canine cognition experts say yes, dogs do love us. Others are careful not to ascribe such an emotion to them. This book leans heavily on science, but rather than try to sort this out logically and academically, I will come right out and admit my bias: Of course dogs feel love.

---

*A note about the rats: These TB-detection rats, along with rats that detect land-mines, are nicknamed HeroRATs by APOPO, the organization that trains them. One of my favorite rat music videos is about the HeroRATs that detect landmines. If you do a search for "hero rats song," it should pop right up. (It's really catchy. Don't blame me if you can't stop singing.)

And if you're holding some shredded chicken in your hand, all the better.

I asked Dr. Wynne for his opinion. He answered: "I think the secret to dogs' success with people is their extravagant capacity for forming strong emotional connections with members of other species. In my scientific writing I call this 'hypersociability' or 'exaggerated gregariousness,' but it is the same thing that laypeople simply call love. Love is the essence of what makes dogs who they are."

PART I

STAYING ALIVE

CHAPTER 1

STOP THE ROLLER COASTER, I WANT TO GET OFF

Dogs and Diabetics

In 1674, English physician and anatomist Thomas Willis was struck by the sweet smell and taste of the urine of people with diabetes. He added the word "mellitus"—whose root is Latin for "honey"—to the disease's name. He eventually devoted a chapter in a book to "the pissing evil" and wrote that the urine of diabetics was "wonderfully sweet as if it were imbued by honey or sugar."

How did he know? By sipping the sweet golden cocktail himself. (From Willis's description, you wonder if maybe he liked it a little *too* much. It sounds like he's describing a late-harvest Semillon for *Wine Spectator* rather than someone's pee.)

Willis wasn't the first doc to tipple tinkle to make a diagnosis. In fact, he was a latecomer to the notion that diabetes can manifest in sweet-tasting and sweet-smelling urine. But he was English, and relatively recent compared with the others, so he got to give it the name it has today.

He probably didn't know that in the fifth century BCE, the Indian physician Sushruta had already used the term "*madhumeha*" ("honey urine") in a medical treatise to identify diabetes. Sushruta described the urine's sweet taste and its ability to—are you ready for this?—attract ants.*

---

*It's easy to imagine one of his patients in ancient India crouching in the dirt to

In the year 643, Chinese physician Chen Chuan once again noted the sweet taste of urine. And there were other notable physicians who made the same observation.

Back in the day, tasting and smelling urine for disease was commonplace. Luckily for busy medieval doctors, there was a tool called a urine wheel, a zodiac-like diagram associating various smells and tastes and appearances of urine with different diseases. So when physicians noted an odd smell in their patients' "water," diagnosing it didn't require reinventing the wheel; they just had to reach out to their own wheel of misfortune.

Happily for modern-day doctors, tests for diabetes no longer involve their noses and taste buds. But it makes you think: If some people can identify diabetes using their senses, it's got to be a slam dunk for dogs and their phenomenal sense of smell.

We don't need to use dogs' talents to diagnose diabetes since simple tests can do that. Far more valuable is the ability of trained dogs to tell their insulin-dependent humans (type 1 diabetics) if their blood sugar is becoming too low and, in some cases, too high.* Their work, when done well, can mean the difference between life and death. All they ask in return is a favorite toy or treat, and some heartfelt words to the effect of "gooooood dawwwwg!"

———

Clay Ronk couldn't get enough to drink. If he wasn't filling up at the sink, he was pouring something from the fridge—usually lemonade, but he really craved Tang. Even in his sleep, his mother heard him calling out, "Tang, Tang, tangy Tang, Mama!" He was irritable, too.

---

relieve her bladder and praying that a fast-responding parade of ants didn't catch up with her midstream. Sushruta's observation still holds true. Ants do seem to like the sweetness of diabetic urine. An article by a doctor in the Philippines notes that ants congregating in unflushed toilets, around splashed urine, or in hampers with soiled underpants "may be the initial sign that blood sugar is abnormally elevated."

*Some organizations will consider training dogs for type 2 diabetes, but since the far more urgent need is for insulin-dependent diabetics, most train dogs only for those with type 1 diabetes.

And losing weight. The seven-year-old wet his bed for the first time since he was out of diapers.

This wasn't how his folks had pictured the end of summer vacation. They figured maybe it was the stress of a new school year, though he wasn't the kind of kid who got anxious about school. He seemed OK otherwise, so they didn't worry that much.

A couple of weeks into third grade, the school secretary left a message at his house saying Clay was sick and needed to go home. His mom, Karin, was working nights as a dispatcher for the Ukiah, California, police and fire departments, and had been asleep just a couple of hours when she heard the answering machine go off. *You're kidding. Something's going around already?* she thought as she zombied herself out of bed and drove to school.

The boy she found in the school office seemed like a different child than the one she'd kissed good night before she left for work. His eyes were sunken like a tired old man's. His skin was gray. The peach fuzz on his face stood out because he was so drawn.

She took him home and tucked him into bed. It was her day off, so she was able to stay home and check on him. A couple of times she found him lying on the floor, barely responding to questions. The next time he'd be back up in his bed. His grandmother came by and was concerned because Clay didn't seem like himself—even a normal sick version of himself.

That night Clay wanted to sleep in his parents' room. Karin made him a bed on the floor next to her. He didn't stir all night. In the morning Karin had a hard time waking him up. This was unusual because Clay was normally an early riser. He didn't seem to notice his dad, Ken, stepping over him as he got ready for work. Ken tried to play with him to see if Clay was OK enough to go to school. Karin could tell he wasn't, and told Ken to let him rest.

Karin had to run an important errand and couldn't leave Clay at home alone, sick, so she brought him with her. She had to help him walk to the car as he leaned against her. Once at the destination, he was unable to get out of the car on his own, much less walk. Karin realized this was beyond the fatigue of a virus. She called the pediatrician and was told to bring him right in.

An "ancient" doctor they'd never seen before hurried into the examining room and told them he was in a rush to deliver breech twins. He pinched Clay's arm and said Clay was extremely dehydrated, ordered blood work, and sent them on their way.

After the blood draw, they headed home. A couple of hours later, Clay was resting on the couch and watching cartoons. The phone rang. It was the pediatrician. He told Karin that Clay's lab work had come back and his blood sugar was 870.

"Do you know what that means?"

Karin did, since a good friend had type 1 diabetes. She knew how dangerously high that number was. She felt a rush of panic.

"You need to get him to the emergency room right away. We'll call ahead and let them know you're coming."

Normal blood glucose is about 70 to 130 mg/dL, a little higher after meals. Levels above 300 are considered much too high. Clay's glucose level, combined with other test results, revealed he was in diabetic ketoacidosis (DKA)—a serious condition that can cause severe dehydration, coma, swelling of the brain, and death.

As soon as Clay and his mother got to the Ukiah Valley Medical Center, Clay's medical team dived in to try to normalize his glucose level using insulin and intravenous fluids. But his veins had collapsed because of dehydration. Clay was already upset by all the painful poking. When a nurse said they were going to have to put a PICC (peripherally inserted central catheter) line in his neck to get the insulin and fluids in and the blood out for testing, he screamed and writhed and had to be held down.

"Can't you say it in a language this poor boy doesn't understand or put the line in his foot?!" Karin said. She asked for the best nurse in the unit. They summoned her, and she inserted the PICC into Clay's foot without much fuss.

They tested his glucose with a finger prick every thirty minutes, but it wasn't decreasing the way they'd hoped. The staff decided to send Clay to the University of California, San Francisco (UCSF) Medical Center. Stat. The Ukiah hospital wasn't set up to deal with this level of diabetic emergency.

Without traffic it's about a two-hour drive—somewhat faster by ambulance—but in the San Francisco Bay Area there's rarely a time without traffic. Karin hoped one of the ambulance teams she worked with would be able to take him. Hospital staff told her if Clay's blood sugar dropped under 499, which was the highest a meter in the emergency room could read, he could go by ground transportation.

Karin phoned work and told her supervisor what she needed. A call went out via radio for the transport. That crew stood by for almost seven hours waiting for his blood sugar to dip below 499, but it never came close.

He needed to go by air. Clay arrived by ambulance at the airport and was transferred to the waiting plane. A doctor and a nurse were aboard, ready to take over his care.

"I can go with him, right?" Karin said. Clay was in and out of consciousness. She couldn't let him go without her.

The pilot told her that the Cessna 414 could take only another hundred pounds. Karin weighed more. The pilot said there was one way around this if she was bent on traveling in the plane.

"Mom, you'll have to sign a form that if the plane goes down, we're not liable."

That didn't seem like a good idea. Her son's blood sugar needed to go down, not his plane. She would drive with Ken. They watched the plane take off. Then they sped to San Francisco, not talking, just trying to get through each interminable minute until they could see their son again.

A roomful of doctors and nurses worked on Clay throughout the night in the pediatric ICU at UCSF. He had been at the edge of the abyss, but by the next afternoon they had pulled him back.

The dramatic beginning of Clay's life with type 1 diabetes

mellitus gave way to a jarringly quiet time. A nurse came into his room with a stack of books on the disease and said Karin and Ken were responsible for reading them while at the hospital. Clay's blood sugar was coming down, and he was sleeping. They had the time they needed to focus on the flood of information they had to digest in order to keep their son alive.

The next day they got a hands-on education in insulin dosing, insulin injection, blood sugar testing, and everything they'd learned in the books. Ken doesn't do well with blood and needles, but he tried his hardest for his son.

The life of a type 1 diabetic is an exhausting continual high-wire act where it's too easy to lose balance. It's a never-ending cycle of blood testing several times a day, calculating how much insulin to give based on carbohydrate intake and activity level. Too much insulin can be just as harmful as too little, resulting in hypoglycemia severe enough to cause seizures, comas, and death. Even with the latest high-tech options of continuous glucose monitoring (CGM) systems and insulin pumps, nothing is predictable or easy in diabetes. What seems to work one day might tank the next.

Most people who see a type 1 diabetic have no idea what's going on behind the scenes to keep him or her healthy enough to function. It's usually an invisible disability, revealed only by a glimpse of a small device attached to someone's body, or a fingertip blood test done as unobtrusively as possible.

Type 1 diabetes is one of the most common chronic diseases of childhood, although it can start well into adulthood. About forty thousand people are diagnosed in the US each year. But type 1 diabetes accounts for only 5 percent of the more than thirty million Americans living with diabetes, according to the Centers for Disease Control. Type 2 diabetes is far more common.

Unlike type 1, type 2 diabetes can often be controlled by exercise and diet. Well-meaning people frequently tell type 1 diabetics about the right kind of diet and exercise that will halt their disease. But type 1 diabetes is not a lifestyle disease. And there is no cure for it.

Clay's parents tried not to feel overwhelmed after their crash course. As they drove home with Clay a few days later, they hoped they would not fail their upcoming real-life tests in Diabetes Survival 101.

Shortly after Clay's eighth birthday, Karin read an article about an organization called Dogs4Diabetics, in Concord, California. The diabetic-alert dogs it was producing seemed like miracle workers. She showed the article to Clay. His eyes grew large.

"Mom, a dog could help me?"

"Yes, I really think so."

She applied the next day and got an immediate reply saying applicants have to have lived with diabetes for a year. Disappointing, but doable. They waited until the one-year anniversary of his diagnosis and applied again. This time they got an email saying the organization had changed its age requirements, and children had to be a minimum of twelve years old to apply for a dog.

Three more years before they could even try. It seemed like an impossibly long time when every day was a struggle. But they would wait. They knew there were other organizations out there, but Karin had done her research and concluded that Dogs4Diabetics was one of the most respected diabetic-alert dog training and placement organizations in the country. Plus the dog would not cost them anything.

Its founder, type 1 diabetic Mark Ruefenacht, makes his living in the exacting world of quality assurance of precision measurements. He runs a measurement standards laboratory, does contract work with NIST, and consults with scientific and forensic laboratories throughout the world.

In 1999 he began merging his volunteer work for Guide Dogs for the Blind with his professional experience to come up with innovative ways to train dogs to detect hypoglycemia in type 1 diabetics. Once he had figured out the best system, he decided to share it with others. He opened Dogs4Diabetics in 2004.

Given his background of perfecting measurements, it's no surprise that the organization's standards are high and read like something out of a statistics course. Dogs4Diabetics kindly supplied me with some basics:

> Our standards are based on statistically reliable levels of recorded performance at all stages of training: A dog is not placed until it reaches a minimum of 80% reliability of identification of hypoglycemic scent in training without a diabetic present. A team* is not graduated until it reaches 80% reliability of alerting on low/high blood sugar in most common environments (home, work, school), based on records of all alerts and lows, recorded and reviewed weekly by D4D staff. There needs to be a minimum of 100 data elements (lows/highs) which averages about 6 weeks of records.

In other words, the dogs and people who make it through the program really know their stuff.

It's difficult to get into the program—Dogs4Diabetics receives a hundred requests for diabetic-alert dogs monthly and can provide only twenty to twenty-five annually. The lucky people who get in have to work hard to graduate. The classes are known for their intensity. And graduating doesn't mean automatically getting a dog. It's common to wait for more than a year for the right match.

Clay was fourteen when he was finally accepted into a class. The family had already made reservations for summer getaways and camps, but canceled everything. He and his parents drove nearly five hours round-trip every Saturday and Sunday from the last week of April through the first week in August. Clay was the youngest in the class.

"It was the most difficult thing I've ever done," says Karin. "There

---

*When the word "team" is used in terms of working dogs, it's usually in reference to the dog and his or her handler. So in this case it would be the dog and the person with diabetes.

was so much emotion we had invested in this, and we worried about the pressures of passing, especially for Clay. I was terrified about us passing. We crammed for the tests together."

They did pass. And then a new wait began. The wait for a dog. They showed up at every training event and watched as newer students were paired with dogs Clay had hoped to get. It was a heartbreaking process for him, but behind the scenes, trainers were in matchmaking mode, looking for just the right dog for each person.

Almost a year after Clay started at Dogs4Diabetics, the program manager asked Clay if he wanted to take a dog home for the weekend just to see what it was like. He was thrilled, but when he and his mom got there, they learned the dog had a slight injury and they wouldn't be able to take her. The program manager didn't want to disappoint them after they'd made the long drive, so she asked Clay if he'd like to take a sweet yellow Lab named Whitley home instead. The tawny girl wasn't the dog they'd had in mind, but at least Clay would be able to experience having a diabetic-alert dog at home.

That weekend, Whitley alerted to Clay. She moved close to him, sat, and stared at him with her huge brown eyes. It was the same sort of expression a dog begging at the table for a crust of pizza or bit of steak might employ. Once Whitley had Clay's attention, she licked him on his arms and went into a downward-dog stretch, front end down, hind end up. She was very casual about it, and if they hadn't known better, they'd have thought she was just getting the kinks out after a nap.

Toward the end of her bow, she dipped her head down and grabbed a durable cloth strip hanging off her collar. The strip is called a brinsel, and Whitley focused her gaze on Clay with the brinsel sticking out of her mouth like a cigar. It's the ultimate signal from a diabetic-alert dog. Something along the lines of *Check your blood sugar because it's not where we want it, and it's going down* [or up, in some cases] *fast*.

Clay and his mom couldn't believe a dog had alerted to him in their house. What they had been waiting for all these years was finally becoming a reality.

This dog who was theirs just for the weekend suddenly became the best dog in the world. They checked Clay's blood sugar, and it was lower than 70. They rewarded Whitley with what they call a party—loud, loving praise and a high-value treat she gets only when she alerts. Clay drank some apple juice to try to increase his glucose, and they checked again in ten minutes to make sure his blood sugar was rising. If Whitley hadn't alerted him, he would have dropped even lower before he felt the symptoms, and it would have been harder and taken longer to get his glucose back up.

On Monday they returned Whitley with heavy hearts, not knowing if they would see her again. But when they came back on Thursday, the trainer had a question for Clay: "I wanted to ask you if you would like to take Whitley home and try a temperament placement test with her? If it all works out, she'll be yours for good."

Clay and his mom couldn't contain their emotions, which ping-ponged from tears of relief and joy to giddy laughter.

Clay's spotless fish tank purred on his desk as the morning sun skimmed through his curtains. He had a mild flu and wouldn't be going to school that day. He hadn't set his alarm, and he slept without stirring. It was easy to sleep late in this room, with its carpet the color of a soft bed of fallen pine needles and its tree-green walls. It always reminded him of the places he loved to fish, hike, and camp.

Whitley had been with him for a few months and was already a combination of second mother, nurse, and best friend. She slept curled on her oversized cushion next to Clay's twin bed. Whitley's nearness to Clay gave his parents an extra level of assurance. He didn't have a CGM system yet, so they were hoping Whitley would be able to alert him if he went low while he slept and didn't realize it.

As Clay slept that morning, Whitley got up and moved to the edge of his bed. No one knows exactly what happened next, but Whitley likely tried to alert to Clay's blood sugar as she normally would. She sat and stared and probably tried to lick him. Maybe she even bowed with her brinsel. But he didn't respond. She had never encountered this situation. Usually Clay woke up on his own when he felt his sugar was too low at night.

Whitley knew what she had to do. She jumped onto Clay's bed and stood over him, paws on his chest, bright pink brinsel in her mouth. She stared so hard it was almost as if she were willing him to wake up.

And Clay did wake up. He felt the weight of her, opened his eyes, and saw her earnest face staring at him, her mouth clutching the brinsel. He knew what he had to do. He doesn't recall walking to the kitchen, but he found himself there. He pricked his finger to test his glucose level. He registered in the low 40s. He was teetering at the edge of severe hypoglycemia.

He grabbed a Hansen's apple juice box—the kind with Clifford the Big Red Dog on the package. (It had been his favorite when he was younger, though at age fifteen he wondered if he was getting too old for Clifford.) He gulped down the juice as fast as its tiny straw would allow. As soon as he felt steadier, he tossed Whitley a treat and told her what a good girl she was.

When Clay's parents found out what had happened, they hailed Whitley as a hero, or something even better. "You are our angel. What a good angel dog you are!" Karin told her. Karin thinks Whitley may have prevented Clay from ending up in a coma, or worse, that morning.

Shortly after that event, Whitley figured out that if Clay wasn't responding to a blood sugar warning, she should rouse his parents. No one trained her. She just Lassied her way to that realization.

"She has changed everything," says Karin. "She gives us a peace of mind we never had before. She is literally a lifesaver."

Whitley has now spent the last four years at Clay's side. She regularly alerts to his hypos twenty minutes before his CGM device does. His parents trust Whitley more than they trust any machine, no matter how high-tech.

"She is always on it," Karin says. "This dear girl has saved him so many times over the years."

Whitley became something of a celebrity on campus during Clay's high school years. She went to most of Clay's classes, tucking under desks wherever he went; she was out of the way at the same time she could keep an eye and a nose on him.

The teachers adored her. "I love Whitley. She is the best-trained dog on the planet," said Ben O'Neill, a teacher in the school's Scrubs and Extreme Responders programs for students exploring health care professions. "Her devotion to Clay is very moving."

I attended a few classes at Ukiah High School with Clay and Whitley toward the end of his senior year. As Clay, who was an instructional assistant in an Extreme Responders class, sat listening to Ben, Whitley watched Clay like a mother monitoring her young child on playground equipment. She was attentive, calm, and ready to step in if needed.

Sometimes she used his feet as a chin rest, and he crossed his ankles to support her head. Even if she couldn't see him, she could smell him—even in her sleep.

Sleeping was the one time Whitley's presence in class could become obvious to everyone. That day Clay's econ teacher was lecturing about supply and demand. As he talked, someone began snoring. It wasn't too loud at first, but the volume quickly increased. I didn't have to look farther than the floor under Clay's table for the perpetrator.

The teacher took it in stride. "I'm used to students falling asleep and snoring in my classes, but this is the first year a dog has done it," he said when he discovered the snorer was under a table, not drooped over it. The students laughed, and Whitley roused for a moment, then settled into a gentler volume.

Whitley's photo appeared in the school yearbook the last two years of high school, just to the right of Clay's photo. She attended a senior prom dinner and photo session with Clay and his date. And at graduation, she wore a purple cap, gown, and Hawaiian-style brinsel. She strode on stage with Clay when he received his diploma, and the audience went wild with cheers.

Whitley has gone with Clay and his family on several trips, including a cross country drive to iconic destinations like the Grand Canyon, Mount Rushmore, and Yellowstone, and a New Orleans river cruise. She accompanied Clay on a graduation-celebration cruise to Alaska. She's regularly his sidekick on fishing and hiking trips. If she could, she'd always be with him. But sometimes, like when he does EMT training, he has to leave her behind.

The result is hard for Karin to watch. Whitley will sit stoically at their pane-glass door, watching, waiting for Clay to come home.

"She pouts, I'm sure because she's worried about him, and she misses him, especially when he's gone for a long time for diabetes summer camp," Karin says. "It's heart-wrenching to see her just sitting there."

Karin and Ken usually manage to distract her after a while and try to help her enjoy her downtime. "We want her to take advantage of just being a regular dog when she has the opportunity," Karin says.

When I last talked with the family, Clay was a couple of weeks away from starting his freshman year at Butte College. He's taking nursing prerequisites and hopes to become a nurse or a paramedic. He is already an EMT, thanks in part to his Scrubs training.

He will be sharing a house with three human roommates and one four-legged one, who will go to classes with him, just as she did in high school. Clay was looking forward to this next stage in his life.

"Whitley has given Clay so much self-confidence to be the adventurous person he is, and to face new challenges head-on," Karin says. "She'll help Ken and me let go of some of the worry as she helps Clay take on his future."

———

It's clear to anyone who watches Whitley and other successful diabetic-alert dogs that some dogs can do this work and do it splendidly.

But studies show mixed results.

In a study published in *Diabetes Therapy* in 2016, dogs successfully alerted to perspiration and breath samples of diabetic hypoglycemia (glucose levels between 46 and 65 mg/dL). The samples were placed inside glass jars, and the jars went into open steel cans. There was no human in the room to cue dogs unintentionally. The people doing the study watched from another room via a video camera. When a dog alerted correctly, he or she received a treat from an automatic dispenser that was remotely activated by a trainer.

Most of the seven dogs did well, but there was one named Isabella who dragged the "GPA" down. She detected positive samples only half of the time, while four of her classmates detected positive samples nearly 88 percent of the time. She may have had a pretty good excuse, though.

The testing took place in an Indiana prison, where the dogs were training to become diabetic-alert dogs. At the time of the testing, the prison was having a sewage issue. The stench managed to work its way into the testing room.

Of course, to dogs, sewage is not a stench. It's a cacophony of fascinating odors that tell stories of the people all around them—stories we can't read and don't want to. So it could be that while the other dogs were focused on the task at nose, Isabella was busy reading the sewage.

That distraction didn't make it into the journal paper. I learned about it from speaking with one of the study's authors, Jennifer Cattet, PhD, founder of the Indianapolis-based organization Medical Mutts. She and the other authors were encouraged by the overall outcome.

"Our results demonstrate that DADs [diabetic-alert dogs] are able to identify Hypo and be trained to alert to its presence," their paper stated. "The results reported here take canine glucose sensing to a new level of sophistication."

But a year later, researchers from the Oregon Health & Science

University published a paper in the *Journal of Diabetes Science and Technology* that evaluated the reliability of eight diabetic-alert dogs (or, as the authors wrote with a touch of snark, "so-called diabetes alert dogs") working under real life conditions with their people. It concluded that there was a high false-positive rate and that continuous glucose monitoring often detected hypoglycemia before a dog.

"The current study," the authors wrote, "helps define the clinical utility and limits of DADs and balances the often sensational reports of DADs in the popular press and social media."

Ralph Hendrix, a longtime Dogs4Diabetics staff member, says he's glad the study acknowledged dogs can detect hypoglycemia, but points out some issues his organization has with the study: Dogs are usually trained to identify rapidly changing blood sugar. They don't wait until the person is already low. Ralph and others I spoke with also wish the study had weeded out poorly trained dogs or handlers instead of relying on patients' statements on their satisfaction with their dogs.

The study's lead author, pediatric endocrinologist Evan Los, MD, wasn't entirely negative about the possibility of dogs as reliable alerters. He told NPR, "Although it appears CGM outperformed trained dogs in this study, it is intriguing that dogs were able to detect some hypoglycemia. Perhaps understanding what factors impact dog reliability could help optimize dog performance."

Those who keep an eye on the literature suggest trying to standardize the training and abilities of diabetic-alert dogs used for future studies. They also hope to see the numbers of dogs in studies increase. A study reported in *Diabetes Care* (by some of the key researchers in the Oregon study) used only three dogs and concluded, "Trained dogs were largely unable to identify skin swabs obtained from hypoglycemic T1D [type 1 diabetic] subjects."

Researchers at the University of Virginia used a larger number of dogs in a study published in 2017. The results showed high variability in the results from the eighteen dogs—all Labrador retrievers bred, raised, and trained by the same organization. The accuracy of dogs alerting to low blood glucose ranged from 33 percent to 100 percent. In other words, some dogs were really good at it, others not so much.

The authors called for larger trials that can help sort out the "factors influencing the complexity of DAD accuracy."

This would be helpful to this increasingly popular doctor dog specialization. Most organizations training these dogs are well-meaning. But the accuracy and reliability of their dogs, and the training given to their people, sometimes falls short. If quality studies can suggest best practices, that could translate to increasingly better generations of these diabetes specialists.

That doesn't necessarily mean cookie-cutter training. There's more than one way to create a top-notch diabetic-alert dog.

———

Young Luke Nuttall and his diabetic-alert dog, Jedi, have a partnership as successful as Clay and Whitley's, but their beginnings couldn't have been more different.

Jedi was three days old when he first smelled the scent of diabetic hypoglycemia. A trainer had thawed out a sample of saliva on a cotton ball from a type 1 diabetic with low blood sugar. With gloved hands, she rubbed it on his mother's belly. As the tiny black Lab and his siblings enjoyed the delectable taste of mother's milk, they also breathed in the scent of hypoglycemia.

This continued until they were weaned. Sometimes the trainers bottle-fed the pups. But even then, they were exposed to the scent, thanks to a little piece of the saliva-soaked cotton placed on the side of the latex nipple closest to their noses as they snortled in the puppy formula.

Later, when the pups played games with people, a prized toy was always paired with the scent of a diabetic low.

It's not like playing Mozart for your newborn in hopes your baby will be smarter. Trainers who use this early-scent-exposure method say it can have a marked effect on pups when it comes to ease of training.

"They learn to associate the smell of low blood sugar with something really good," says Crystal Cockroft, founder of Canine Hope for Diabetics, which supplied Luke with Jedi. "It becomes something they're always wanting to find, something they know deep down."

Jedi hadn't been born when Luke was diagnosed with type 1 diabetes at only two years old. The toddler had been under the weather. He was lethargic, itchy, crying through the night, and had an insatiable thirst. At one point he woke up screaming and gulped six baby bottles of water until he fell asleep from exhaustion two hours later.

He was going through diapers at an alarming rate—a red flag to his mom, Dorrie, who teaches child development at Pasadena City College. She took him to the doctor, who ran some tests and gave them the bad news.

The intensive, round-the-clock work of keeping Luke alive after his diagnosis became crushing for Dorrie. Luke was the youngest of three boys, and between working and parenting, Dorrie was already busy nearly 24/7. She was desperate for anything that would help ease the load.

When she learned about diabetic-alert dogs, she imagined how one could come into their lives and make things as close to normal as possible. Dorrie and her husband searched for an organization that would provide a young child with a dog. There weren't many. They found one across the country that promised a dog would solve their problems and claimed 100 percent alerting rates for high and low blood sugars. Dorrie checked out their dog graduates and found a couple who were doing good work. The Nuttalls sent in $2,000 as a down payment for a $22,000 puppy.

But while they waited, Dorrie learned about problems with some of the dogs. That they weren't reliable. That they arrived as puppies and the organization expected families to train them from scratch, with almost no support. That even those families that managed to train the dog to occasionally alert ended up with fearful or aggressive dogs. Some families were suing.

This was not what Dorrie needed. She knew she couldn't get the deposit back. A couple grand was a lot of money for them, but they couldn't take the chance on a dog who might make life harder.

Dorrie continued searching for a better organization. A year after Luke's diagnosis, she found Canine Hope for Diabetics, which was only about seventy-five miles from their Glendale home. Crystal told her the organization didn't normally provide dogs for young children, and gave her a much more realistic view of what to expect from a diabetic-alert dog. She told her how much work a dog would be, that training never stops, and that no dog alerts to every low or high.

Canine Hope was putting out only four or five dogs a year and spending a great deal of time on each dog. Dorrie didn't want to wait for a trained older dog. She wanted the chance to train the dog herself, with the support of the organization.

She knew it would take time, and probably more training expertise than the family could muster. The Nuttalls had three dogs already, and those guys didn't even know how to sit on command. How could they train a diabetic-alert dog? But there was something about this idea that spoke to her. She was determined they would work hard and succeed.

Crystal had done a puppy placement like this once before, and it had worked out well because the family was "100 percent dedicated." She saw the same qualities in Luke's family. She picked a sturdy black pup she sensed would be a good match for Luke: The pup had a great nose, a strong drive to work for food, and was calm enough not to get flustered by the chaos of a family with small children and other dogs.*

The Nuttalls, self-described *Star Wars* nerds, knew what they were

---

*Jedi's success as a diabetic-alert dog placed as a puppy is probably an anomaly. Crystal's organization placed a few more pups as DADs-in-training after Jedi, but the families weren't able to put in the immense effort the Nuttalls did, and the dogs didn't live up to their potential. Since then, Crystal has provided only trained adult dogs.

going to name Luke's partner: Canine Hope's Master Jedi Knight, or Jedi, for short.

Crystal told Dorrie there was no guarantee. At worst, Jedi would be a great pet. He joined the family when he was twelve weeks old.

Jedi proved to be an enthusiastic, talented student. A typical Lab, he was as food-driven as Crystal had described. And since he'd been exposed to the scent early on, it was easy to get him to show that he smelled a diabetic low by offering a small reward for certain actions.

"He will do anything for a piece of kibble or slice of tangerine," Dorrie says.

Whenever she tested Luke's blood sugar—up to a dozen times a day—she made sure to bring little Jedi. "He's low! He's low!" she'd exclaim when Luke had hypoglycemia. For high blood sugar readings, she'd enthusiastically say, "He's high! He's high!"

With occasional intensive training weeks at Canine Hope, Jedi was able to show he recognized the scent of Luke's lows at six months old. He'd smell Luke running low and run to the fridge for a treat, knowing he was due for a reward. The family found this adorable and endearing. By the time Jedi was a year old, he was alerting consistently to Luke's lows. Soon after, Jedi could reliably alert to Luke's highs.

Jedi's alert for low blood sugar is like Whitley's. But instead of showing Luke the alert, he goes to Dorrie. He stretches with his front end down and hind end up, and grabs a brinsel—either the one on his collar or one she always has hitched to her belt loop. When Dorrie wants to know if it's a low or high, she'll ask Jedi. If it's low, he'll bow again. If it's high, he'll give Dorrie a high-five with his paw.

The body language couldn't be clearer, she says. Jedi is remarkably accurate and doesn't overalert. And he's only improved with age.

"No dog catches absolutely everything. But Jedi's alerts beat the meters and CGMs almost every alert. Especially after almost six years," Dorrie says. "Once in a great while we get an alert to something we can't figure out—very rare or maybe it's me. I get low blood sugars sometimes. But usually it's just an early alert way before the meters catch it."

She says Jedi usually beats the meters by fifteen to twenty minutes, allowing Luke to avoid big lows and highs. Since getting Jedi, Luke no longer reaches the point where he passes out. His A1C level, which reflects his average blood glucose levels over the past three months, is usually around 5.5, with a standard deviation in blood sugar of 28 mg/dL. These are excellent values, on par with a person without diabetes.

Luke doesn't have to be near Jedi to alert to him. During training he responded from the distance of a football field away when the wind was blowing in his direction from Luke. And at home, Jedi can be inside and smell Luke having a blood sugar issue when he's outside playing with friends.

Jedi has alerted to thousands of highs and lows. "He makes us all a little more relaxed, a lot more happy," Dorrie says. "He makes everyone feel loved. He's not just another tool against diabetes. He's an extremely special part of our family."

Jedi starts the night in Luke's room, then moves to his parents' room after his first alert of the night. But that doesn't stop him from waking up to Luke's lows or highs. His parents' bed is a testimony to Jedi's nocturnal alerting: The baseboard is covered in scratches from his nails as he tries to rouse them.

Dorrie has a popular blog and Facebook page about Luke and Jedi. People come to her to try to find out more about getting a diabetic-alert dog. Despite how much Jedi has done for their family, she says she spends most of the time telling people they should think twice about getting a dog.

"People are like we were, desperate, looking for something to make life easier. A good dog is an amazing help, but it's not just a machine on autopilot that will be the answer for busy families," she says.

She doesn't want anyone to get ripped off, or to get in over their heads. She tells those who contact her how much work dogs are. She explains that dogs will wake up parents at night, when monitors might not, so they often get less sleep, not more. And there's poop and walking. And constant training and reinforcement.

She lets them know that yes, Jedi has saved Luke's life, and she's grateful for Jedi every day. But a dog isn't the magic answer. The work, day and night, of having a child with type 1 diabetes doesn't disappear when a dog walks into your life, she tells them.

You can feel her exhaustion in a blog post from Valentine's Day 2018:

> Every single night before bed I test his blood sugar. That is about 2,340 nights that I've found my sleeping child's hand under the covers and pricked his finger to get a drop of blood big enough to get a reading.
>
> 2,340 nights that I've looked at a number and decided what I needed to do next. What alarm to set, what dosing to adjust, how much insulin or glucose to give with full understanding that my decisions directly impact him.
>
> 2,340 nights I've made decisions a pancreas should make, or maybe next in line doctors, without a meticulous degree and through trial and error I've decided what to do next, I've considered his exercise his recent patterns his dinner and nutritional contents to decide how much insulin his body will need.
>
> 2,340 nights I've set alarms, plugged in equipment, inserted pumps and needles.
>
> 2,340 nights I've thought of families and children who do not have supplies or insulin or life expectancies longer then a year.
>
> 2,340 nights I've wandered through my dark house searching through supplies and doing calculations in my head wondering how many people would support us in our fight for a cure if they knew what diabetes really was. I've wondered how compassion could be lost for so many that

go through so much because their diagnosis has the word "diabetes" in it.

2,340 nights I've prayed for a cure and thanked god for the science and miracles that have kept him here with us.

2,340 nights . . . that will be forever for Luke unless there is a cure.

#weneedacure please help us tell the world it's time.

———

People have been training dogs to alert to diabetes for a couple of decades, but dogs have been freelancing for far longer. When I was a kid, my parents told me about their friend's little dog who would scratch at her leg at odd times. It annoyed the woman until she realized the dog was doing this shortly before she started feeling "off" from her diabetes. Once she understood what her dog was trying so hard to tell her, she listened, and ended up with far fewer distressing episodes of low blood sugar.

Companion dogs have surely been sensing changes in the odors of their people way before my childhood, but the science didn't start looking at this phenomenon until relatively recently.

A case study published in *BMJ* (formerly the *British Medical Journal*) in the year 2000 reported with charming enthusiasm that some pet dogs provide "a novel alarm system that can detect hypoglycaemia before the patient notices any symptoms and that operates robustly in a uniquely, patient friendly fashion."

The authors reported on three pet dogs, two of whom routinely detected the hypos of their companions and "then undertook further corrective action by waking them to eat—thus going further than any available glucose sensor."

The study's conclusion may have inspired some early diabetic-alert dog training: "An extended healthcare role should now be considered for man's (and woman's) best friend. Research is urgently needed to determine whether dogs can be trained to recognise and react to early signs of hypoglycaemia. Hypoglycaemia alarm dogs could provide an important aid to patients with poor awareness of symptoms, particularly those prone to nocturnal episodes or who live alone."

And it's not just dogs. It appears there are some talented doctor cats out there as well. In 2011 a Queen's University Belfast researcher reported on five people whose cats woke them up when they had hypoglycemia. One particularly determined cat with chronic arthritis in her paws managed to get past her pain to scratch at the bedroom door until she woke up her person. In all cases of kitty alerts, their people checked their glucose and found they were very low. The researcher concluded that "other species, such as the cat, may also have a role to play in the detection of certain underlying physical ailments."*

And there was this unintentionally amusing proviso: "Whether this species offers the same ease of, or degree of flexibility in, training [as dogs] is still unknown . . ."

For now, dogs who sniff out diabetic highs and lows probably don't have to worry about job security.

A study of 212 insulin-dependent diabetics with pet dogs found that almost two-thirds of the dogs often reacted to their hypoglycemic episodes. They barked, cried, licked, nuzzled, jumped up at them, and stared at them. A few sensitive souls showed fear—trembling, moving to another room, and/or hyperventilating.

The most promising finding was that one-third of the diabetics said their pet dogs reacted *before* they were aware of their own low blood sugar. People like my parents' old friend would not be surprised by these findings. And neither would a diabetic doctor I visited in his office about ninety minutes north of San Francisco.

---

*If you poke around the internet, you'll find plenty of people talking about how their cats alerted to their low blood sugar. A news report on YouTube features a man who says his cat, Oz, saved his life three times, including the time he was in a diabetic coma on the living room floor. Oz ran and woke up the man's girlfriend, who called 9-1-1. Despite the cat's lifesaving acts, the man told the reporter that Oz is not the "brightest brick in the wall." In the video, Oz didn't so much as give him a dirty look, much less scratch him.

The patient examination rooms at the Sutter Pacific Medical Foundation in Santa Rosa, California, contain all the usual trappings: a state-of-the-art computer, tongue depressors, an otoscope, gauze, boxes of examination gloves, a red biohazard wall bin, a shiny reflex hammer, and other tools of the trade. The rooms used by Steve Wolf, MD, have one extra feature: a dog bed.

Every day a medical assistant checks which rooms the family medicine doctor will be using and sets up a dog bed in each one—usually tucked against a wall next to the computer where Dr. Wolf types in patient information, a few feet away from the patient.

Dr. Wolf, now fifty, has been dealing with his own type 1 diabetes since two weeks before he took the Medical College Admission Test (MCAT) that would help determine if he'd be going to medical school. He had been feeling miserable for weeks, with fatigue and weight loss and extreme hunger and thirst. He chalked it up to a bout of bronchitis mixed with the stress of preparing for the exams.

On the day of the MCAT, he walked into the testing room with a couple of gallons of water and an ice chest jammed with food, and was trying to fit it under his desk when the proctor approached him. The proctor firmly told him that he could only bring two pencils and his ID. All food and drink needed to be left in another area. He could eat and drink during breaks.

He ran out to his stash at every chance and slammed down food and chugged as much water as he could, then continued the test. By the time he was down to the last twenty-five or so questions of a section, his bladder was competing with his brain for attention.

Two days later, he was diagnosed with type 1 diabetes.

Since then, he has used every tool at his disposal to help him manage his condition. He started using insulin pumps when they were the size of a paperback* and tries to keep up with the latest technology for pumps and for monitoring his glucose levels.

But there's something else in his arsenal that most diabetics don't have. Something with no digital readouts and dials and doohickeys: Kermit, his deeply devoted diabetic-alert dog.

The yellow Labrador retriever was slated to be a guide dog, but every time the trainers at Guide Dogs for the Blind put the harness on him, he froze and wouldn't move. A guide dog who can't wear a harness has to find another career. Kermit ended up with Dogs-4Diabetics, the same organization that trained Whitley.

Kermit isn't Dr. Wolf's first foray into the world of diabetic-alert dogs. In the early 2000s he had a boxer named Graham who somehow trained himself to alert to Dr. Wolf's hypoglycemia. Graham would paw his leg and whine at certain points throughout the day, and it didn't take long for Dr. Wolf to realize what Graham was doing. He encouraged his dog to continue alerting by giving him love and attention every time he alerted.

Graham saved his life on a few occasions. One time Dr. Wolf was sleeping and his blood sugar dropped into the 20s. He is sure it would have been "the big sleep" if Graham hadn't been fiercely determined to wake him up. His recollection of the event is hazy because of his condition at the time, but he remembers Graham barking in his face on the bed and eventually rearing up on his hind legs and body-slamming him.

"I thought maybe he was telling me about a robber, but first I checked my blood sugar and realized I was in trouble," he says.

He had fruit snacks and a juice box close at hand and had barely finished them when he noticed Graham was already curled up on the bed, mission accomplished.

---

*He's lucky he didn't need an insulin pump in the early 1960s. The first portable insulin pump was worn like a backpack, and had so many dials and switches and tubes that it looked like a space-age jetpack. Its inventor wears it in an old black-and-white photo, and he looks like he's going to blast into outer space. It was clunky, but cutting-edge at the time. Today's insulin pumps are about the size of small cell phones.

After Graham passed away in 2010, Dr. Wolf couldn't think about getting another dog. About a year later, though, he was shopping at Costco and ran into someone with a diabetic-alert dog. He struck up a conversation and found out that the dog was trained at Dogs4Diabetics, which was located only about sixty-five miles southeast of where he lived. He applied the same week, was accepted quickly, and began the rigorous program.

The trainers there had to be especially choosy when selecting a dog for Dr. Wolf. He has an active lifestyle involving outdoor sports, so the dog had to be high-energy. At the same time, the dog also needed to be calm and gentle enough to sit through a doctor's encounters with patients, including newborns and the elderly. And the dog needed to be able to greet patients and welcome their attention, if there was attention, while still remaining focused on Dr. Wolf's glucose levels.

When Kermit got through training, they knew he was the dog for Dr. Wolf.

Kermit goes almost everywhere with his man. When Dr. Wolf walks into an examining room to meet a patient, Kermit walks right in with him. The doctor introduces him, then it's "Go kennel!" Kermit finds his bed and lies down for the duration. When the appointment is over, he and Kermit walk side by side back to Dr. Wolf's office—colleagues in the war against illness.

During Kermit's early days visiting patients with Dr. Wolf, he was reluctant to alert. "He could see I was conducting business and didn't want to interrupt," Dr. Wolf says. "I had to encourage him when I could see he was fighting the urge to alert." The doctor carries dog food with him whenever he visits a patient with Kermit in case he has to reward him.

As important as Kermit is to his well-being, Dr. Wolf doesn't always bring Kermit with him when he's doing medical procedures. Until recently Dr. Wolf delivered babies. Kermit would be in the nearby call room or at the nurses' station while Dr. Wolf was helping bring new life into the world. But sometimes Kermit would get up and scratch on the call-room door or try to pull away from the nurses' station. When that happened, someone would knock on the delivery-room door and let Dr. Wolf know what Kermit was doing so he could check his blood sugar. Sure enough, Kermit usually had a reason to be concerned.

One of the few times Dr. Wolf doesn't bring Kermit into an examination room at Sutter is when his staff informs him the patient is a heavy smoker; he's concerned about the scent interfering with Kermit's sense of smell. He'd also respect the wishes of someone who is allergic to dogs, but in all his years as a family practitioner, he's run into only one patient with this allergy. She said it was OK to bring Kermit in, though, and she ended up petting him because she couldn't resist. (She washed her hands immediately.)

Only a few patients have expressed a fear of dogs. Kermit seems to know, and usually goes straight to his bed and doesn't try to get a pat or a hug. Dr. Wolf believes that Kermit, like other dogs, has a sixth sense about people who are scared and gives them space. But if someone is seriously fearful, he respects the fear and leaves Kermit in his office or with a staff member.

While I was spending the afternoon with them, Dr. Wolf got called to a room to do a laceration repair. He could have taken Kermit in, but instead left him in his office with me, with the door open.

I thought I would keep Kermit company and we'd be grand old friends while Dr. Wolf was out. After all, Kermit and I had already enjoyed playing with his favorite toy—a red lobster with googly eyes. And he seemed to like my ear rubs, leaning happily into them while I was talking with Dr. Wolf earlier.

Besides, dogs love me, and this dog would surely rather hang with me than just wait for Dr. Wolf.

I overestimated my curb appeal.

After a minute or two of halfheartedly playing with Mr. Lobster and me, and not seeming all that interested in belly or ear rubs, Kermit took his place on his green bed under Dr. Wolf's desk and peered out the door down the hall. He lay there staring with tender brown eyes, waiting. He was a picture of patience. And he looked concerned, like someone in a hospital waiting room gazing in the direction they imagine their loved one is having surgery.

I took a few bites of my sandwich, and he didn't give it a sideways glance. When I came back from washing my hands, he didn't seem to notice me passing in front of his field of vision. He looked right through me as if I were invisible.

I clearly didn't have a ghost of a chance with Kermit while he kept vigil for Dr. Wolf. We waited for him together, with only the low thrum of the office ventilation system and the patter of April rain to break the silence.

Months later (in Kermit time), Dr. Wolf returned from the procedure down the hall. Kermit stood up and waggled a greeting that seemed to be both joy and relief, all the while looking at his face intently. If he could talk, he would likely say something along the lines of *Thank goodness you're back! You don't know how I worry about you when I can't be near you!*

Not that Kermit needs to be close to Dr. Wolf to sense he's heading for trouble. Kermit has accurately alerted when he was outside and Dr. Wolf was inside—as Jedi has with Luke.

"The most impressive [time] was when I was at a friend's house watching the Super Bowl," Dr. Wolf recalled. "Kermit was outside being a dog, playing with his best dog friends. At some point we heard kind of a knocking at the back door of the house. It was Kermit pawing at it to tell us he wanted to come in. My friend let him in and Kermit came right over to me and alerted. I was dropping low and I had no idea.

"He's the best sensor," he said. "I trust Kermit implicitly."

Kermit had been dozing next to his toy lobster as we spoke, but when he heard his name, his ears kicked up and his eyes instantly opened.

"It's OK, Kermit, I'm just talking about you, not to you," Dr. Wolf reassured him and smiled.

Dr. Wolf continued. "My dog is more accurate than my sensor.

Dogs can alert within five seconds of a drop because you're already breathing and sweating out the scent from the liver," he said. "The best sensors currently measure interstitial glucose [the fluid between cells] every five minutes and average the measurements over thirty minutes. So sensors can be thirty minutes behind real-time change in blood glucose. Dogs are almost immediate.

"Plus, beyond their alerting, dogs have intangible benefits for diabetics, like getting us out for exercise, decreasing isolation and depression. A diabetic-alert dog has the combination of being able to save your life at the same time as giving unconditional love.

"All this fancy equipment I have can fail. Technology is susceptible to battery problems, a transducer can come loose. The transmitter of my current pump isn't working without a good signal. I can lose a connection. Kermit never loses connection."

But Kermit and other well-trained alert dogs are not infallible. When Kermit accompanied Dr. Wolf to New Orleans, he wasn't catching his lows. It turned out he was panting so much from the heat that his nose wasn't at its most efficient.* Dr. Wolf got around this by having Kermit lick his skin so he could taste and smell his sweat.

Another time that Kermit's nose didn't work was during the wildfires that decimated giant swaths of Santa Rosa in 2017. Kermit couldn't smell Dr. Wolf's lows or highs, and didn't alert for the three days he was in the fire zone. Dr. Wolf was concerned about the toxic smoke permanently damaging Kermit's nose, so he had a friend who lived farther away pick him up and keep him until the smoke cleared.

It's not just environmental factors that can make a medical alert dog less efficient. Without constant reinforcement of their training, their skills can get rusty.

And dogs do cheat.

---

*Kermit is in good company. This happens to military working dogs who find themselves in places like Iraq and Afghanistan in the blaze of summer. Their handlers have to be vigilant about keeping their dogs cool enough so they can sniff efficiently, and also, of course, so they don't suffer a heat injury.

Dogs who alert are godsends, but they're not always angels. If there's a faster way to get a treat, many will take the quickest path to the reward until told otherwise. In my years writing about dogs who use their nose to save lives in war, or protect presidents, I've heard all kinds of stories about cheating dogs. Some dogs figure that if they get rewarded when they appear to smell an explosive, they may as well act like they smell explosives as much as possible.

It's human nature.

Kermit doesn't cheat. Not really. But on occasion, when he's being talked about, he'll alert. To give him the benefit of the doubt, this may be because Kermit is used to giving demonstrations of his skills. During demos, Dr. Wolf talks about Kermit and calls on him to show what an alert looks like. Kermit is probably like the *Far Side* comic dog, hearing "Kermit blah blah Kermit blah blah blah." When there are enough "Kermit blah blah" statements, he may know a request to alert is coming up. Sometimes he jumps the gun.

I watched Kermit alert for real partway through our afternoon together. He stood up and casually dipped into a downward-dog position while staring at Dr. Wolf. Kermit has been trained to grab his brinsel after he does his downward-dog, but the bow-and-stare method is shorthand he and Dr. Wolf understand.

Kermit, like many diabetic-alert dogs, alerts to a blood glucose level drop of 10 percent or more within a ten-minute period. Dr. Wolf checked his glucose level: 182 mg/dL. We talked for twelve minutes and checked again: 106 mg/dL, a big drop.

"GOOD BOY! Nice!" Kermit's tail lobbed back and forth. "Now he gets a treat and I get a treat," he told me.

He gave Kermit a few pieces of chicken jerky and looked for a snack for himself. An extra desk next to his computer was covered with food: a bag of tangerines, a plastic container of chocolate-covered blueberries, and a paper plate with an orange, a lollipop, a big red pear, and an apple. A metal cabinet above his desk was like a mini-mart for diabetics, with a neat line of canisters containing cookies, dried figs, chocolate-covered sea salt caramels, jelly beans, and an assortment of other foods that can rapidly stop a drop or treat a low. It may sound like junk food, but it's essential to consume a relatively simple sugar that can be absorbed quickly.

He downed a handful of Jelly Belly jelly beans, and we continued talking. In a few minutes Kermit stretched and bowed and stared again. "Are you really alerting?" Dr. Wolf checked his blood sugar. It had increased and seemed to be on an upward trajectory.

Kermit took another bow. He was like an actor coming out for one more curtain call when most people have stopped clapping. Kermit, though a highly skilled medical alert dog, is still a Lab. And as we've already seen, Labs tend to be food-motivated. Kermit occasionally tries to get an extra treat by alerting after an alert. Dr. Wolf changed the subject, and the bowing stopped.

A medical assistant popped her head in the door and told Dr. Wolf a patient was waiting. He checked a pocket to make sure he had some treats in case Kermit alerted in the examining room. Kermit looked at Dr. Wolf and looked at me, then back at Dr. Wolf. I could almost hear Kermit thinking.

You're not gonna leave me with her *again, are you?*

"Let's go!" he told Kermit as he strode out of the office. Kermit wagged and joined him for their next appointment.

———

"What do you call a diabetic-assistance dog in Rome?"

"I don't know."

"Very rare! Ha-ha!"

So begins a conversation with Italian dog trainer Paolo Incontri. It's a cool November morning, and we're sitting at an *alfresco* table of a café across the street from the Colosseum. We couldn't get much closer to the Colosseum unless we were in it.

Cigarette smoke from a table of boisterous Italian men in black suits floats relentlessly to our table. Paolo gives them the best glare he can and waves his hand in front of his nose, but it's not getting the message across. So Valentina Braconcini, founding president of

L'Associazione Italiana Cani d'Allerta Diabete (IACAD), walks over and asks them to keep it down and to blow their cigarettes away from our table.

She's petite but packs a punch. She returns to our table, and they pipe down and puff in the opposite direction until they get animated again, which takes all of about ninety seconds.

"This is one thing that would keep me from giving someone a diabetic-assistance dog," Paolo says, nodding in their direction.

"Loud people?" I ask.

"No, smoking. Smoking is bad for the dogs. They can't smell the diabetic changes." (Kermit would concur.)

Paolo is founding partner and national training manager for the association, which he began under a different name in 2015. He's sixty-one, with a shaved head, a tight goatee, and wire-rim glasses. A soft wool coat and a scarf keep the chill off his slight frame.

There's something about him this morning that reminds me of the "job" he had for several years before devoting himself full-time to training dogs: Paolo had been a Buddhist monk.*

He traveled to Nepal and Sri Lanka, helping the poor, but spent most of his time as a monk in Italy. "The romantic vision people have about monastic life doesn't correspond to the truth," he says. "It is a simple life to be lived among the people and not in some kind of cave or a monastery on top of a mountain."

Paolo has one of the more interesting and indirect career paths of anyone I've met in the dog world: Before he was a dog trainer or a monk, he'd had a long career in Italy's Arma dei Carabinieri—a national police force older than the country of Italy.

Dogs have been part of his life ever since one followed him home before Christmas when he was a young boy. "I've always been

---

*Not long after we met at the café, Paolo would become a Buddhist monk again. In late 2018 he received the renewal of his monastic ordination and will be known in certain parts of his life as the Bhante Upali. The dogs and their people will still know him as Paolo.

able to communicate with dogs," he says in his excellent English. "I feel like I am a translator of human language and dog language."

He had been working as a trainer on and off, but in 2010, he felt a calling to work with dogs on a more regular basis. When he learned about diabetic-alert dogs, he was drawn to the idea that they can save lives. He thought it would be especially helpful to train dogs for children with diabetes.

"I always wanted to find the halfway point between helping the sick and working with dogs," he says. He got some training in diabetic-scent detection from an American organization and started working with families.

Paolo believes it's important to custom-make a relationship between a dog and a person or family. He explains it in his poetic manner: "One size does not fit all. Every family is different. Everything has to be in the mind, heart, and hands of the trainer from the beginning, as a tailor that first helps choose the most suitable fabric, then takes the measurements, then starts the work, then he checks and corrects and eventually you wear his work."

There aren't many diabetic-alert dogs in Italy. Paolo hopes that will change so anyone who really needs a dog will be able to get one.

For now, Paolo is helping families see if their own pet dogs can be transformed to become reliable diabetic-alert dogs. He looks for certain characteristics—calm yet inquisitive dogs who enjoy easy and fun scent-detection games he sets out for them. Then he works with the family and the dog, using positive reinforcement, never stressing the dog. "It must be great fun for them, or it's not going to work," he says.

He and Valentina are making plans to train specially bred litters of puppies for this work once the group gets a more robust library of diabetic hypoglycemic scents and a little more funding.

"We want to help as many people get good, reliable dogs for diabetic assistance as we can," Paolo says. "There's such an unmet need in Italy. People and the government don't understand what these dogs do. We want to help families suffer less, and children be healthier, and Italy learn about medical alert dogs as service dogs."

The pain of having a diabetic child is the same everywhere in the world. Several months after we met at the Colosseum café, Paolo put me in touch with a family he'd been assisting in the southern city of Reggio Calabria, located in the toe of the Italian boot.

"When we were told our son had diabetes, I stopped breathing," said Lidia Calabro, whose son Matteo was diagnosed with type 1 diabetes at the age of six. "I also stopped thinking about how I felt. I just had to be his support and learn how to handle insulin, measure blood sugar, get over my fear of needles, and at the same time give him courage. It was such a sad feeling for him that he was going to be affected by this terrible disease for the rest of his life."

She said Matteo is intensely curious, and that his mind "was in turmoil for days after his diagnosis." One day he walked up to her and her husband and said, "Mamma, Papà, I *must* have a dog for my diabetes. I saw in a documentary that some dogs can help people with diabetes."

They had a miniature schnauzer named Frida. When they found out about Paolo, they contacted him.

"Paolo warned us that it would not be a walk in the park. You put your personality into play, you put on the field emotions, skills, motivation, patience, hope, frustration, uncertainty, and a thousand other things, and you have to manage them. It is not easy, but it is very worth it."

A few months later, Frida is alerting to Matteo's hypos with an accuracy that thrills the family. When she senses something is off, she runs to Matteo and pokes him with her nose. Paolo's interpretation of what she is saying: *Something is wrong inside of you. Listen to me!* If Matteo doesn't acknowledge her the first couple of times, she licks and wags and does anything to get his attention. Then she runs to get his parents or grandmother and pokes at them and runs back to Matteo. They check his blood sugar. The whole time her tail is a blur of wagging. She loves this game.

And it gets even better for Frida when Matteo's glucose monitor shows he is too low or high. "Brava, Frida! Brava!" the parents, grandmother, or Matteo—or all four at once—enthusiastically tell the little dog. She gets a treat or two as a reward.

"We love this exciting, exhausting, and beautiful experience," Lidia explained. "Frida is Matteo's greatest, most helpful, precious, faithful, and loving friend for life."

Paolo told me that during his years as a monk, he felt exceptionally happy when helping people but that his work with dogs and diabetics has proven even more fulfilling. "It is a joy to watch how dogs can reach across species so gently and tenderly and transform lives. We don't know exactly how they're doing it, but we don't really have to know, do we? It's working."

Of course, some of us just can't help wondering exactly how they do it . . .

———

Before it became clear that scent is how most dogs seem to alert to diabetic events, researchers also postulated that body language, tremors, more rapid breathing, or changes in behavior or demeanor might be the ways some dogs sense trouble with blood sugar. It wouldn't be surprising if these also play a role since dogs are so attuned to how we act and look, but they seem to be secondary to scent.

The authors of a 2008 case report in the *Irish Journal of Medical Science* broached an unusual idea. They suggested a dog alerting to hypoglycemia could be picking up on "energy wave changes in a person's electrical and/or magnetic fields."

The *BMJ* case report on the three dogs also offered an unorthodox possibility: "We are attracted by the notion of the 'sixth sense' with which dogs are commonly credited, but acknowledge that this will need to be substantiated by further research."

The idea of dogs being able to use intuition or energy-wave detection might be kind of cool and heartwarming. But at this point, at least, it's not terribly scientific.

The best explanation to date is that dogs are detecting the volatile organic compounds in exhaled breath that change with large fluctuations in blood sugar. A 2016 report from the University of Cambridge and University of Oxford used soft-ionization mass spectrometry to measure VOCs in breath. The researchers found that the common breath VOC isoprene rose significantly during hypoglycemia. But there was no correlation between isoprene and other levels of blood sugar. And it was the only VOC they found that greatly increased during hypoglycemia.

The authors wrote that they didn't know how hypoglycemia could cause an increase in isoprene. But they did suggest that measuring breath VOCs like isoprene might one day be a noninvasive alternative to finger pricks for monitoring diabetic blood glucose changes.

It would be pretty convenient if diabetics could, say, blow into a tube and check their VOCs for accurate and real-time glucose levels. But would this put dogs out of business? Maybe one day—if technology like this gets ridiculously good and easy to use.*

But as much work as it can be to keep diabetic-alert dogs in top form, they have so much more to offer than their alerts. Studies list numerous psychosocial benefits of diabetic-alert dogs, including significant improvements in quality of life, decreases in anxiety about hypos or hypers, decreases in visits to the hospital, and greater independence.

Then there are the intangibles that studies aren't really designed to describe. They're like the benefits most people derive from their pet dogs, only perhaps even more intense because of the life-and-

---

*And then there are betta fish—the popular, colorful fish that are usually kept by themselves in relatively small aquariums. A study of twenty-eight adolescents showed significantly improved glycemic control among those given a betta fish to care for compared with the control group, which didn't get fish until after the study. This is an age when there's often a deterioration of diabetic control because of normal feelings of invincibility and independence. But associating diabetes self-care tasks with other routine daily activities—like feeding a fish in their room—"may be another tool in the diabetes educator toolbox," the study concludes.

death element: The sense of having a devoted partner who is always looking after you. The unconditional love of someone who keeps you from grave danger. An understanding soul who lifts your spirits when your condition feels overwhelming.

No machine could ever do that. Most people can't even manage it.

These qualities aren't unique to diabetic-alert dogs. Most people who depend on their service dogs treasure the caring, loving nature of their dogs—even if they can't always express how they feel about their canine caretakers . . .

CHAPTER 2

IT'S ABOUT TO HIT THE FAN

Seizure-Alert Dogs and the People They Love

An enthusiastic greeting from a dog is the same around the world. There's no translation needed for the blurred metronome tail, the wiggling body, the dancing paws, the eyes gazing up at you with a mixture of joy and *iloveyoupleasepetmewowicantbelieveyouareHERE!*

So when a black Lab named Nina gave me this kind of welcome when I entered her house in Zagreb, Croatia, it was refreshing to be able to communicate with her. I didn't have to keep my *molims* and my *hvalas* straight. I didn't fret about whether I was saying *"drago mi je"* ("nice to meet you") the right way or in a way that had been making the local taxi drivers smile politely and nod silently.

With Nina, I could just talk dog. Which meant, in my case, talking to her in English, supplemented with the common body language of people who love dogs: arms wide, smiling mouth open in the style of amazed babies on viral videos, eyebrows raised high. It was pointed out by my daughter when she was a mortified teenager that when I meet a happy dog, I also bobble my whole upper body from side to side.

In other words, I arrived at Nina's house and promptly looked like an idiot.

But the human members of the Kobešćak family are as polite as my cab drivers, and they smiled broadly and nodded and ushered me in. I was relieved to find that Matea Kobešćak speaks English so well that she sounds downright Australian. She works in nautical and adventure tourism around the world and has probably met her share of boaters from the land down under. She introduced me to her mother, Sanja, a special education teacher, and her father, Zdravko, an IT consultant.

As we stood in the cheerful chartreuse kitchen, I noticed they were all glancing behind me toward the floor of the next room. I looked over my shoulder and saw a figure sitting on the floor, slumped against a wall. It was Davor Kobešćak, the man I was here to see.

"Oh no! Is he OK?"

"He had a seizure, just before you rang the bell," Matea, his sister, explained.

Davor's head drooped, and he was struggling to raise it. His father excused himself and knelt in front of Davor. He spoke gently to him, in words I didn't know. In the universal language of father and ill son, you don't need to understand the words.

I watched the scene while mindlessly giving an ear rub to Nina, who was still wagging at my side. Then something occurred to me that made me yank my hand back.

"Wait, isn't Nina supposed to be helping Davor?"

Nina is Davor's lifeline. She can often predict seizures, and once Davor has one, she helps him recover. Had I been preventing her from doing her job? Was Davor suffering needlessly because the Kobešćaks were too polite to tell me to keep my hands off his service dog? It hadn't occurred to me that even without her vest, and even with her friendly greeting, she was on the job.

"No, it's OK, she already did help," Matea said. She explained that several minutes before I arrived, Nina had told the family that Davor was going to be having a problem. She did this by crying and whining around Davor, and then doing the same around the other family members. Even though a lifetime of seizures has caused profound neural damage in his brain, Davor still knows Nina is alerting. He understands everything, his mother says.

For Sanja, that's the most heartbreaking part. Her son knows what is happening, but it's hard for him to act, to move, to speak so that people outside the family understand him. She's grateful that Nina knows what's going on with him.

Matea told me that when Nina whined to the family before I arrived, Zdravko walked over to him and tried to guide him to the couch in the living room. They never know how much time will pass between Nina's warning and a seizure. It could be a minute; it could be twenty minutes.

But Davor wanted to look at his father's hand instead. He likes to study hands and the items they're holding. He can inspect hands for a long time. He also talks about one thought, over and over. Lately he has been obsessed with a memory from childhood: a boat they were pulling on a trailer while driving to the coast. His parents and sister don't know how it got stuck in a crevice of Davor's mind and keeps resurfacing. But they like to hear him talk, even if the words come out slow and mangled.

Zdravko had caught Davor as he collapsed, balancing him in expert hands and using the wall to guide his son to a sitting position. Nina, who had been watching this from a few feet away, ran over to Davor and licked all around the perimeter of his face. This was tricky because Davor's head was hanging over his chest. But she got right in there and did her job with no prompting.

Depending on the type of seizure, when Nina licks the edges of Davor's face, especially around the jawline and ears, he often starts to come out of it. A neurologist told his parents that this acts to stimulate the vagus nerve, which helps pull him out of a seizure quickly. Some people with epilepsy have vagus nerve stimulators (VNS) implanted, but the Kobešćaks say they have a four-legged VNS with no side effects.

If Nina can get to Davor and lick his face within five to ten seconds of his collapse, she can prevent his seizure from going further. It may take him a while to recover, so she'll let him have some time.

She may go in another room, or lie on his legs, or tuck herself behind him if he needs support.

When I arrived, Nina had completed the first part of her job and was waiting for the next phase. I hadn't prevented her from tending to Davor. But now it was time for her to get to work again.

Sanja walked toward her son and tapped her thigh. "Ninaaa," she sang out. The dog jogged in, licked Davor gently a few times on his cheeks and on his nose, and sat facing him. Almost immediately, Davor lifted his head. He saw his dog and stared at her for several seconds. Then he leaned down and placed his hands on the floor, trying to push himself up on all fours. He couldn't steady himself and tipped backward into a slumped sitting position again.

He looked up and saw his father's arms extended toward him. Zdravko crouched low in front of his son, reached around him, and pulled him up, slowly, carefully, his face showing the strain, and something else: the determination to make his son as OK as he could. Once Davor was standing, his father helped him over to the couch and settled him in, telling him something gently, tenderly.

Zdravko is not a large man. But he is a strong man. He has had twenty-six years of trying to help his son fall without hurting himself, of lifting him back up after a seizure, of muscling him up the stairs to their home and acting as his brakes going down the stairs. At first it wasn't so hard because Zdravko was younger and his son was smaller. As Davor grew and took on a bulky physique, it became more difficult for Zdravko. Really, for all of them, because anyone who is around Davor helps him. But Zdravko tends to be the foreman of the lifting crew, and he lives in pain he doesn't like to discuss.

"It is nothing compared with what Davor has been through," he says.

Davor had his first seizure somewhere between air-raid sirens, on November 7, 1991. He was five years old. It was a stressful time in Zagreb. The Croatian war for independence had begun earlier that year. Air-raid sirens wailed with distressing frequency.

One afternoon less than a month after the Yugoslav air force had bombed the presidential palace only three kilometers from the Kobešćak house, Davor slumped over in his chair and fell to the floor. He was briefly unconscious, and afterward it took him twenty minutes to get back to normal. Two hours later he collapsed and fell down the stairs. The family rushed him to the emergency room.

His parents say Davor was always a sensitive child. They realize the war didn't cause his epilepsy. But they still wonder if the noise and the stress could have had some effect since stress can be a trigger for seizures—if the perfect storm of conditions within his body and outside his body converged to activate something that might have otherwise lain dormant.

He was eventually diagnosed with Lennox-Gastaut syndrome—a complex and severe form of epilepsy that usually begins in early childhood, typically at three to five years of age. Children with Lennox-Gastaut often have several types of seizures and experience them frequently.

Worst for Davor and his family are the tonic-clonic seizures (previously known as grand mal seizures). They're not usually a common type of seizure with Lennox-Gastaut, but they've hit Davor hard. He loses consciousness, and if he's standing, he'll fall. His body goes stiff, and he convulses for a couple of minutes as his muscles tighten and relax. These seizures leave Davor depleted for hours.

What had felled him before my arrival was probably an atonic seizure, also known as a drop attack. They're characterized by a loss of muscle tone and can involve a loss of consciousness. They're generally brief, lasting under fifteen seconds, but Davor's tend to last several minutes without the dog's help. Even with Nina there to help him, it takes a while for him to pull out of it. His parents think it's because his brain is badly damaged from so many seizures for so many years.

Sanja can tell you about almost every seizure Davor has had in the last couple of decades. She has a master's in special education, and a few years after Davor got sick, she put on her researcher hat and started keeping journals. She has been tracking the dates, times, numbers, and every detail she can of his seizures, his medicines, his injuries from falling. She writes in script, usually in pencil. Her accounts fill twenty-one big black hardcover journals. They're clustered on three shelves in the living room, among binders and envelopes crammed with decades of medical records. Sanja hoped that by keeping track she could spot some kind of order in the chaos, discover a pattern, find a solution, a way to get her son back from this hell.

"You must do something or you lose your mind," she says.

It was around journal number eight that Sanja's entries changed. The frequency of Davor's seizures decreased. His injuries were fewer. And there was this fluffy puppy who had made her way onto the pages. Her name was Frida.* She was a black Lab they'd bought from someone who normally breeds guide dogs for the Croatian Guide Dog and Mobility Association. Sanja had asked for the organization's help when Davor turned seventeen. The trainers, who had never trained a dog for someone with seizures, guided the family on how to encourage Frida to help Davor.

Frida proved to be a natural. Even as a pup, she ran to Davor and licked his face when he was felled by a seizure. This was without any training. To the family's amazement, Davor would often become aware again. If he was unconscious and she got to him quickly enough, he wouldn't descend into the abyss. It was as if the puppy was throwing a lifeline to him.

"She loved him from the beginning. She could sense he needed her, and she knew what to do," Sanja says.

They encouraged this. They'd hand Davor a treat to give Frida

---

*I wish the little Italian Frida had a different name because now I have to make a footnote to say, "Not the same Frida as the previous chapter's Frida." The Croatian Frida was named after the song "Frida" by the Croatian pop-punk group Psihomodo Pop. The family had to come up with a name that started with *F* since all the pups of the litter were supposed to get names starting with *F*. As Matea was thinking of a name, she heard the song, which starts with lyrics that translate to "Frida was my queen." "I knew Frida was going to be so important to us, like a queen, so it was perfect," she says.

when he regained consciousness. If he couldn't manage, they'd give it to her and praise her like she'd just done the best thing in the world.

Because, of course, she had.

Frida learned other ways to decrease the length of Davor's seizures. She'd hurry over with a toy and get in his face so he could see it. She'd paw at him. Anything to get his attention on her. If he was holding something in his hands, she might take it away.

Maybe she was just trying to get him to play with her. But the Kobešćaks think Frida knew what she was doing.

It got to the point where he would sometimes regain awareness just by hearing the *tap-tap* of Frida's nails on the floor as she headed his way. Was it a conditioned response or just the distraction of his canine caretaker? His parents think it had something to do with the love Davor felt for his dog.

She was his only real friend. He attended programs outside the house and interacted with other people, but the Kobešćaks had never heard Davor call anyone a friend. When he told them, "She is my friend," it was an emotional moment for them. It still gets them choked up to realize that Frida, a dog, was the only one who made him feel this way.

The Kobešćaks describe Frida as an emotional dog. She was highly attuned to people, and if someone looked distressed, she would run to his or her side. This would even happen with strangers. A runner leaning over with his hands on his knees at the park would get the "Frida checkup." "She always cared how people were feeling," says Sanja.

Frida was only two years old when she began alerting to Davor's seizures. It wasn't a trained alert. It was more like a concerned friend who could see something was happening and wanted to let others know. At first the Kobešćaks couldn't figure out what was wrong. She would run around crying and whining in a desperate manner.

They quickly noticed a pattern. Usually within twenty minutes of Frida starting to cry, Davor would have a seizure. They couldn't believe it. Maybe it was a fluke. They timed it. Again and again, the pattern held. How could she have learned this on her own? As soon as they realized the connection, they rewarded her with loving praise and little bites of food.

Before Frida joined the family, Davor had been having about 340 seizures a year, including forty-two tonic-clonic seizures. Two years later he was down to half the number of seizures. The family didn't and still doesn't know why. It wasn't a change in medication. They attribute part of the remarkable decrease to Frida's halting many of his seizures early. They're also sure it also had something to do with Frida's love for her young man.

"It was his feeling of being loved unconditionally by someone other than us—the feeling of safety and caring," says Sanja. "You can't measure empathy or love or the connection. You can just observe the results."

Frida was so connected to Davor that when he was in his room and she was relaxing in the garden, she'd bolt inside and alert if she sensed trouble. She stayed with him until he sat or lay down, and she'd go to another family member if no one was close by. At times like this the family realized Frida was observing something other than some slight changes in Davor's manner. It had to be a scent. And it had to be a strong enough scent that she could catch some molecules as they wafted through an open window or door.

By helping Davor, Frida took some of the load off of the family. "She brought us more laughter. She had us talking to each other and others more," Sanja says. "We opened up about how we were feeling. She got us into the fresh air and introduced us to people with similar issues."

Frida couldn't detect every seizure. When Davor was having frequent seizures, she would miss some. The Kobešćaks think it had to do with the diminishment of whatever olfactory signals Frida might detect. She alerted best when the seizures were less frequent.

When Frida was eight, her health started going downhill. She had a genetic problem with her retina that was slowly causing her to go blind. She was diagnosed with a thyroid issue and was put on a

couple of medications. She slept far more than normal. And her al-
lergies were getting the better of her, causing ear infections and skin
infections that were uncomfortable and difficult to eradicate.

"A situation like this—everyone, we all age faster, we wear out,"
Sanja says.

Here's how Matea explains it: "Frida loved what she did, but it
took a toll on her. She absorbed everyone's stress and Davor's problems like a loving little sponge. She was one hundred percent dedicated to helping everyone, but we needed to give her a rest."

Frida had walked in on puppy feet and quickly changed their
lives. And now they were facing the reality anyone who has ever lost
a dog has had to face: Dogs never live long enough.

They decided to try to phase her into retirement so she could enjoy
a little downtime, and to get another puppy to train for Davor's seizures. They ended up with another black Lab they got through the
guide dog association. She came with the name Nina, and they
thought it fit her, so they kept it.

At first the Kobešćaks were concerned that maybe Frida had been
a fluke, one dog in a million. They worried that Nina wouldn't tune
into Davor's seizures as naturally, or that she'd never learn the job.

But Frida made sure that didn't happen. As soon as Nina arrived,
she became Frida's project. Nina watched Frida help Davor, and with
encouragement from the family, she began to lick his face after seizures. She watched Frida alert, and in time, it rubbed off on her.

"Frida was a brilliant model and teacher," Matea says. "Nina was
a good student."

The Kobešćaks showed me a heart-melting video of Nina as a
fuzzy little puppy lying in the grass next to Frida. Nina watched as
Frida held a stick between her paws and gnawed on it. Nina had a
stick, too, and was chewing on it in the same fashion as Frida. At one
point Nina got up to sniff the camera, then saw Frida steadfastly
gnawing her own stick, so ran back to join her again, a miniaturized
mirror image of her role model.

Frida also passed down her love of the scent of impending rain.

Nina would often follow Frida to the balcony before a rain. They'd lie next to each other and wait for it. When the rain started, they'd stay until it got too wet for them. You could almost predict the weather by watching them, Sanja says.

Nina even learned an amusing sleeping style and location from Frida: upside down, near the entry to the pantry where the dog food is kept, a front paw against the tile wall, a rear paw against the cabinet for balance. Nina did this for a good hour during my visit.

Frida died at age ten in their summer home on the Adriatic coast of Croatia. Her ashes are in a little box on a shelf in the living room of their Zagreb home, close to all of Davor's files and medical journals. Beside it is a candle and a photo of Frida as a young pup with a red Christmas ribbon around her neck.

Another photo of Frida—a large, framed, and matted black-and-white—hangs above the dining table. It's the first thing you see when you walk in the main part of the house. The photo had been tweaked to look soft and gauzy, as you'd imagine a dog from heaven might look. Frida is gazing upward, with her head slightly tilted as if listening to someone intently.

Zdravko walks into the room and looks up at Frida's image.

"She is always with us," he says, and joins Sanja and me at the table.

Nina walks outside to the balcony and lies down. We drink our hot coffee and wait for the rain to fall.

Davor is one of many epileptics who have experienced a dramatic decrease in seizures thanks to a dog. A study published in 2002 in the journal *Seizure* followed ten people with tonic-clonic seizures for forty-eight weeks as they got paired with dogs who learned to alert to their seizures. Their overall seizure frequency dropped by 43 percent. A 1999 study by the same lead researcher described similar positive results when she and her colleagues paired six people with dogs who alerted to their seizures. (They didn't report the percentage of decrease in this study.)

They posited that dogs who act as an early-warning system may decrease anxiety. Anxiety, they wrote, had been linked to seizures in a troubling reciprocal relationship: the more anxiety, the more seizures, and the more seizures, the more anxiety. The unpredictable nature of seizures can lead not only to anxiety but also depression. A dog who could tell someone of an oncoming seizure even just a few minutes ahead could significantly reduce anxiety and increase overall quality of life.

"Some of our subjects have told us that gaining the ability to predict their seizures has allowed them to engage in more activities than before, and has reduced some of the fear of the condition," the authors wrote in the 2002 paper.

In their earlier study they concluded that "the reduction in seizure frequency suggests that these specially trained seizure-alert dogs may be considered as a potential and additional treatment for people with epilepsy."

This was exciting stuff with big promise for follow-up research into the benefits of seizure-alert dogs. But you may have noticed that these are not new studies. There's been scant research on dogs and their effect on seizures since shortly after the turn of this century. This may be partly because of three small studies that came out a little later.

In a study published in 2005 in *Epilepsy & Behavior*, researchers evaluated two seizure-alert dogs whose people were inpatients at an epilepsy care unit where they had constant EEG monitoring. The result: "The dogs' performance in alerting before a seizure was poor for patient 1 and misleading for patient 2," the authors concluded. "In our limited but objective experience, the 'seizure dogs' were not as effective as previously thought in predicting seizure activity." (They did recognize that the hospital setting might affect the dogs and the patients, and called for greater numbers of patients and dogs for future research.)

Two short papers about seizure dogs published in *Neurology* in 2007 lent support to the negative view of seizure alerting. The researchers in the two small case studies found that dogs were sometimes alerting to psychological seizures—seizures with no evidence of a neurological basis. One takeaway was that people need better diagnoses before investing in seizure dogs because psychogenic non-epileptic seizures (PNES), also known as pseudoseizures, are often treated with psychiatric evaluation and behavior therapy—not the medicines for epileptic seizures. Another concern was that the dogs of people with PNES might actually be *causing* the seizures if they developed a conditioned response to "stereotypical dog behaviors."

After these papers, with the exception of a couple of systematic reviews and a groundbreaking scent study you'll read about later, it's been pretty much crickets in the science-journal world.

Despite the promising early studies that reported on the dogs who were trained to alert to their people, the consensus in some circles is that dogs cannot be trained to alert to seizures in the same way dogs can be trained to alert to diabetes; that they can only be encouraged if they show signs they can tell a seizure is coming. (This is what Davor's family did once Frida and Nina showed concern about his seizures.)

A PBS *NOVA* article from 2017 stated that "there is no proof that dogs can be trained to detect seizures, let alone predict their onset far enough in advance to tell humans about it."

The Epilepsy Foundation's website features an article entitled "Seizure-Alert Dogs—Just the Facts, Hold the Media Hype":

> "Seizure-alert dogs, save lives." . . . while it makes for a great headline, it also makes for a grave misrepresentation of the truth. The truth is, seizure dogs can not be trained to "alert" a person of an oncoming seizure.

Don't tell that to Bud, the black Lab who was trained to alert to Leslie Fong's seizures before he even met her. Leslie, who lives in Santa Rosa, California, suffers from epileptic generalized seizures, including tonic-clonic seizures, as well as occasional nonepileptic seizures. Her neurologist talked to her about how seizure-alert dogs can help. She says he recommended she check out Little Angels Service Dogs in the San Diego area.

The organization, which trains several types of service dogs, doesn't make a guarantee about dogs being able to alert to seizures. Its founders think there are certain conditions that make it harder for dogs to detect seizures ahead of time. For instance, if someone's seizures strike quickly with no change showing on an EEG reading beforehand, that person might not be a good candidate for an alert dog. Those whose brains show precursor activity even though they may not be aware of any change could be more likely to produce signals a dog can recognize. It's all conjecture, based on years of experience with clients and neurologists. The organization may soon be involved in a study that explores this.

Little Angels has produced twenty-eight seizure-alert dogs since it started in 2006. Most of the dogs are successful alerters. Leslie was willing to take the chance that her seizures might not elicit a response. At worst, she figured, she'd have a dog who could help her during and after the seizures.

Leslie sent Little Angels the requested samples of saliva on gauze pads and cotton, and other gauze pads swabbed on her palms. The samples needed to be collected and sealed in separate containers immediately after a variety of seizures. Since she has no warning of her seizures, her husband, an EMT who is becoming a nurse, helped her with the samples as soon as she was stable.

Down at the other end of the state, trainers at Little Angels had selected a dog they thought would have a good chance of becoming a seizure-alert dog. Bud, who was a rescue from a trainer's neighbor who didn't take such good care of him, was observant and focused— important qualities for a dog who's going to be on the lookout for whatever he senses before seizures. He was highly food-motivated, and the trainers were able to teach him basic obedience skills easily.

They worked with Bud on a sequence of alerting: When a trainer said "alert," he would go to the person standing in as the epileptic, tap her with his paw, run to another part of the room and push a life-alert button, then zip over to get an emergency pouch with medicine and bring it to the faux epileptic. He loved doing this. It was his joy—a big, fun game—and he got amply rewarded for it.

What happened next provides a fascinating look at how modern-day doctor dogs are starting to be trained.

One of the trainers in the large room quietly, subtly opened a screw-top jar containing one of the gauze pads with Leslie's saliva. The trainer couldn't make noise or big movements because she didn't want the dog to associate Leslie's "seizure scent" with the jar. Once the jar was open, another trainer put Bud through the alert sequence. The idea was that over time he would come to associate the smell of Leslie's seizure with the need to alert.

When Bud was deemed ready, Leslie headed down to Little Angels headquarters in the hills about twenty miles east of San Diego. She would be there for two weeks of intensive training with Bud. When she arrived on the property, a trainer brought Bud out to meet her. Leslie later sent me a video of their first encounter. It shows Bud catching a whiff of her as he approaches, and even though other new people are around, she's the one he recognizes.

"He had been smelling her saliva this whole time, and all good things came from when he smells her saliva," says Judy McDonald, one of the trainers at Little Angels. (You'll meet Judy again later in a very different chapter in her life.) "All the rewards and happiness were associated with her, and here she was in *person*."

During their second week of training, Leslie got to take Bud back to her father's house, where she was staying at night. On Bud's first night with her, she was sitting on the couch and Bud walked up to her and pawed at her.

"I didn't think anything about it," says Leslie.

"Next thing we know, she was seizing," says her husband, Brandon. "It was a grand mal seizure."

Bud did the best he could to lie on her, but the shaking was too much. He put his head in her lap and kept it there after the seizure

ended. Her seizure lasted about two minutes. Afterward, Brandon—
dumbfounded that Bud had alerted to this seizure—gave him a delectable treat and a lot of love. When Leslie came out of the worst of
the postictal state about fifteen minutes later, she realized what Bud
had done. "He is the greatest gift," she told her husband, choking
back tears.

That was in 2015. Bud has been a devoted friend and caretaker
ever since. He still sometimes tries to lie on Leslie during a tonic-
clonic seizure, as if trying to stop it from taking hold of her, but these
days he usually helps by fitting himself under her head, like a big
furry brown pillow. He figured that out himself. After her seizures,
he stays right next to her. Leslie often comes out of a seizure and
finds Bud's head and paws on her chest.

"It helps keep me calm until I'm more stable," she says.

She and Brandon continue Bud's scent-sample training to keep
him in top form. He usually alerts between thirty seconds to ten
minutes ahead of her seizures—tonic-clonic or otherwise. Bud even
wakes up from naps to tell her she's going to seize. He's not perfect.
He misses a seizure every once in a while. But he has helped give
Leslie back the ability to do the simple things, like take a shower
without fearing she'll collapse in the tub with no warning.

Bud isn't a fluke. I visited Little Angels and watched a yellow
Lab–golden retriever mix named Dexter do the same alert training
Bud had done. He also adored the game. He didn't seem to notice
when a trainer silently opened the jar labeled "Natalie." He just kept
alerting with big strides and a wagging tail.

Natalie Tapio is twenty-two and has had intractable epilepsy for
the last four years. Her focal aware seizures—also called simple partial seizures—aren't dramatic to witness. She looks like she has frozen
in place for ten seconds up to three minutes. On the inside, though,
she feels dread and fear. She is aware during the seizure, but can't
move. Even her eyes freeze in place, although she can blink. She feels
trapped in her body. If she's holding something, she will probably

drop it. If she's standing, she may fall. The seizures can happen at any time, typically about ten times a week. She has no warning of them.

Natalie had been sending cheek swabs and palm swabs to Little Angels from her home in Washington State. A few weeks after my visit, Dexter was ready to meet her. Natalie traveled down with her parents. They trained two hours a day together for two weeks. On the first day, she didn't have a seizure during training. But on the second day, Dexter ran over to her and put his paw on her leg and looked at her earnestly. Everyone in the room cried—the trainers, Natalie, her parents. Could the training be working so quickly? Three minutes later, Natalie had a seizure.

I spoke with Natalie and her mother, Lisa, several months after they took Dexter home. Dexter has been "the most amazing, amazing addition to the family," Natalie told me. He has never had a false alert, and he has missed only a few seizures, including a couple when he was sleeping, although he usually wakes up from sleep to warn Natalie.

Like many other medical alert dogs, Dexter doesn't have to be near Natalie to foretell a problem. One time Lisa and Dexter were sitting in the waiting room at the doctor's office while Natalie was in the examination room behind a closed door, down the hall. "We're sitting there, and all of a sudden he looks up at me, and he looks down the hall, and he looks at me and he paws me," Lisa said. She was stunned. Sure enough, a couple of minutes later, Natalie had a seizure in the room.

At this point it's rare for organizations to use scent to train seizure dogs to alert. Most train dogs to be seizure-response dogs who can summon help, get medicine, and stay close to their people during and after seizures. Some of these organizations teach recipients how to recognize signs that a dog is aware of seizures before they happen.

At Canine Partners for Life, in Cochranville, Pennsylvania, trainers employ a unique way to gauge their dogs' potential to recognize seizures before they occur. Candidate dogs each spend a few nights with one of their nearby graduates who has multiple seizures a day. He looks for any signs: barking, staring, not listening to any commands. If dogs show a propensity, trainers will work with them to bring out the alerts. "If it's the right dog, they just have to witness a seizure a couple of times to get it," says Tonya Guy, associate director of communications. When the client arrives at the campus for three weeks of intensive training, the alerting behavior is fine-tuned.

Even when a dog seems to have potential, trainers don't make promises about the dog's alerting ability. But all is not lost if the dog doesn't prove to be an ace alerter. At the very least, the dog will be a responder—an important job. Seizure-response dogs can be life changing. A study from 2008 in *Epilepsy & Behavior* found that 82 percent of the twenty-two people who acquired seizure-response dogs reported "major" quality-of-life improvements, and the rest had moderate improvement.

Seizure-response dogs are in high demand. Organizations that train these dogs often have long waiting lists. Georgia-based Canine Assistants has a whopper of a waiting list: more than two hundred people for seizure-response dogs. Some of the demand may be from its partnership with the global pharmaceutical group UCB, which funds the training and lifetime costs of food and vet bills for qualified people with epilepsy. But even before UCB's sponsorship of dogs, the organization couldn't keep up with demand.

Canine Assistants doesn't train its dogs to alert. "It is a natural ability of the dog that scientists still do not understand and one that cannot be trained or selected," its FAQ page states. But the organization reports an incredible statistic that made me do a double take to see if I had misread it: 87 percent of its seizure-response dogs "go on to PREDICT or react in ADVANCE of a seizure."

The 2008 *Epilepsy & Behavior* study found that 59 percent of the seizure-response dogs they followed had developed spontaneous alerting behavior. That was remarkable enough. But almost nine out of ten Canine Assistants being able to alert is a phenomenal success rate.

The percentage of pet dogs who learn to alert is far lower, but still impressive.* Not surprisingly, there's a dearth of studies on this, but a 2003 paper in *Seizure* reported that of the dogs of twenty-nine epileptics, three dogs (about 10 percent) alerted their humans to seizures.

And a year later, a pediatric neurologist with Alberta Children's Hospital at the University of Calgary reported that 15 percent of pet dogs living with epileptic children predicted their seizures. And not just every so often. These dogs reportedly alerted to 80 percent of seizures, with no false positives. "Anticipatory behaviors were never demonstrated without a subsequent seizure," he and his colleagues wrote in the journal *Neurology*. The dogs usually acquired this ability within the first month with the family, after watching just one seizure.

Talk about fast learners. And the actions of these dogs were often noble and heroic. One would "forcibly sit on her toddler and not allow her to stand prior to a drop attack," the authors wrote. One pushed a young child away from the stairs shortly before her seizure.

A family in the study had two children with seizure disorders. The dog would follow the three-year-old around the house for hours before the child had an episode, and wouldn't eat, drink, or go to anyone else. When the eight-year-old was ten minutes from a focal aware seizure, this same dog would find her and "forcefully lie" on her. The dog seemed to know that if she wasn't standing, she couldn't get badly hurt.

Dogs like these not only sense trouble brewing but also act with what seems to be an understanding of the serious nature of this condition. A dog in Minneapolis embodies these qualities. Plus he has

---

*Not all pet dogs react well to seizures. A report in the journal *Seizure* from the year 2000 noted that some dogs "may resort to a survival strategy: flight (run away, withdrawal, escape, avoidance), fight (attack, aggressive defence, protective behaviour), freeze (tonic immobility) or appeasement (conflict behaviour, vocal distress, submission or flirtatious play). Any of these behaviours will be based on a fearful and basic survival strategy." Although it is extraordinarily rare, sometimes people get hurt—or even killed. In August 2018 a Cincinnati woman's mixed-breed dog mauled her to death during her seizure. In 2016 two German shepherds killed a man who was having a seizure in his home near Cairo, Egypt.

a secret weapon against seizures on his collar. I'd like to introduce you to Brody. But first, let's meet the woman he lives for.

———

Terri Krake wanted to be a cop ever since she was a young girl. She liked to play army games, and later changed to cops and robbers—fake handcuffs and all. Friends nicknamed her "Bullet" because of this and because she ran faster than most of the kids. She looked forward to the day she could pack a pistol and put the bad guys in their place.

There was only one problem. She had never heard of a woman police officer. Then in 1974, when Terri was sixteen years old, along came Angie Dickinson in the TV series *Police Woman*. Dickinson's groundbreaking Suzanne "Sgt. Pepper" Anderson character made Terri realize she had a chance in law enforcement.

Three years later Terri was accepted into a police academy west of New Orleans and then landed a job at the sheriff's office. It provided excitement, but the jurisdiction wasn't so big that it was overwhelming. "It was a new adventure every day, and I loved it," she says. "I could finally help people and make a difference."

One summer evening in 1982, she was dispatched to a suburban neighborhood where a tank-truck driver had gotten lost, driven up a residential street, and made a left turn in such a way that the tanker overturned. The containment doors at the top of the tank weren't locked. They sprang open, and gasoline poured into the subdivision, which housed mostly older residents.

A fellow officer monitoring the scene shared his concern with Terri: "Something could happen. This could ignite from a pilot light or anything, and we're going to have a lot of hurt here."

As soon as he said this, she heard someone shouting, "Run! Run now!"

Terri wanted to know why she was supposed to run, and in which direction. She turned around to see a thin blue streak racing from a house to the overturned truck. Before she had time to process what could be going on—that a pilot light had lit the fumes—she felt intense heat and saw flames.

There was a loud *boom*. Terri rocketed into the air. A manhole cover had blasted off because of the pressure from the fire underground. As she shot up, close to the utility wiring, she thought, *Is this how I'm going to die?*

A few seconds later she crashed back down and landed on her head. She was dazed, but braved it out. She felt OK other than a loss of hearing. Everything was muffled as if she were underwater. She kept working, trying to get people out of their houses and to safer ground. Manhole covers exploded, but she barely heard them now. Gasoline snaked its way through grass and flames followed.

A few hours later, the fire was out, and everyone went back home. But Terri's life would never be the same. When she crashed to the ground, she had suffered a brain stem injury. A couple of days after the incident, she had her first seizure of a lifetime of seizures that would follow.

The worst were debilitating tonic-clonic seizures that came with no warning. Sometimes they hit her one right after another, causing her to seize far longer than the average single tonic-clonic seizure, which is usually over in a matter of a few minutes. Her partner, Lora Kennedy, would watch helplessly as Terri stiffened, lost consciousness, and thrashed and spasmed on the ground. All she could do was try to roll her on her side, get something soft under her head, and cover her with a blanket. "She truly was like a fish out of water. It was so frightening," Lora says.

Terri would never go back to the police work she loved so much, but eventually, with the help of medicines and physical therapy, she was able to find less demanding work. For more than a decade, the medicines kept the seizures under control—maybe just a couple of seizures a year, and she could sense them coming. She had a good run. But gradually the medicines lost their effectiveness.

In the late 1990s the seizures took over her life.

She became depressed and was scared to leave her house. Once highly social, she became isolated. She would go out only for doctor's appointments.

Some days she had three tonic-clonic seizures. She could drop anytime, anywhere. The seizures left her debilitated and foggy for hours after.

Terri learned her triggers for seizure onset. Pain is one of them. The seizures themselves can cause pain from sore muscles, which can bring on another seizure. But worse was the toll that falling to the ground took on her body.

All told, Terri's falls have resulted in thirty-five concussions, ten knee surgeries, three broken-nose surgeries, a broken wrist and several broken fingers, a sprained back, broken ribs, and a few shoulder dislocations.

In 2008, her neurologist suggested she try VNS therapy—sometimes described as a pacemaker for the brain. A device about the size of a silver dollar is implanted in the chest wall. Thin wires from the device are woven around the left vagus nerve in the neck. When the VNS is activated, it sends electrical impulses up the vagus nerve to the brain stem, which sends signals to areas of the brain involved in seizures.

Just what it does in the brain is still something of a mystery. "We don't know exactly how VNS works," states a page about VNS on the Epilepsy Foundation website. But in some people it can dramatically decrease seizures.

Terri figured she had nothing to lose but seizures, so she opted for the implant. Her neurologist worked with her in the following months to figure out the best rate and level of the electrical impulse. The sweet spot seemed to be an impulse every five minutes.

When it goes off, Terri knows. VNS devices can affect the voice and cause a slight choking sensation. When she talks during an impulse, she sounds like someone has a hand around her throat—and she says it feels like it, too. That sensation lasts thirty seconds. Every five minutes. All day, all night.

She's learned to live with this because it's minor compared with her seizures. VNS isn't a magic bullet against seizures. It doesn't always work. And even if it does, users still have seizures. The idea is that they won't go on longer than the interval between the electrical pulses. Those lucky enough to sense a seizure before it begins can take advantage of a special magnet that comes with most VNS devices. They can swipe it over the implant and may be able to prevent the seizure from starting. Since Terri could never tell when she was going to have a seizure, this feature didn't help her.

The magnet can also be used to stop a seizure once it starts by having someone else place the magnet over the device. That works if others are around, but Terri was often alone since Lora worked long hours as a data-entry specialist. While the implant was reducing the impact of the seizures, Terri was far from seizure-free.

She was resigned to living the rest of her life as a recluse. Her only companion during the day while Lora worked was their old rottweiler, Izabeaux, or Izzy for short. When Terri had seizures, Izzy often lay by her side. When Terri came to, Izzy would lick her hand and face. Terri found it comforting that this dog was so devoted. It made her feel less horribly alone and scared when she woke up disoriented and in pain. And Izzy's licks seemed to help her come through the fog more quickly.

When Izzy died of cancer in 2009, Terri felt more alone and despondent than ever.

A neurologist had told her about dogs who help people with seizure disorders. When her grief over Izzy's death lifted a little, she started doing research. It turned out there was an organization only eighteen miles away that trained these dogs. Besides general service dog skills like opening the refrigerator or drawers to retrieve items, the seizure dogs could fetch medicine and a phone, and summon help by pushing a big life-alert button on the floor. They were also trained to lie next to their person during a seizure, or on their lap. After a seizure, dogs would lick their person on the hand or face.

This sounded awfully familiar to Terri, who realized Izzy had really known what she was doing.

Terri applied to Can Do Canines and got called in for an interview. By now she *really* wanted a seizure service dog and was nervous about how she'd do at the interview. She had to scrape the rust off her ability to speak with people other than doctors and family. She didn't want to screw up.

She didn't have to worry. Trainer Mona Elder liked her immediately. "She was warm, smart, sincere, and truly in need of one of our dogs," she says. "And she had a really interesting idea."

Terri asked Mona if it would be possible to train a service dog to use the VNS magnet. Mona didn't see why not. The magnet is a little larger than a quarter, and with some ingenuity, it could be attached to a dog collar. Since the organization already trains its seizure dogs to lie next to their clients during a seizure, it probably wouldn't take much tweaking to get a dog to lie with his neck to Terri's chest.

Mona had a dog in mind for Terri: a big black Lab named Brody. She hoped they'd be a good match. As soon as Terri saw him from the other side of the training room, she knew he was the one. "I was smitten," she says. "My heart just melted."

The feeling was mutual. Brody ignored the little treats Mona tossed to him and headed straight for Terri. She bent down to say hello and he licked her all over her face. Then he stopped and sat and stared at her with his deep brown eyes for a long time. She says she knew what he was trying to tell her.

I'm here for you and I know you're the one I'm meant to be with. I've got you, don't worry.

Over the next months, she learned all the ways Brody could help her. He had trained with people acting as if they were having a seizure—not with people having real seizures. The transition usually works out, but only time would tell.

Early in their training together, Terri got to bring Brody home for a weekend. He was fifteen months old. She was just supposed to play with him and hang out. She was ecstatic about being able to spend a whole weekend with him. Friday was fun and games. On Saturday, Lora went to work and it was just Brody and Terri.

Terri doesn't remember falling. But she does remember that when she came out of the seizure, Brody was with her. She couldn't move much yet, but she could see he was lying right next to her, flanking her side. She felt a surge of warmth and relief that he was so close to her, and that she wasn't alone.

Then she felt something else. Something sharp in her side and something odd on her chest. Once she regained use of her arms, she propped herself up and saw that she was buried in dog toys.

She realized that while she was seizing, Brody had brought all the toys he could find, plus some hand weights that held his toy box in place. He even brought over the "Brody phone," the big life-alert button he hadn't quite learned to use yet.

"When I saw all he had done to help me, I just cried and hugged him tightly. He won my heart that day, forever," she says.

Mona soon added a new task for Brody: the snuggle. He quickly learned that when Terri said, "Snuggle," he needed to get his collar over the left side of her chest, above her heart. This would get him in the right position for the magnet to activate the VNS.

While snuggling with Brody made Terri happy, she says the electrical impulse triggered by the magnet "felt like a karate chop to my Adam's apple."* Afterward she always coughed. The cough was Brody's signal to lie on her legs to keep her from standing until she had recovered.

Getting out of the house was an essential part of the training. At first it was disconcerting, like coming out of a dark room into the bright light before your eyes have adjusted. But Brody and Mona guided Terri through the rough spots, and soon she was walking with confidence into places she'd never dreamed she'd go again.

The three of them took field trips to grocery stores, restaurants, movies, parks, and malls. It was the standard public-access training all the organization's dogs get, but for Terri it was much more than that. It was her baptism into the world she had left behind.

---

*It would later turn out the electrode was anchored in a place that was causing a far more dramatic reaction than most VNS users experience.

. . .

Brody had been living with Terri for only ten weeks when he began alerting to her seizures. At first it wasn't a clear alert. He would get agitated, pace, not listen. Sometimes he head-butted her legs. She couldn't figure out what was going on, but pretty much every time, she'd have a seizure a few minutes after this odd behavior.

It wasn't hard to correlate his behavior and her seizures. Soon Terri learned to read his body language, and would lie down and ask him to snuggle. His magnet would set off the electrical impulse, *boom*, and she wouldn't seize. It took about a year to fine-tune their communications about this matter, with Brody pawing at her thigh until she paid attention.*

The first year they were together, he activated the VNS device sixty-nine times. The second year, he was up to ninety-nine times. These days he alerts more than a hundred times a year; Terri has just a few seizures a month because he's able to prevent the bulk of them.

Before she got Brody, she was raced in an ambulance to the emergency room up to three times a week because of injuries or overly long seizures. In the eight years she's had him, she's taken this trip fewer than twenty times. She attributes 30 percent of this success to VNS and 70 percent to Brody.

"It's like having my own personal EMT 24/7," she says. "An EMT who snuggles and lets me hug him and is my best friend."

When I visited Terri in her three-story home in the Longfellow neighborhood of Minneapolis, Brody greeted me at the door, wagging his tail in goofy circles and licking my face when I reached down to rumple his ears. He was graying under his eyes and along his chin, but his black coat gleamed as it must have in his youth. I

---

*The magnet is a strong one. So strong, in fact, that Brody once got stuck to the refrigerator door and couldn't pull himself away until Terri found him and coached him on how to get out of the embarrassing predicament. She says that since then he has been more careful about opening and closing the fridge while fetching her items, and that when he does get stuck on occasion, he can extricate himself without too much fuss.

fell for this older gentleman immediately, and could imagine how Terri must have felt when she first met the young dog who would end her time as a reluctant recluse.

Terri made her way to the living room, limping slightly and walking slowly. "This is what happens when I don't listen to Brody," she said.

She sat on the floor with her back against a couch. Brody immediately left my side and walked over to Terri. He looked at her closely, lay down perpendicular to her leg, and rested his head on her shin, facing her. It would be his vantage point for much of our interview. His eyes shifted from Terri to me and back as we talked, following the conversation as if it were a Ping-Pong game.

Brody can alert Terri to most of her seizures, even if he's sleeping. But sometimes she's not paying enough attention. Maybe she's in a rush or too focused on something else to notice. A few days before I arrived, Terri and Brody were leaving the house to go to breakfast with a friend, who was waiting in her car in front of their house. Brody kept stepping in front of Terri. He blocked her path on the stairs and got underfoot.

"C'mon, move, Brody, I'm hungry!"

This wasn't like him. Normally Brody is a gentleman, always walking beside her, checking in with her to make sure she's doing OK. And here he was, almost tripping her. "Brody, that's annoying," she said. It's the last thing she remembers before her seizure.

She dropped hard. She injured her knees and dislocated her right shoulder. "You'd think I'd learn my lesson," she said. "You do not ignore this dog."

One time she was at the top of the stairs and seized and fell backward to the bottom. Brody had been trying to tell her, but she figured she just needed to get up to her bed. She broke some ribs in addition to two banister spindles and ended up with a concussion. Brody ran over and activated her VNS, then raced to the "Brody phone" and slammed it with his paw. As Terri was emerging from the seizure, she heard the emergency responder's voice crackle on the other end: "Brody, I'm going to stay right here with you. Help is on the way."

Brody doesn't need to be near Terri to sense a seizure coming on.

Sometimes he's on one floor of the house and she's on another. He'll thunder up or down the stairs, skid to a stop next to her, and alert. She'll get her chest close to him and *bam*. Seizure prevented.

Even though Terri wasn't able to walk long distances when I visited, she still got Brody out for long walks. She'd sit on her motorized scooter and hold the leash as they meandered through the neighborhood.

Brody gets to enjoy the big backyard whenever he needs to. And once a week he and several other service dogs come together for playtime. Terri imagines they probably swap stories and give one another advice, but to the humans it looks like it's all about running around and having a blast.

She enjoys seeing Brody cutting loose like this. She says he's a workaholic. This dog was not content to be just a seizure savior. At some point, he branched out into several other specialties.

A few years back, Brody developed an odd obsession with Terri's neck. He sniffed and nudged it with his nose several times a day. She thought maybe it was his new way of connecting with her. But after several weeks, she noticed that when he bumped her in certain parts of her neck, it hurt. She decided to bring it up to her doctor when she went in for something else.

The diagnosis: medullary thyroid cancer.

Brody, the oncologist.

"Brody knew it all along," she said. "He was just trying to get me to figure it out. He saved my life—again."

Brody stayed by her side through medical tests, and as soon as she was out of surgery and the hospital staff gave the OK, he jumped up to the foot of her bed, lay down, and curled up tight next to her feet. She wasn't fully conscious, but she learned later that her feet moved toward him as soon as she sensed he was there. He rested his chin on her ankles, sighed, and went to sleep. He stayed with her around the clock as she recovered.

Since the surgery, Brody hasn't paid any attention to her neck.

Terri still gets checked every six months, just in case, but she's pretty sure she'd hear from Brody if anything was wrong.

But her medical issues weren't over. Besides her "pacemaker for the brain," Terri ended up getting a heart pacemaker because of severe irregular heartbeats. It doesn't do the job she hoped it would, and she frequently experiences atrial fibrillation and tachycardia episodes.

Guess who usually tells her about them before they happen?

Brody, the cardiologist.

When he senses heart trouble coming, he won't let her move. If she gets up, he stands in front of her. If they're walking, he'll stop and look at her.

"I finally learned it's the way he says *DANGER!*"

And then there's Brody, the endocrinologist. Lora has also had significant health issues over the last few years. On top of her own heart problems, she developed diabetes. Brody will tell her when her blood sugar is off. He places his head on her lap and won't move until she checks.

"He's been right every single time," Lora said. "I thought he couldn't possibly do more than he already is, and he took me on, too."

Dr. Brody's patient list is never closed.

The only problem with Brody is that he's ten years old. Terri knows Labs have a shorter shelf life than smaller dogs, and she worries about what will happen when she loses him. Two of his littermates, who were also service dogs, have already died. Another one had a massive stroke.

She doesn't want to think about the heart-shredding pain of his death. She's afraid that without him, she'll plunge back into the darkness. Maybe there will be another medical alert dog for her one day, but she's sure there will never be another dog remotely like Brody.

"We're so melded together. This hand is the dog who saved me," she said, making a small arc motion with her left hand. "And this hand is me," she said, drawing her right hand and wrapping her hands in a tight ball. "We're like one heart beating together."

━━━

How do dogs like Brody, Frida, Nina, Bud, and Dexter detect seizures? A review paper published in *Epilepsy Research* in 2011 concluded that "the consensus . . . is that dogs probably alert to specific and subtle human behaviour." For years it's been thought that dogs are sensing subtle changes in facial expressions, breathing, heart rate, and body language, or that dogs might be detecting unusual electrical signals from the brain.

I put the question to Nathaniel Hall, PhD, director of the Canine Olfaction Research and Education Laboratory at Texas Tech University, when I met him at a conference in Arizona in 2017.

"We really have no idea. It hasn't been researched to any degree," he told me. "The dogs may be smelling a biochemical change if there is one, but no one has shown this."

The theory that scent could play a role in alerting is becoming more accepted as we learn about the power of dogs to sniff out disease. Our understanding is limited, but two studies are beginning to shed light on what's going on.

The English charity Medical Detection Dogs is probably the world's foremost center for training dogs to sniff out the scent of disease. The organization is working with Ghent University Hospital in Belgium "to show that seizures have an odor, just like the other diseases," says Claire Guest, the organization's cofounder and chief executive.

The hospital has been sending Medical Detection Dogs samples from people in pre-seizure mode—probably around the time a dog would be able to smell something if there is a scent. One year of the three-year study has been completed. Claire wasn't at liberty to say much about the results because they were preparing to publish a paper, and the results have to be hush-hush until then.

"I can say that it's going very well," she told me.

The other study paired a team from the University of Rennes 1 in

France with Medical Mutts, the organization that did one of the diabetes studies cited in the previous chapter. Medical Mutts, like Little Angels, trains its seizure-alert dogs to alert to the scent of its epileptic clients.

The samples for the study were all collected in the hospital. The researchers swabbed the skin of patients during seizures, during "normal" time, and during exercise. (The patients also blew breath into a plastic bag in which the samples were stored.) Five dogs who had been trained on samples from other people during their seizures successfully alerted to the seizure samples only. The samples they alerted to represented a variety of seizures.

"We are thrilled to finally be able to scientifically show what we've known for a long time," said Dr. Cattet of Medical Mutts.*

Maybe one day dogs will help researchers find out what scents they're detecting before seizures manifest. This could aid in the development of a device that could be used by anyone to "sniff" and alert before a seizure felled them.

Researchers around the globe are already following dogs' noses to uncover the hidden scents of one of the leading causes of death. Cancer strikes more than 1.7 million Americans each year and seventeen million people worldwide. What our canine research partners are helping us learn may lead to more of us surviving the "emperor of all maladies."

---

*She was also thrilled when, in spring of 2019, a paper about the study was published in Nature.com's *Scientific Reports*, and made headlines around the world. But since this book was nearing completion at my publisher, I wasn't able to go into the details of this exciting, late-breaking development.

CHAPTER 3

A DOCTOR DOG IN THIS FIGHT

How Canines May One Day Help You Survive Cancer

Baby Boo was an unassuming medium-size dog with ears that flopped out sideways and rotated forward like small triangular satellite dishes. When she trotted down the sidewalk of her leafy London neighborhood, they flapped like the wings of a happy cartoon bird. Her saucer eyes conveyed more emotion than the average dog's. Every time she looked slightly to the side, the whites showed, giving her the appearance of intelligent concern.

She had the sleek black-and-brown coat of a Doberman pinscher. But the eyes were definitely and intensely border collie. One darting glance would deflate a rebel sheep's fantasies of breaking from the flock.

Baby Boo was the daughter of a border collie–ish dog named Frisky Fru. The Whitfield family had adopted Frisky Fru when their neighbors moved and didn't want to take her. The Whitfields didn't realize Frisky Fru was pregnant. They were able to find homes for all but one pup—the runt of the litter. One of the children, smitten with her from the moment she was born, called her Baby Boo. It stuck.

A caring soul from the start, Baby Boo was always tending to Frisky Fru and the other family dog, Lucy Lou, who happened to be a kleptomaniac. Lucy Lou, a retriever-Dalmatian mix, lived to escape from the house or yard and dash off to nearby shops, where she would pilfer whatever she could get her mouth on. Usually it was small items, like cookies or little cakes, but once she brought home a can of baked beans.

"Oh no! Why do you steal things, Lucy Lou?" her family asked. But Baby Boo didn't care that her housemate was a thief. She groomed her and watched over her almost as much as she looked after her own mother.

Then an odd thing happened when she was about two. Baby Boo took an interest in a spot on the leg of Bonita Whitfield, who was forty-four. As Bonita washed dishes at the sink, Baby Boo would walk up behind her and sniff the back of her left thigh for several seconds until Bonita shooed her away. This went on for a few months, with Baby Boo snortling into the back of Bonita's thigh whenever opportunity allowed, even when Bonita was wearing slacks.

Bonita found it annoying, but what could she do? Dogs will be dogs.

One warm summer afternoon, on a day off from her banking job, Bonita decided the outside of the house's windows needed cleaning. She changed into shorts and brought her supplies and a ladder to the yard. The dogs followed. Partway through her task, she came down from the ladder, and sweet, gentle, caring Baby Boo jumped up and bit at the back of her leg. She did it again and again. It was the same spot she'd been sniffing all along. The nips didn't draw blood, but they hurt. Bonita couldn't figure out what had gotten into her.

Later that day, Bonita was changing into a skirt when she touched the spot that had so interested Baby Boo. It was raised. She twisted around and saw it was a fairly large black bump. She had never seen it before.

She brought it up to the bank's secretary, who had once worked at a skin clinic in Canada. The secretary took a look and insisted Bonita call her doctor immediately. The doctor saw it and sent her to King's College Hospital in London. A doctor there excised the lesion and sent it for a biopsy.

It turned out to be a melanoma, the deadliest form of skin cancer. They'd caught it just in time. The doctor told her that in another year, the cancer would have spread throughout her body.

Baby Boo became the family hero, getting extra treats and hugs all the way round. With the mole gone, she no longer examined Bonita's leg. Her discovery would have just been another interesting family story if not for a young researcher named Hywel Williams.

Dr. Williams was training to become a dermatologist at King's College Hospital. While reviewing more than two hundred cases of malignant melanoma from previous decades, he came to Bonita's file. He noticed that someone had written, "Dog sniffed at mole!!!"

"I laughed it off, but that night as I drove home, I kept thinking about it. I called her the next day and learned her fascinating story," Dr. Williams, MD, DSc, told me when I got in touch twenty-eight years after it happened.

"One could say this dog literally saved her life."

He wrote about the case with dermatologist Andres Pembroke in a letter to the editor of the prestigious general medical journal the *Lancet*. It appeared in the April 1, 1989, issue. The doctors told the patient's story (not referring to Bonita or her dog by name) in a couple of paragraphs and suggested that this might be worth exploring scientifically.

"Perhaps malignant tumors such as melanoma, with their aberrant protein synthesis, emit unique odors which, though undetectable to man, are easily detected by dogs with their well-developed rhinencephalon."*

The letter concluded, "We have not as yet proceeded to a trial of sniffer dogs in our melanoma clinic but the adjunctive use of animals with highly developed sensory modalities in cancer diagnosis is worth considering . . ."

The letter was one of forty letters published that week. It livened up the space between "Warning against Use of Intrathecal Mitoxantrone" and "Immunosuppressive Properties of Cyclosporin Metabolites."

---

*"Rhinencephalon" is a somewhat awkward-sounding word for the part of the brain that deals with smell. Sometimes it's just called the "smell brain," which sounds like something my brother and I called each other as kids.

"Sniffer Dogs in the Melanoma Clinic?" was the least scientific-sounding title in the journal that week, unless you include "Impregnated via a Bullet?," which you probably should.* But it's likely that it got far more publicity than any of the other letters or articles.

The Associated Press picked up the story, and reporters from around the world sought interviews with Dr. Williams, and sometimes with Bonita. The story appeared in different versions in media outlets around the globe, from respected newspapers to the *Weekly World News*, which added dramatic flair with the headline "PET DOG SNIFFS OUT GAL'S CANCER *and saves her life!*" The half-page piece appeared after a full-page article entitled "SPACE SHUTTLE ATTACKED BY 200-FT. UFO!" with the subtitle *"Bug-eyed aliens invaded Discovery & terrified crew."* (If you had read about Baby Boo in that article, you could not be blamed if you didn't believe it.)

There had been anecdotes of people's dogs detecting their cancer before, but nothing had appeared in a scientific journal. This gave legitimacy to the idea. Still, the science world took much longer than mainstream media to warm up to it.

Dr. Williams tried to get funding for cancer-detection dog research after the *Lancet* letter, but couldn't. "I think there was a lot of skepticism in the scientific world, and we were just in the wrong place at the wrong time," he said.

For years, there was no news of any research in the field.

Then, in the mid-1990s, a Tallahassee, Florida, dermatologist took an innovative approach to dogs helping with cancer detection. Armand Cognetta, MD, who specialized in skin cancer, was frustrated

---

*"Impregnated via a Bullet?" was a one-paragraph letter to the *Lancet* that referred to a case report published in the same journal in 1875: Back in the American Civil War, a seventeen-year-old girl was watching a battle (people used to do this) when she was struck in the abdomen by a Union soldier's bullet that had somehow gone through a Confederate soldier's left testicle. She became pregnant and later married the Confederate soldier. (But son of a gun! I looked it up on Snopes, which reports that the story had been printed as a bit of fun in the *American Medical Weekly* in 1874. Journals that subsequently reprinted portions of it as fact did not catch the gag. If nothing else, the name of the "doctor" reporting it—L. G. Capers—should have been a hint.)

that one in five melanomas was not discovered in time for the patient to survive.

"I literally go to sleep sometimes thinking, 'What's a better way?'" Dr. Cognetta said in an Associated Press article.

He had heard a radio report of a dog who sniffed out a body in a lake and wondered if it would be possible for a dog's great nose to be used for cancer detection. A search of the scientific literature led him to the *Lancet* letter. He asked local dog expert Duane Pickel if he thought a dog could be trained to detect cancer. Duane, who had handled and trained dogs in the military and was retired after twenty-two years in the Tallahassee Police Department's K-9 unit, told him what he'd hoped to hear:

"A dog can be trained to find anything you need it to find."

Duane volunteered his dog George for the cause. George was a standard schnauzer he'd already trained as a bomb-detection dog. Duane developed a fun way for George to want to sniff out cancer: He hid test tubes containing melanoma samples around a room and asked George to find them. When he did, Duane rewarded him. George was always happy to find a test tube with melanoma. The next phase of training saw George alerting to a test tube with the melanoma in a rack with other test tubes that didn't contain a malignancy. He did extremely well over repeated trials, with a reported accuracy of 99 percent.

Then George went from detecting melanoma *in vitro* to doing it at least somewhat *in vivo*. A nurse with a family history of skin cancer volunteered to wear dozens of bandages, one of which would have a melanoma sample sealed under it. Would George know melanoma without the test tube? They waited as he circled her and sniffed.

He seemed attracted to one of the bandages. He sniffed it extra hard. Then he sat and looked at it. Nailed it!

Later he would be trained to gently touch the spot with his paw. They did more than forty trials in a year and reported that George again reached nearly 100 percent accuracy. When it came to real patients with melanoma, George met with seven over a couple of years and correctly identified a malignancy in four of them—maybe five, depending on how you interpret it. It wasn't anywhere near 100 percent, but Dr. Cognetta and Duane thought the misses could have happened because George had been trained on the nurse, who always showered first, washed her clothes with scent-free detergent, and didn't smoke. Patients probably had many olfactory distractions.

Dr. Cognetta's study was understandably rudimentary, but it was a brave foray into the idea proposed by Dr. Williams and Dr. Pembroke. He had no question that dogs *can* detect cancer. But how accurately?

"That's for the next phase, done elsewhere," he said in the AP article.

It would be several more years before there was serious research on cancer-detection dogs. This new phase may have been kicked off, yet again, by another letter to the editor of the *Lancet*. It was coauthored by none other than Dr. Williams, and entitled "Another Sniffer Dog for the Clinic?"

Dr. Williams and Dr. John Church, a retired orthopedic surgeon, reported on a sixty-six-year-old man whose Labrador retriever, Parker, kept pushing his nose into his man's thigh. It was a spot the man had been treating as eczema for eighteen years. But after two years of his dog hounding him, he gave in and went to the doctor. In September 2000, the lesion was removed and turned out to be basal cell carcinoma. After it was gone, Parker showed no more interest in the spot.

This letter to the *Lancet* concluded with a call to arms:

Although all these data are anecdotal, we believe that the phenomenon of some dogs seeming able to detect unique odours of certain skin cancers worthy of investigation in rigorously controlled experiments. Whether they can detect odours associated with other specific diseases such as tuberculosis or Ebola virus should also be investigated to aid early detection.

The letter was published in the September 15, 2001, issue—a mere four days after 9/11. It could easily have gotten lost, buried under the rubble of the tragedy that gripped the world. Mainstream media didn't give the letter much attention. Reporters had their hands full.

But in a switch, this time it was science that took notice. The seed had been planted by the first letter, and after a long period of dormancy while conditions for its survival were improving, the idea was ready to germinate. In 2003, Dr. Church held a conference in the United Kingdom about ways to use dogs for studies on cancer detection. Among the speakers at the packed event were Tadeusz Jezierski, PhD, DSc, a revered canine-olfaction expert from Poland, and Michael McCulloch, PhD, who had begun his own cancer-detection dog study in California.

The conference helped launch a new field at the intersection of science and dogs. It was the beginning of the golden age of research on cancer-detection dogs.

Funding and studies would take time. One study here, one study there, a year or two or three in between—like a promise of rain after a drought. Even now, there's not a deluge of studies, but the number of researchers using dogs to sniff out cancer continues to increase.

Most of the published studies mention the 1989 *Lancet* letter as the starting point for science acknowledging the possibility that dogs can detect cancer. So do the mainstream articles that report on these studies.

Even though Dr. Williams—with the help of Bonita and Baby Boo—had kicked off this new field, he would be involved in only one study of dogs detecting cancer. He has moved on to other areas of dermatology research and practice.

He's now a professor of dermato-epidemiology at the Centre of Evidence Based Dermatology, University of Nottingham. He is also the director of the National Institute for Health Research's Health Technology Assessment Programme. It's a big-deal national job. As he wrote me in an email: "Basically I am in charge of most of the major publicly funded trials happening in the UK NHS today (around 400 studies worth around £1/2 billion). I am the first dermatologist to hold such a post and it is a great honour. I remain director until Oct 2020, then I shall fall in a heap." He still does research (he has published more than five hundred papers) and has a weekly clinic in pediatric dermatology.*

He fancies whimsical bow ties and speaks in a charming, sing-songy South Wales accent. His report on Baby Boo's feat is still a highlight of his storied career.

"I look at it with fondness, especially to see some good research eventually developing that might help cancer patients in the future," he told me. "It was quite a risky thing for me to report at such an early stage of my training, but we felt it was important to suggest the scientific idea so that others could make a judgment for themselves.

"It showed me that research isn't linear. Sometimes it's enough to have an idea and let others test it out."

He said of all his patients, in all his years of practice, Bonita was the one who had the most effect on his work.

"It taught me the importance of listening to patients. They are often right about things even though we might not have the technical and scientific knowledge to explain everything when we first encounter them."

I wondered what had become of Bonita. I looked for her and didn't find any contact information. I feared the worst. Maybe another melanoma had eluded Baby Boo.

---

*As busy as Dr. Williams is, he writes autoreply emails that are something of a legend among his many correspondents. When I tried contacting him in late December 2017, I got this response:

Some of you have already started to send me sneaky emails in the hope of getting one of my draft autoreplies. I am not sure how to take that, but no chicken stories this time. But talking of emails, I just am wondering how long it will be before I get one of those invites to be a keynote speaker at an obscure meeting on a topic I know nothing about? Do you get lots of those?—I get around 12 a day. They usually start off telling me about the nice meeting location and then throw in the names of some important-sounding people, giving you the illusion that you are someone special being invited to give a keynote. Sometimes, I am tempted to say that I will come, but I know it would all end in tears, and in me parting with lots of money for nothing in return. That is their purpose after all, so I should not complain.

But when I poked around social media, I found her on Facebook. There hadn't been any activity for a long time. I reached out to her and, just in case, to her daughter, Jane, hoping they wouldn't think I was a creepy stalker. A couple of weeks later, I heard from Jane. She told me that Bonita is alive and well and would love to speak with me.

Bonita is seventy-five, a great-grandmother, and an animated talker. She has no more dogs. Frisky Fru died at eighteen, tended to more tenderly than ever in her dotage by daughter Baby Boo. Lucy Lou also passed on at an old age after a life of debauched thievery. Baby Boo lived to be nineteen years old. They are all buried in Bonita's yard. The only pet she has now is a cat named Bert who likes to drink water from the tap.

"I know I wouldn't be here today if it weren't for Baby Boo," she said. "Since that time, I always listen to my pets. They talk to you. You just have to be able to know what they're saying."

Bonita didn't seem to realize what Baby Boo's actions had started. I told her about the many studies and articles that have referred to the *Lancet* letter, and the current state of research involving dogs detecting cancer.

"Oh, that's lovely, isn't it?" she said. "It's her little legacy. Baby Boo would like that."

——

Claire Guest bursts into her small office at the headquarters of Medical Detection Dogs with four dogs in tow. "I'm terribly sorry for keeping you," she says, wiping a streak of dog slobber from her leather riding boots with something she pulled from her vest pocket. "They needed a walk and it always takes longer than you think it will."

Medical Detection Dogs is involved in several important national and international studies. Camilla, Duchess of Cornwall, and her husband, Prince Charles, are patrons of the nonprofit. British press reported that the duchess got emotional at a demonstration in which she and the prince watched as three Labrador retrievers detected cancer samples with ease.

Claire has even met with Queen Elizabeth II on a couple of occasions.

But today Claire is sitting on the floor of a small office that now smells of dog breath, and brushing burrs out of the fur of two panting English cocker spaniels.

Medical Detection Dogs is located in the midst of rich green swaths of farmland in the village of Great Horwood, about ninety minutes northwest of London. It's glorious countryside, but during certain times of year, the burrs seem to Velcro themselves onto the dogs, especially the ones with the more resplendent coats.

As we talk, and Claire picks at the more stubborn burrs, people dash into her office every few minutes to ask questions, or take dogs for training, or tell her about upcoming appointments. She's used to multitasking. She's busy nonstop these days.

"It's never-ending," she says. "I love the energy and the excitement because the world is really finally taking it seriously that dogs do seem to be able to detect cancer."

The organization officially started in 2008, but its roots go back to 2003, when Claire and Dr. Church—the coauthor of the second *Lancet* letter—collaborated with several others on a study to find out whether dogs can detect cancer. (This is known as a proof-of-principle, or proof-of-concept, study.) Six dogs—including a wee papillon—were trained to detect the scent of bladder cancer in urine in a lineup of six healthy subjects. They were successful 41 percent of the time—not stellar compared with today's standards, but a statistically significant success rate compared with the 14 percent expected by chance. It was an exciting result because it was a scientifically rigorous study.

The study was published in the *BMJ* in 2004. It proposed the idea that tumors release volatile organic compounds that have distinctive odors dogs can detect even in small quantities thanks to their "exceptional olfactory acuity."

"The results we achieved should provide a benchmark against which future studies can be compared," the authors wrote, "and we hope that our approach to training may assist others engaged in similar work."*

Even more intriguing than the dogs' overall success was when all six dogs appeared to fail. They all "unequivocally" alerted on what had been deemed a control—a urine specimen declared negative for bladder cancer based on cystoscopy and ultrasonography. The paper explained what happened next: "The consultant responsible for the patient was sufficiently concerned to bring forward further tests, and a transitional cell carcinoma of the right kidney was discovered."

In other words, the dogs beat the doctors and their sophisticated equipment. And they detected a cancer they had not been trained to detect.

The study, as predicted by the researchers, helped inspire more canine cancer-detection work around the world. "For me," says Claire, "the paper was the moment when I knew that this work must continue." The research led to the founding of Medical Detection Dogs. Claire had worked for Hearing Dogs for Deaf People for twenty years when she left to cofound Medical Detection Dogs with Dr. Church. It was harder to get backing—financial and otherwise—than they'd anticipated.

"There was huge skepticism to overcome and it took us considerable time to build support and then register the charity," she says.

In 2009, Claire's fox red Labrador retriever, Daisy, was among the dogs being trained on cancer samples. She had been acting strangely around Claire. One day, while Claire was letting her dogs out of the back of the car at a park, Daisy just sat and stared at Claire. Claire thought she looked anxious. Then Daisy smashed her nose into Claire's chest a couple of times, prodding her hard. That evening she felt that area of her chest. There was a lump.

Claire knew many stories of dogs detecting cancer in their own

---

*By coincidence, two months later, *Applied Animal Behaviour Science* would publish a study by Duane Pickel and his group on their latest findings on dogs detecting melanoma. It's not every day a retired K-9 officer and military dog handler gets top billing on a scientific paper.

people. She figured it was nothing, but just in case, she made an appointment with her doctor. The lump she felt was a harmless cyst, but deep behind it was something the doctors thought needed further investigation. After a mammogram and core biopsy, she was diagnosed with breast cancer.

She had a lumpectomy, several lymph nodes removed, and five weeks of radiation, and has been cancer-free since. "Because the tumor was so deep," she says, "the doctor told me by the time I discovered it on my own it may have been too late. Daisy saved my life."

As Claire tells me the story in more detail than I had already read in her book *Daisy's Gift*, the star of the book is lying in a cushy dog bed. She is thirteen and has arthritis in most of her joints. She looks frail, but she is alert as ever, with her large brown eyes trained on Claire. Someone walks in the office.

"Time for PT, Daisy! You ready?" Daisy lumbers out of her bed, stretches, and wags down the hall for physical therapy.

"Daisy is everything to me. She saved my life, she's my best friend and confidante, and she helped give me hope to keep going with detection work despite all the skeptics," she says. "I dread the day she won't be with me anymore."* She tries not to think about it. Focusing on the organization helps keep her mind from the inevitable.

Medical Detection Dogs has about thirty biodetection dogs on its team these days. Most work in cancer detection, and some others are in pilot projects for detecting other diseases. All of the dogs live in homes and come in a few days a week for training or working.

With just a couple of exceptions, that's the setup for almost all cancer-detection dogs in the world. They spend most of their time with their families—often fosters taking care of them during their couple or so years of work. Training is fun and reward-based, and working periods are kept short.

---

*Daisy passed away about four months later, at fourteen. "Her work persuaded many of the possibilities of a revolutionary way to detect cancer," Claire wrote on MDD's website. "Her legacy will live on in the work of the charity and will lead to advances never thought possible." I feel lucky to have met the old girl.

Medical Detection Dogs is involved with two large cancer studies. One is a breast cancer study with rigorous protocols—so rigorous that the study had been paused shortly before my visit. The dogs had already completed work on breath samples from one thousand patients, but the amount of breath in the tubes was not consistent enough. The trial had been kicked back to research and development. It's not the first breast cancer study to use the noses of dogs, although when it proceeds, it will be by far the most comprehensive.

A groundbreaking study by Dr. McCulloch, Dr. Jezierski, and colleagues published in 2006 found that dogs could distinguish between exhaled breath samples of women with breast cancer and healthy women. The dogs demonstrated 88 percent sensitivity (the ability to detect the disease, a true positive) and 98 percent specificity (the ability to identify samples without the disease, a true negative; in the case of dogs detecting cancer, that means ignoring the negative sample rather than alerting to it). But the results of another study published two years later were disappointing. None of the six dogs performed better than chance for detecting the positive samples, and only two out of the six dogs showed specificity better than chance.

In a promising study in 2017 by the Curie Institute in Paris, 130 women with breast cancer kept a square of gauze, held in place by a clean bra, against their affected breast overnight. They sealed the square in a sterile jar, and the samples were later sniffed by two Belgian shepherds. The dogs had a success rate of 90 percent on the first trial and 100 percent on the second trial. (No figures are available on false positives.) The institute hopes to start a three-year clinical trial to test the feasibility of this technique for cancer screening.

The other cancer work that's keeping the dogs at MDD busy is a proof-of-principle study on prostate cancer, with dogs looking for cancer in urine samples of three thousand participants—the largest of any such study so far. In initial training trials, the dogs had an impressive 93 percent reliability rate. Four previous prostate cancer studies by others have ranged from a low of 13 percent sensitivity and

71 percent specificity to a high of 99 percent sensitivity and 97 percent specificity.

Claire has no doubt dogs can accurately detect cancer. Not usually, at least.

"Some nights I wake up in a hot sweat," she says. "What if I made this all up? Then I watch the dogs alerting to cancer, working so well, and all is well."

The two cocker spaniels Claire had been grooming during our conversation pass her inspection. One lies down on a chair; the other pads off to a dog bed on the floor.

"Excuse me just for a second," Claire says. She brings over a handheld vacuum, gets on her knees, and hoovers the crimson carpet of all the burrs and fur. I want to grab the vacuum and do it myself. "*You* shouldn't be doing this," I would tell her. "You know the queen of the United Kingdom!"

But before I can get the words out, she's done.

"So much to do, so little time. The clock is always ticking."

———

Lives are on the line. People around the world are dying from cancers they might have been able to survive if detected earlier. Too often, the tests available today don't find cancers until it's too late. Or they're invasive or expensive, or both.

Some researchers would like to figure out a way to have dogs screen large numbers of patient samples quickly and reliably in laboratory settings. Having dogs screen patients in person is not the goal of serious scientists.

"That would be rather like the grim reaper, wouldn't it?" says Claire. "We don't want dogs to become that."

Besides the bad PR of having dogs giving dire news by offering a paw or sitting and staring, most researchers say there are too many confounding factors to ever have dogs examine people in real life. They want this to be science, not educated guessing. It's challenging enough to get accurate results with dogs in a laboratory setting for one specific cancer, much less on a whole person for many types of cancer.

"The doctor dog will see you now" is not a likely phrase you'll hear at your physical in the future, despite occasional news headlines about dogs performing "PET scans."* The dogs who may one day help save lives will likely remain behind the scenes.

So far, dogs have been trained with varying degrees of success to look for breast, cervical, colorectal, lung, stomach, liver, ovarian, prostate, skin, and thyroid cancers. Trained dogs have sniffed for cancers in more than a half dozen sample types, including blood and sweat, urine and feces (no dog would complain about this assignment), and tissue samples and breath.

Dogs seem to be able to detect cancers across all four stages—not just when cancer is advanced.† That's exciting news, and encouraging. Early detection not only would save lives, but also could make treatment far less debilitating or prolonged.

Good science takes time. Proof-of-principle studies are going on around the world. Ideally, science learns from its mistakes. The authors of papers often write about ways to improve future research. The authors of the breast cancer study where dogs didn't perform better than chance, for instance, suggested that "better management of urine samples and a more stringent training protocol during our study may have provided new evidence as to the feasibility of using canines for cancer detection."

Yet even studies that seem to be glowing successes can have flaws

---

*Not to mention cats doing "CAT scans." The idea of cats sniffing cancer may not be far-fetched. I've come across a few accounts of cats reportedly alerting their people to cancer. One, a rescued Oregon cat named Mia, made her person aware she might have a problem in her right breast. "All of a sudden out of nowhere she just got up on my chest and she sniffed that breast and then looked in my face, sniffed the spot again and looked in my face," Michelle Pearson said in a radio interview. "I tried to shove her off and she came back up and just laid down on that right breast. And she looked at me like, *I'm trying to tell you something.*" Michelle went to the doctor and was diagnosed with Stage 2 breast cancer.

†Some researchers think it may even be possible for dogs to detect precancerous cells, but precancer is a tricky topic, and much more research needs to be done.

that aren't apparent until later research fine-tunes techniques. What researchers have learned during these studies highlights the intelligence and remarkable senses of canines.

In some of these studies, handlers have been in the same room and visible to the dogs. It may not be a big deal, but it could be a confounding factor—something researchers try to pare away to get to the purest and best results.

The problem is that dogs can be so attuned to our body language—sometimes even the subtlest shift in expression—that they may be taking unintentional cues from the person in the room. It's a phenomenon known as the Clever Hans effect.

Hans was a horse who lived in the early 1900s and wowed crowds with what seemed to be his mental prowess. It looked like he could tell musical notes from one another, read, spell, do simple math, compute fractions, tell time, and identify dates on a calendar. He answered spoken and written questions by tapping numbers or letters with his hoof. Even biologists, doctors, and psychologists believed he could do these feats.

A commission in his native Germany was set up to figure out what was going on, and determined it wasn't a hoax. But shortly after, a biologist and psychologist figured out that Hans *was* very clever, although not in the way everyone—including his human partner—had thought. He concluded that Hans was so observant that he could read the "almost microscopic signals" in his owner's face.*

It has become more common—almost standard—for handlers to be hidden behind a screen or in another room during studies of dogs sniffing for disease. I watched dogs who sniff for colorectal cancer in a pilot study in the Netherlands burst with wagging tails through a little doggy door into a room with the samples on a scent carousel as

---

*After this, Hans's reputation went down the drain. He met a tragic and undeserved end. I'm a softy, and it's too hard for me to write it in my words, so I'll quote from a paper in the *Communicative & Integrative Biology* journal: "At the beginning of World War I in 1914 he was drafted as a military horse and was killed in action in 1916 or was consumed by hungry soldiers."

researchers observed from a large one-way window. The handler was hidden in the room behind a white box with a little one-way window for observing, and popped out to reward the dog for correct answers.

One of the dogs in the study was a Belgian Malinois. I've never seen this hard-core breed doing work other than for the police or military—tracking bad guys, taking them down, or sniffing for drugs or bombs. Seeing the same breed of dog brought by Navy SEAL Team 6 on the Osama bin Laden compound raid now checking for colon cancer in a neat Dutch lab gave me an even greater respect for this breed's capabilities.

Cancer studies have used many breeds of dogs—including Labrador retrievers, German shepherds, poodles, dachshunds, golden retrievers, Large Munsterländers, rottweilers, schnauzers, cocker spaniels, springer spaniels, Havanese, and Portuguese water dogs—and mixed breeds as well. The breed of dogs doesn't seem to matter as much as the dog's drive for a reward.

If a dog isn't toy- or food-driven, he or she won't have much motivation to work. As much as we'd like to think otherwise, dogs are not doing this work to benefit mankind. They're doing this for a ball or a special toy or a tasty snack, mixed with sincere praise for a job well done.

But just because dogs have good noses and are happy to work for rewards doesn't mean all dogs will be great at detecting the scents we ask them to find. Dr. Angle, the Auburn University researcher we met in the book's introduction, says this is one reason he and his team use several dogs in each study. Even though the dogs they work with come from the CPS breeding program, which is on its seventeenth generation of Labrador retrievers bred to be top-notch sniffers, not all the dogs are going to be able to do the job.

"We can have ten dogs on a study. Maybe eight can detect something, and the other two can't detect it at all," he says. "It's a physical capability like in humans. Same breeds, same bloodlines, but very different results."

It's kind of like how some people, thanks to what may be a genetic variation, can't smell the odor asparagus gives urine.

If someone runs a cancer study using only one or two dogs, and those dogs happen to be the ones who can't detect that scent, it could lead to unfortunate outcomes. Along the lines of that soon-to-be-tired analogy, you'd hate to run a study with humans sniffing the urine of people who recently ate asparagus, and inadvertently use humans whose sense of smell can't pick up the scent.

In general, though, dogs are masters at finding most scents.

"If there's an odor, we can train them on it," says Cindy Otto, DVM, PhD, founder and executive director of the Penn Vet Working Dog Center at the University of Pennsylvania. "They're heroes without knowing how important they are."

But how do dogs even get to the stage where they can detect cancer? No one knows what the volatile organic compounds of cancers are, so researchers can't simply whip up a soup of known VOCs to train a dog. The dog has to be a sleuth and put together an olfactory picture from the VOCs in samples presented to him or her. Considering there are hundreds of VOCs in even healthy samples, it's a mind-boggling feat.

Dr. Otto likens it to people learning to find Waldo on a page of a *Where's Waldo?* book—without knowing what Waldo looks like. They can't even exclude objects while they search. They may point to the woman in the bathing suit, the striped umbrella, the piece of cake, in their attempt to find out what a Waldo is. But eventually they will find Waldo, and *boom!* From then on, the happy, nerdy fellow with the red-and-white-striped shirt, matching hat, and blue pants is the guy they'll pursue.

It's more complicated than that in cancer detection. Dogs may be sniffing for patterns of VOCs. There is no one Waldo.

In most of this research, dogs are looking for the common odor within one type of cancer. It's believed that each cancer has a scent that's unique to it and it alone. Lung cancer may have its own scent, and breast cancer may have its own. Researchers are asking dogs to find the fingerprint scent.

But an important question remains: Does cancer itself have an overall common odor—something shared by most or all cancers?

It's not a question most researchers have tried to answer yet. But thanks to anecdotes about cancer-detecting dogs being able to find more than one kind of cancer, many in the field are willing to conjecture there may be a generalized cancer smell.

"It may be like listening to a piece by Mozart," says Claire. "It's complex, but every so often you come across a bar of music that repeats. It could be like that with cancer. There could be that repeating bar, that one small common factor."

She's careful when she talks about this idea, though. "There's no published evidence that dogs can detect different cancers by one scent. Stating this as fact could result in discrediting the work, and there's some fantastic work being done."

Claire has had personal experiences with a dog being able to detect multiple types of cancers, but she tries not to let it get in the way of pure science. Daisy, credited with detecting Claire's breast cancer, has also successfully sniffed a few types of cancer at Medical Detection Dogs. She had originally been trained on bladder cancer for a study. But she later rooted out samples of prostate cancer and kidney cancer.

It could be that Daisy learned to differentiate cancers by their individual, unique scents. Or maybe she discovered a general scent that cancers have in common. Claire sometimes wishes Daisy could talk. "Oh, the things she could tell me!"

Researchers are in awe of the odors dogs can detect, but it's a double-edged sword. Canine olfaction is so keen that it can end up being frustrating when trying to do real science.

While dogs are figuring out what they're supposed to be finding in a study, they may choose samples based on the location where the samples were obtained. Dogs have picked up on hospital disinfectant odor and alerted to that. They've even selected samples based on the person preparing the samples.

Dr. Angle says since people shed so many skin cells—thirty thousand to forty thousand per *minute*—dogs have alerted to the person dealing with the samples, even though the person is wearing gloves.

"Dogs are natural biosensors. They track things," he says. "They're innately able to pick up on a human odor, so you have to have this in mind when conducting studies."

Researchers continue to try to improve the ways dogs can detect cancer. There are dozens—sometimes hundreds—of details they need to consider when putting together a strong study that might make it into a peer-reviewed journal to further the science. What's the best way of training the dogs? Who will collect the samples? How should the samples be stored? How long should detection sessions be?

A more recent question—and a vital one: Can we get enough samples so a dog doesn't have to sniff the same sample twice?

It turns out that dogs have really good memories for smell. "Their olfactory memories are crazy!" says Dr. Otto. Dr. Angle seconds that. "Dogs can remember samples for *years*," he says. "We've pulled synthetic odors from old projects years later, and the dog still alerts to it as if they'd been trained on it yesterday."

That's good, in a way. That might be part of the reason dogs may be able to zero in on "Waldo" so well. But there's a flip side to this great memory: Dogs have been known to memorize the sample itself instead of responding to the cancer in a sample.

"They basically learned *that* odor of *that* sample, not of ovarian cancer generally," says Jennifer Essler, PhD, a postdoctoral fellow at the Working Dog Center.

It would be as if you were in an experiment where you have to push a button every time you see an image of someone with earrings in order to get a reward. The images are random and can be shown more than once. Eventually you might take the shortcut, and instead of looking for the earrings, you might recognize the person wearing the earrings. So every time you see, say, Emma, with her curly brown hair and wide-set eyes, you'll push the buzzer. You don't have to go to the trouble of looking at her ears to see if there are earrings anymore.

With dogs, it's much the same. The scent of a sample might be stronger than the scent of the cancer. If dogs have enough repetitions of a sample, they might end up having a hard time generalizing the odor for the cancer in their study.

"Dogs cheat," says Dr. Otto. "They love to do this, and if you put a shortcut in inadvertently, they will take it. They don't have any skin in the game."

Samples are already like gold. As common as cancer is, researchers in the field have to work hard to get adequate numbers of samples. When the dogs' memorization skills became apparent, it created a new challenge. Scientists need to figure out ways to get more samples, or get creative.

Dr. Otto and her team are trying to do both while training dogs to detect ovarian cancer. Since their approach is unique, and since I have a personal interest in this particular cancer, I thought a visit might be in order.

———

Dr. Otto, her training manager Pat Kaynaroglu, and I are in stealth mode. We're hiding behind a one-way mirrored window in a large storage room of the Penn Vet Working Dog Center, waiting quietly. We're about to see if Osa, a German shepherd, can alert to blood plasma samples of ovarian cancer.

We don't want her to know we're there. She's been training nearly a year for this day, and if we do more than whisper, she'll hear us and might get distracted. I even have to be careful about flipping the pages of my reporter's notebook because the sounds travel from our area to hers almost as if we're in the same room.

A few dogs at the center can already detect ovarian cancer in plasma. But this is Osa's first time trying. Until now, Osa has been trained on ovarian cancer cell lines. Cell lines, which you may have learned about in Rebecca Skloot's book and the subsequent movie, *The Immortal Life of Henrietta Lacks,* if not in Biology 101, keep dividing and growing in the laboratory and are widely used in cancer research. They can be bought online from laboratories around the world.*

If Osa could alert to the plasma of women with ovarian cancer, it would be a big deal. Not only would it mean that the dogs are alerting to the actual cancer, and not the body's reaction to cancer, but it also would mean the team might not have to "waste" as much of its precious store of ovarian cancer plasma samples during training. Dogs could initially train on the cell lines, then switch to plasma, and more samples could be reserved for studies.

Osa strides into the detection room, and I hold my breath. She walks quickly around the scent carousel, sniffing at samples in each port at the end of eight steel arms. She doesn't alert anywhere.

But the next time she goes around, she stops and sniffs one of the samples for a couple of seconds. We hear the *click* of the training clicker, and she runs to the next room for her reward. The handler, with changed gloves, puts a new sample in another port and we wait.

This time, Osa stops and sniffs the port with the new sample. It's not a full alert, but it's close enough. *Click!*

"She's really telling us something!" Dr. Otto exclaims in a whisper while Osa is out of sight enjoying her reward. Dr. Otto is beaming. Osa goes around one more time, stops at the correct port, and is done.

"She has *so* found a Waldo!" Dr. Otto says. "She did it!"

---

*You really do just go online and put cancer cell lines in your shopping cart. I randomly selected a life sciences company that sells three hundred thousand products, found the cancer cell lines, selected ovarian cancer cell lines from two dozen types of cancers, then clicked on three different cell lines, adding them to my cart as I would do with books or socks on Amazon. They were about $300 each. I clicked my cart and had to register. I stopped there because (1) I would rather buy socks and books than ovarian cancer cell lines, and (2) I'm pretty sure that at some point I was going to have to prove I was a scientist qualified to buy such items. But it was fun to see how easy it is for real researchers to purchase them for studies.

. . .

I learned that day that scientific discovery is not always glamorous. It can be three people hiding like Peeping Toms, silently thrilling to a dog's slight change of behavior. It was exciting to be a witness to something that could make a difference in how dogs detect ovarian cancer in the future.

The day before, I'd watched a mostly black shepherd named Bobbie as she got ready to sniff diluted blood plasma from someone with ovarian cancer. She had already been trained to detect a single drop of undiluted plasma. Now she had advanced to a one-to-one ratio, half plasma, half saline. Researchers had mixed one drop of plasma and one drop of saline, then extracted one drop of this mixture as the sample for detection.

Keep in mind this isn't whole blood. Plasma is just one part of blood. It's the yellowish clear liquid that carries red blood cells, white blood cells, platelets, and other components of blood. That a dog can detect a single drop of plasma is remarkable. That a dog can detect plasma diluted one to one with saline is extraordinary. Some dogs at the center had even been alerting to a one-to-two ratio.

It's a scientific limbo dance with cancer scent, seeing how low it can go before it's too low for the dogs to be able to smell it. The diluted plasma wasn't riding the carousel by itself that day. The other ports contained controls, including plasma from women with benign ovarian tumors, plasma from women with no known tumors at all, saline, and ordinary items like paper clips and latex gloves.

Before starting, Bobbie trotted over to a large bin of dog toys in the room adjoining the detection room. "Dogs get to choose their own paychecks here," said Dr. Essler.

Bobbie dipped her nose into the bin and selected a rubber bone-shaped toy and walked off with it. Dr. Essler was surprised. "That's not her normal choice," she told me.

Bobbie stopped and seemed to think. She walked back to the bin and returned it. She chose a blue rubber ball instead. "Ha-ha, that's her usual choice!" Dr. Essler said. Bobbie is a dog who knows what she likes. The hope was that she would also like diluted plasma from ovarian cancer patients.

The first time around the scent wheel, she missed the diluted plasma. A handler switched the positions, but she missed again. I wondered if the scent could have become too low for Bobbie. Was a one-to-one dilution too much?

She took a third stroll around the carousel. This time she alerted to port six.

Yes! Click, cheers, the bounce of a ball. Next time she found a new sample in port eight. After that, she nailed it every time.

If Henry Higgins had been in attendance, he would have had occasion to exclaim, "I think she's got it! By George, she's got it!" As it was, the room of researchers and handlers let her know she was a very good girl. After each alert, she chomped the ball and wagged her tail and reveled in the praise.

The only times Bobbie didn't alert were when there was no plasma from ovarian cancer patients. This wasn't an error; it's called a blank. In a blank, all arms of the carousel hold some kind of scent, but the cancer is left out.

When a session is blank, dogs shouldn't alert. In fact, dogs are rewarded for not alerting. They always have to have positive feedback for the right answer. If there's nothing in a particular round and dogs have been trained with the expectation of always finding something, they'll often "find" something anyway just to get a reward.

In other words, they'll cheat.

So they need to learn that it's OK if there's nothing. They should find a cancer sample only if it's really there. That's pretty obvious, but until recently, blanks hadn't been commonly used.

Blanks are important if the science of sniffing cancer is to go beyond studies of known cancer samples and move to actual screening for cancer in the real world. In cancer screening, no one knows if a sample is positive or negative. Dogs have to be able to slog through round after round, and possibly come across no positives for several sessions. If they don't get rewards, they could start alerting to cancer that isn't there. That's a problem. Even worse would be if a dog were bored or distracted or overwhelmed and missed a positive sample.

Researchers at Krems University Hospital in Austria set up part of a lung cancer study as if it were a screening. "To imitate a real-life situation, the dogs were not rewarded during the actual testing," explains Klaus Hackner, MD, coauthor of the study. "We did not want to reinforce a possible wrong result." The handlers also didn't know which—if any—of the five samples of breath during each detection round was from someone with lung cancer.

In traditional studies, someone is in the know, and the dog is rewarded. But in this screening-like study, Dr. Hackner says, "the lack of feedback was very stressful for both the dogs and the handlers."

Dr. Hackner, a dog-lover himself, notes that the dogs didn't end the test days stressed. "They were treated with much care, and 'after work' they were of course rewarded." (It's what he'd want for his own dog, a beloved decade-old beagle mix named Pauli. "He enriches my life every day.")

At the end of the testing, the dogs recognized 78 percent of the samples that were positive for lung cancer. But they "diagnosed" 66 percent of healthy samples as cancerous. (In the scientific parlance introduced earlier, that's 78 percent sensitivity, 34 percent specificity.) If this had been a real screening, it would have resulted in quite a few sick people not being diagnosed, and a lot of worried, healthy people being flagged for potential cancer.

In their paper in the *Journal of Breath Research*, Dr. Hackner and his coauthors concluded that "canine scent detection might not be as powerful as is looked for in real screening situations. One main reason for the rather poor performance in our setting might be the higher stress from the lack of positive responses for dogs and handlers."

In other words, without a regular paycheck, dogs may not be reliable. The authors suggested "positive feedback mechanisms for future study designs. In fact, it seems to be favourable to confront dogs relatively often with the pattern odours." Adding positive samples during screenings may help dogs remain accurate and inspired.

Most researchers in the field agree that, so far, dogs seem to be good at detecting cancer in a laboratory setting where someone knows if a sample is cancerous or not and dogs get rewarded when correct. As methodologies improve, so should accuracy.

But will dogs one day be able to reliably screen samples from patients whose cancer status isn't known? I had heard of only one scientist in the world attempting to screen the public.* I wanted to know more—to see what this would look like in real life. I packed my bags and headed west. Way west. The story of doctor dogs took me to a beautiful community far beyond anything I expected.

It is a challenge to get to the town of Kaneyama, in Japan's Yamagata Prefecture. First there's the trip to Tokyo. If you're leaving from San Francisco, as I did, it's a ten-hour flight across the Pacific Ocean, over features like the Chinook Trough, the international date line, and the massive Hawaiian-Emperor seamount chain. You can't actu-

---

*That's not to say no one is screening people. Glenn Ferguson, a former kayak instructor, has been screening American firefighters for cancer with five dogs, mostly beagles, for a few years from his Gatineau, Quebec, town house. Firefighters, who are at higher risk for certain cancers, wear a surgical mask for ten minutes, pop it into a vial, and their department mails the masks to him via his organization, CancerDogs. Glenn trained his first dogs from samples he collected in shopping malls and at cancer runs and walks. But he says the dogs' repertoire has increased to include most cancers. When I spoke with him he was up to ten thousand firefighters annually. He charges $30 each. That's a pittance for a diagnostic test but adds up to a handsome piece.

His dogs always have a positive sample planted among screenings of seventeen masks at a time to keep up morale, and they alert to samples frequently. Average fire departments have about a 25 percent positive rate, and a couple were at 50 percent. (Glenn says one of those was redone with better collection and storage practices on the firefighter end, and the rate dropped to 25 percent.) The positive results leave firefighters concerned and scrambling for further testing. For those who test positive, Glenn recommends a plant-based diet and, for starters, getting a skin checkup, a colonoscopy, and, for women, a mammogram. "These can be done relatively inexpensively and rule out a lot of cancers," he says.

At press time a startup in Israel was inviting people to send in saliva samples for its dogs to sniff for cancer, claiming a 95 percent success rate, "including early detection." The cost was 400 Israeli shekels, or about $110.

ally see most of these except on your seat-back monitor when you get
tired of hopelessly cramming essential polite expressions you should
have learned weeks ago from your Japanese phrase book.*

Then there's the Shinkansen ride out of Tokyo. It's best to spend
some time in Tokyo before embarking on this journey. Getting to the
high-speed rail for the big trip is an adventure of its own; the Tokyo
Metro subway map looks like a plate of spaghetti someone has
dropped on the floor. Once finally on the Shinkansen—the best form
of public transportation you will ever take if you like cleanliness,
pleasant and on-time service, and sweet chiming arrival and depar-
ture tunes—you bullet your way north.

Eight stops and 272 kilometers later, you arrive in Fukushima,†
where the Shinkansen becomes more of a local train. It slows down a
little, which is good, because you'll soon be streaming through some
of the most beautiful scenery in the world. Rice fields flash by, gold,
green, then soba fields with their white blossoms. Gold, green, white,
gold, green, white, backed by rich green pyramids of hills and mountains, each with its own faithful entourage of bright white clouds.

In ten more stops, you reach Shinjo, the end of the line. You are
now 421 kilometers north of Tokyo. But you're still about fifteen
kilometers south of Kaneyama. There's a nearby bus that can get you
there. It takes about thirty-five minutes. Or you can rent a car if
you're confident about driving on what Americans tend to call the
"wrong" side of the road.

Luckily for my trip, Akiei Shibata, a Kaneyama town clinic official, was waiting at the station. He would escort me along with Masao Miyashita, MD, PhD. Dr. Miyashita had joined me on the
Shinkansen in Koriyama, the stop before Fukushima. He had spent
the morning at a hospital there performing endoscopies—something

---

*Not that I'm speaking from personal experience or anything . . .

†The train doesn't stop anywhere near the site of the Fukushima Daiichi nuclear
disaster. It's about a ninety-minute drive from Fukushima to the nuclear plant of
the same name, not that you will be driving to or from there. And anyway, it's
decommissioned.

he does once a week on a "day off." Normally he works at the Nippon Medical School Chiba Hokusoh Hospital, in Inzai, Chiba Prefecture, east of Tokyo. He's a busy guy—deputy director of the hospital and head of digestive surgery there. He's also a professor at the med ical school, and involved in several research projects.

The doctor's pet project was the reason I had made this trip. Several years ago, after reading studies from around the world about dogs and their cancer-detection capabilities, he wanted to explore the possibilities himself. Anything that could help with early cancer detection sounded good to him. He'd seen too many deaths, watched too many patients and their families suffer.

He knew there was a dog available for some studies he wanted to do, thanks to an earlier study by Hideto Sonoda, MD, PhD, from the Department of Surgery and Science at Kyushu University in Fukuoka, Japan. Dr. Sonoda's team reported in the journal *Gut* that the sole dog in the study was highly accurate at detecting colorectal cancer from breath and stool samples. It seemed the dog could even detect early-stage cancer.

Dr. Miyashita met with Yuji Sato, who runs St. Sugar Japan, the cancer-detection dog training center used by Dr. Sonoda. He was impressed by Marine, the black Labrador retriever who appeared to be a one-dog cancer-detection unit as she sniffed out several types of cancer. Dr. Miyashita and other researchers from Nippon Medical School ended up working with St. Sugar on two studies—one on breast cancer, one on cervical cancer. Marine worked on the cervical cancer study, and a dog trained specifically for breast cancer was the sole dog in the other study.

After Marine died, Sato-san brought on a few other Labrador retrievers he had been training to detect the scent of cancer.* Dr. Miyashita was happy to see that these dogs, like Marine, appeared to be able to detect more than two dozen types of cancer—almost any cancer presented to them.

---

*This section uses last names followed by "-san" for most of those without MDs or PhDs. It is the polite and acceptable way in Japan, and it wouldn't do to call them by their first names in this book.

"There seem to be common VOCs for all or most cancers," he had told me on the train, "and I think each cancer might also have its own unique VOCs. Of course, much more work will need to be done, but I find it amazing."

In a way, Dr. Miyashita came to Kaneyama because of horses. A few years back he was looking into offering horse therapy at his hospital for patients and staff. The expert he was working with knew a man who does horse therapy in Kaneyama. In addition to his work with horses, Wataru Inoue produces a lecture series. He invited Dr. Miyashita to see the horses and give a seminar on any topic.

Dr. Miyashita's topic was "amazing animals"—"the super abilities of whales, dolphins, owls, and butterflies," he told me, "and of course, cancer-sniffer dogs." After the talk, Inoue-san brought the doctor into town and introduced him to Mayor Hiroshi Suzuki.

Mayor Suzuki was troubled. A thick issue of a magazine had recently been published listing cancer mortality rates and numbers in Japan. Of Japan's 344 "secondary medical districts," Mogami—the rural area that includes Kaneyama—had the highest mortality rate for stomach cancer in women. The ranking for men's mortality from stomach cancer was 22 out of 344.

Areas of northern Japan are known to have high rates of stomach cancer. Dr. Miyashita and other gastric cancer specialists say there are probably a number of causes, including high intake of salt from the pickled and preserved foods common to the region, genetics, an aging population, and infection with the bacteria *Helicobacter pylori*.

The mayor was worried about the health of Kaneyama's citizens, and embarrassed by the ranking. He asked the doctor for advice. Dr. Miyashita went over all the usual causes of stomach cancer. Mayor Suzuki wanted to know if there were easy, noninvasive screening tests. There are not.

Dr. Miyashita told him about his work with cancer-detection dogs. He explained that the dogs haven't ever screened for cancer, just worked in studies. He couldn't make any guarantees, but it would be interesting to see if the dogs could succeed. He thought they'd have a good chance.

Mayor Suzuki was excited about the possibility of the residents receiving screenings that could detect cancer early and save their lives. He brought it up at the next town council meeting.

The council voted to spend 11 million yen ($98,000) annually to conduct a screening study of up to 1,000 of its 5,600 residents. The members approved the project for three years, but funding would have to be approved each of the following years. People who signed up would be tested for cancer—cancer in general, not just stomach cancer—by submitting a urine sample, which would be frozen and sent to the Chiba hospital, then brought to St. Sugar. Results would come back within three months, and anyone who tested positive through the dog analysis would receive medical consultation and further testing through traditional methods like endoscopy and CT scan.

It had been four months since the start of the study when I arrived at the Shinjo train station with Dr. Miyashita. He was scheduled to give a talk to Kaneyama's residents that evening, updating them on the results of the screening so far. The dogs had screened about 250 samples and alerted to five samples. Dr. Miyashita and a local doctor would be meeting with these men and women the following day to discuss options and quell fears.

Shibata-san drove us to Kaneyama as opera music from a Verdi CD filled his Honda. The farther we got from Shinjo, the more spectacular the scenery: cedar forests, streams, rivers, traditional old Japanese houses, colorful rectangular fields of vegetables and grains almost ready for harvest, mountains shrouded in mist.

It was hard to believe that this pristine paradise could be so high up on the cancer-mortality list.

When we arrived in Kaneyama—whose name means "golden mountain"—school was getting out. Dozens of uniformed elementary school students were walking home. They smiled and told us "*Konnichiwa!*"

Many children seemed surprised to see me. Tall Caucasian women with wavy hair made unruly by the September humidity are not common in these parts. A few, with big grins, carefully practiced their English: "Hello! How. Are. You?" I smiled back. "I'm doing great, thank you! How are you?" They laughed and gave me thumbs-up or peace signs.

Shibata-san told me (through Dr. Miyashita, who would be my translator for the duration) that it is "very, very uncommon" to have Western visitors here. And yet at least one of its brochures is in both English and Japanese—just in case foreign tourism ticks up.

In a little park in town, next to a mountain stream burbling with big and colorful koi, sits a monument commemorating British explorer and writer Isabella Bird. She steamed to the area in 1878 and traveled Japan by train, foot, horse, "man cart," boat, and, once or twice, a cow. She briefly mentioned Kaneyama in her book *Unbeaten Tracks in Japan* when describing the area's stunning mountains, which seemed to block her northward progress: "At their feet lies Kaneyama in a romantic situation, and, though I arrived as early as noon, I am staying for a day or two, for my room at the Transport Office is cheerful and pleasant, the agent is most polite, a very rough region lies before me, and Ito has secured a chicken for the first time since leaving Nikko!"

I wondered how much the area had changed since she passed through. Several large old homes and buildings in the main part of town appear quite old, but I don't know if they could have been around when she was here.

They look as if a Swiss Alps architect and a Japanese architect had gotten together long ago and designed a new breed of mountain structure. Their outer walls are thick and smooth, and coated with bright white paint. Dark brown cedar roofs with steep slopes jut far past the walls, protecting them from the deep snows of winter, and other wooden "mini roofs" shelter every door and window. Shibata-san said that long ago, these had been miso storage buildings.

One of these buildings now houses a gift store that specializes in cedar products, made from local wood that is a backbone of the economy here. You walk in and are greeted by the fresh woodsy scent of cedar emanating from the cedar walls and from all the items for sale. While I shopped, Enya's *Shepherd Moons* album was playing, and a light rain pattered against the thick windows upstairs.

The mayor was expecting us, so I made my purchases, which the shopkeeper wrapped in white paper marked with little koi and green mountains.

We arrived at the office of Mayor Suzuki. A tall, elegant man with light steel-colored hair, he was wearing no-rim glasses and a crisp blue-striped shirt. His secretary served us tea in locally made ceramic cups set on cedar saucers. Dr. Miyashita briefed him on the project so he'd know what to expect at the town meeting. I asked questions here and there, as the doctor translated for me.

Mayor Suzuki stated that he was "embarrassed and concerned that the mortality rate for stomach cancer is so high. We need to help the people in whatever way we can to keep them healthy.

"We hope and believe the dogs can succeed, because people will be happier to have the easy screening of the dog than the usual methods."

Mayor Suzuki said his mother had died of stomach cancer fifteen years earlier at the age of eighty-two. Her doctor didn't tell her she had terminal cancer. This wasn't unusual. In fact, it was the norm. Until the early 1990s—or, in some cases, much more recently—it was a long-standing custom in Japan for doctors not to tell patients the truth about their cancer diagnoses, especially if they had a terminal illness. A 1988 UPI article stated that eight out of ten doctors said they lied to their cancer patients.

The patient's immediate family members, if there were any, would be told, and it would be up to them to tell the dying loved one. But chances were that the dying family member would not find out. Another survey, reported in 1989, said that only 21 percent of people would pass along a cancer diagnosis to their sick relative.

Until the late 1980s Dr. Miyashita himself often used to withhold the truth because it was viewed as something that would be upsetting to the patient. People with hopeless gastric cancer might be told they had an ulcer.* Even Emperor Hirohito, who was diagnosed with duodenal cancer in 1987, was apparently never told of his diagnosis. He died in January 1989, after a dreadful last few months. It was only after his death that his cancer was announced to the public.

Gradually Japan changed, and patients are now told if they have cancer, no matter how bad it is. Some more traditional rural areas came along more slowly, which is why Mayor Suzuki's mother, who died in 2002 three months after her diagnosis, did not know.

And now, with this study at hand, people would not only be learning if they had cancer, but the news would be coming, indirectly, through dogs. I found the residents' ability to not only embrace the times but try to race ahead of the times admirable.

That night about 250 people gathered in a large meeting hall to hear Dr. Miyashita discuss the progress and to ask questions. The faces were serious as he went through a PowerPoint presentation showing dogs and statistics.

For some reason I was seated at a table in the front of the room next to the stage. The mayor had introduced me to the audience. I knew this when I heard my name and something like the words "American journalist."

Several TV and newspaper reporters, including an NHK news crew, filmed or took notes as Dr. Miyashita spoke. I understood nothing he said except "cancer-sniffing dog." Those words brought me back to a road trip I'd taken with Dr. Miyashita a couple of days earlier to meet one of the cancer-sniffing dogs on the project. Since I had nothing else to do, I jotted down some extra notes I hadn't had time to write from that day.

On the two-hour drive from Dr. Miyashita's hospital to St. Sugar, it became clear that he is someone who thinks outside the box—a

---

*If you want to see a powerful, haunting film about this, watch the 1952 Akira Kurosawa movie *Ikiru* ("To Live"). You may look at life a little differently when you are done.

quality that goes along with his willingness to screen a remote town for cancer via dogs.

Shortly after we started our drive, he connected his mobile phone to his SUV's radio and played an album in the background. I didn't pay much attention to the music since I was busy interviewing him. But after I began to feel carsick from taking notes on winding roads, I took a break from the interview. With a lull in the conversation, I listened to the music.

After a couple of minutes, he asked if I liked it. I did. I told him it reminded me a little of the early Beatles.

He beamed. "Ha-ha, that is *me* singing! I remastered it last year!"

He explained that he and his friends had recorded the music when he was twenty. One friend had written the lyrics, and young Masao was the music and voice and guitar talent. It was the year 1973, just before he was going to start medical school.

They sent the tapes to several US studios and waited. His dream was to be a singer, or write music, or both. If there had been interest, he would have dropped the idea of going to medical school and focused on his musical career. "I thought maybe I could be the fifth Beatle," he said, and laughed heartily.

But they never heard back from anyone.

With plan B dashed, he stuck to plan A. It wasn't a bad plan. I asked him why he had wanted to become a doctor.

"You will laugh, but it's true. I was inspired by American TV shows I watched when I was young."

First was *The Fugitive*, which ran in the US from 1963 to 1967, although he watched it a little later in reruns. It featured David Janssen as the devoted Dr. Richard Kimble, convicted of a murder he didn't commit and hunting down the real murderer while trying to stay a step ahead of the law. It impressed young Masao that the TV doctor would always stop to help people along the way. He admired the doctor's devotion to aiding others, even if it meant the doc's life would be harder because of it.

But his greatest role model came along a couple of years later with

Medical Center, a series that aired in the US for seven years starting in 1969. Masao idolized Dr. Joe Gannon, a dashing and sensitive young heart surgeon who worked at a fictional hospital in Southern California. He was so influenced by Dr. Gannon that he visited UCLA's teaching hospital during a summer break from Nippon Medical School to get a feel for where his hero worked.

Dr. Miyashita pointed out that neither TV doctor used dogs in their practice.

"If someone had told me back in medical school that one day, when I was much older, I'd be trying to find cancer by using dogs, I would have laughed," he said.

We arrived at St. Sugar, in the coastal city of Tateyama, Chiba Prefecture. The training building is close to Sato-san's house. Both are powder blue and flanked by palm trees. They look out onto the Pacific Ocean across the road. A bright yellow memorial to Marine stands at the entrance to St. Sugar. Sato-san, a slight man with silver hair, greeted us and ushered us into the training center. We exchanged our shoes for slippers at the entrance, and he brought us to a small training room.

There I met the current star of the training center—a slender yellow Lab named Bea (short for Phoebe). She immediately ran to me for a snuggle. I had been missing Gus and was happy to be with any dog, especially another yellow Lab. After a couple of minutes of hugs and pats, Bea sat and gave me her paw.

Again. And again. And again.

"Um, is she trying to tell me something?" I asked Sato-san.

If Stewie had done this back in Chico, I would have made an appointment with my doctor, stat. But Sato-san assured me that Bea doesn't alert to cancer on people, and that this isn't her signal anyway. This was just the universal dog signal for "Please?" or "More?" It made me feel better when she headed over to Dr. Miyashita and gave him her paw several times as well.

Sato-san called her to one end of the room and tossed the ball for her a few times. It was her warm-up, a little thank-you, a down payment before her detection work began. "Let's go and smell," he told her quietly in Japanese. Today's demo was on urine samples. One test tube contained urine from a woman with breast cancer, the rest contained specimens from women without breast cancer.

Rows of test tubes were lined up on the floor in wooden boxes with screened tops. Bea walked from one to the next. She seemed tentative sometimes, not quite sure. It wasn't the quick confidence I was used to with detection dogs. But judging by her reward—the tossed ball—she had gotten it right. Sato-san changed out samples while she wasn't in the room and did it again. She alerted accurately again.

This was just a demonstration. During studies, Sato-san is not in the room, although the experimenter handling the dogs is. I wondered if this could somehow influence the dogs, even though the experimenter is blind to which sample is positive.

He says the dogs work fifteen minutes, three times a day at most. He wants to keep them well rested and not overworked. To this end, after the demo on the way back to the car, we walked by a long in-ground swimming pool under construction in front of the training center. Sato-san said he was having it built for the dogs, as an extra-special treat in the hot, humid summers.

"They work hard. They deserve to play hard," he said.

Dr. Miyashita wrapped up his forty-five-minute talk to the people of Kaneyama just as I ran out of details to write about our trip to St. Sugar. A town official moderated a question-and-answer period. I heard him say "Maria-san" a couple of times toward the end. Heads turned toward me, and I smiled and nodded dumbly. I vowed to myself that if I ever came back, I would know a lot more Japanese.

I spent the night in a cozy Alpine-style hotel in Kaneyama that serves as a ski lodge in winter. Its German name, Hotel Schönes Heim, surprised me, but inside, Japanese hospitality flowed, as did the water in the hot onsen spa bath.

The next day, Dr. Miyashita and Shibata-san picked me up and drove me back to the cedar gift store. Upstairs, we met with a seventy-seven-year-old woman, Eiko Tan. She sat on a bright orange couch next to Dr. Miyashita and told me about her late husband. "Everybody loved him and he loved everybody. He was always so happy. He would play golf in the rain and come home smiling and wet," she said. A tear came to her eye and she blinked it away.

She said that even the dogs of the town loved him. When he walked around town, it was like a parade behind him. He was the pied piper of dogs in Kaneyama.

They were together for forty-nine years. When doctors discovered his stomach cancer, it was too late to do anything that would save him. His doctor was honest with him and told him he should spend as much time with his family as possible. His widow said she wishes the dogs were sniffing cancer when her husband was alive.

"Maybe the dogs can save other people in the future," she said, smiling at Dr. Miyashita.

"I hope so, very much," he said. "We are working so hard on this."

We spoke with other older residents whose spouses had died of stomach cancer. Some had given urine samples in hope of helping advance science so others wouldn't have to succumb to the disease. Others didn't want to. They felt it was too strange.

Our last stop was a traditional old Japanese home, with tatami-mat floors and sliding rice-paper doors called shoji. Four generations reside there. The oldest is eighty-two-year-old Tsuruko Chigahara. She smiled with her whole face and seemed delighted as she welcomed us into the large home she shares with her son, daughter-in-law, granddaughter, grandson-in-law, and great-granddaughter. We took off our shoes, and she ushered us to a nearby room to sit on floor cushions around a low circular black table.

Chigahara-san adjusted her floral bib apron and asked if we'd like some food. She and her son brought in several plates of fresh, home-grown edamame, strawberries, apples, pears, tomatoes, and some fruits I didn't recognize. They laid them on the table next to our teacups and a pot of green tea.

We wiped our hands with hot, wet washcloths and enjoyed the bounty as she told us about her husband, who was diagnosed with stomach cancer five years earlier. He used to smoke and drink—both risk factors for stomach cancer—but he hadn't for years. He had had *H. pylori*, but it was long ago eradicated. He didn't want surgery or chemo. He was eighty and had lived a full life. She said he didn't want the pain and problems caused by interventions. When it was his time, he would go.

Chigahara-san had married him when she was twenty-one years old, after relatives set them up. "It was the only way, back then." She laughed, and her eyes smiled. She said her husband was a group leader in construction, and was a little rough around the edges, but always tried to make her happy.

"Later in life he became kind and gentle naturally, to everyone," she said.

Her husband lived five years after his diagnosis, and only had noticeable problems at the very end. He went into the clinic because he got a little wobbly the week before he died, but he came home and was talking with his family until the night before he died.

He had passed away in this house a little more than three months before my visit.

Chigahara-san brought me over to a large altar on the other side of the room. It seemed to be made of mahogany, or some other deep, smooth wood, and had multiple levels. On top in the center a golden Buddha statue sat in prayer, under two round lanterns. Golden vases with golden metallic flowers sat on both sides of the altar, and on a shelf below, golden platters held three oranges each. There was a book of some sort, with family names. Maybe a family record of births and deaths, Dr. Miyashita later told me.

On the shelf below was an assortment of wrapped snacks—her husband's favorites. I noticed that the yellow gift bag containing a box of special chocolates I'd brought from San Francisco had been placed there. It was touching to see how she had automatically put a gift on his altar, as if to let him enjoy it, too. Candles, papers, fresh flowers, a small gong and wooden hammer, and bowls with incense lay at the altar's base. In front of the altar was a framed photo of her husband of sixty-two years. He was probably in his midsixties in the photo, clad in a formal black robe with a white lining around the neck. His mouth was set in a serious pose, but his raised eyebrows gave the impression that he may have been amused by all the fuss of taking a formal photo. It seemed like an expression he'd picked up from his wife.

As she walked us to her door at the end of the visit, Chigahara-san giggled at the idea of dogs helping people know they have cancer. "Dogs are good animals. Please wish them good luck."

Dr. Miyashita and a young clinic doctor, Kyoichi Seo, were meeting that afternoon with the five people the St. Sugar dogs had indicated were positive for cancer. They told me the people were understandably concerned. Dr. Miyashita said he would discuss their cases individually, suggesting various medical follow-ups, and letting them know that the dogs are good but aren't perfect. He would explain that this is the first time for such a screening, and it's a time of learning and refining, and he'd reassure them that they'd be carefully monitored.

These were private patient meetings, so I decided to go for a walk. Shibata-san joined me because he wisely thought it was best to have a guide, even though he didn't speak more than a few words of English.

It was drizzling, so we spent a little time enjoying the natural beauty of the town, and more time inside buildings: A children's library above the post office. A sumptuous old café decorated with antiques and featuring a variety of typewriters. Another converted miso storage building. I couldn't tell what it was now, but it looked interesting and smelled a little like a bonfire.

The door was open, so we walked in.

A man welcomed us to Miura Pottery. Its main room stood two stories tall, not including the peaked roof of the building. Coffee-colored wood beams contrasted with the clean white walls. It was a perfect backdrop for the traditional pottery and paintings around the gallery. The bonfire smell I'd caught outside had come from a hearth, called an *irori*. Three women sat around it, drinking tea from a cast-iron teapot kept warm in the embers.

The man, Seitero Miura, didn't speak English. But thanks to a couple of different mobile apps, and with Shibata-san helping with apps of his own, we were able to communicate.

I told him why I was visiting Kaneyama. He typed something and showed it to me when it came out in English.

"My father died of stomach cancer."

I typed on my app: "Oh I am so sorry! When did he die?"

"I was 11. I am now 28. 17 years ago."

"You were so young. Did he live a long time with it?"

He brought over his mother, Sanae Miura. He said something to her, and she spoke into his phone as the app translated.

"We thought it was colon cancer. He had pain in his lower belly. He had stage 4 stomach cancer."

I learned that she and her son had moved the gallery to this building a few years ago, but had always lived nearby. They are both artists.

I looked around at the pottery and asked Miura-san if his father, Masashi Miura, still had any pottery there. He showed me three large vases. I asked if there was something smaller. He brought me to a table with several miniature cups that looked like large sake cups or miniature teacups.

Of all of them, only two had been made by his father. Each year, there is less of his father here. I bought a single cup. It has a base of bare clay, and the rest of the cup is painted deep brown with a glazed rim the color of milk chocolate.

The cup made it through the rest of my travels in Japan. Every time I drink from this little cup, I think of its creator and his family, and all the people in the Mogami district lost to stomach cancer. I say a toast to them, and I wish the dogs good luck: *Ganbattene!* A lot of people are counting on them.

It has been a year since my visit. The second year of screening has been approved by the town council, even though the first year ended with disappointing results. Of the 924 samples collected, dogs alerted to nineteen as positive. Of those positive samples, so far only one person has been found to have cancer. Among the 905 "negatives," five residents have been diagnosed with cancer.

Dr. Miyashita does not blame the dogs. He says the failure is all human—part of the learning curve. "It is a matter of learning how to help the dogs do this consistently and better. We are all a little frustrated by the results but still optimistic to believe the dogs' ability to sniff out cancer samples. The question is how to design the screening test."

There could be many explanations for the results. Maybe looking for all cancers at once is too much. If the dogs had been specifically trained on gastrointestinal cancer only—almost all studies have focused on one cancer—maybe they would have been more successful.

Dr. Miyashita thinks one reason for missing the positives was the size of the test tubes (tiny, and tops screwed on tightly). He says that once they moved new samples to larger test tubes with tops screwed on but less tightly, the dogs alerted to each of the five they had missed.

As far as the nineteen people the dogs alerted to, he said it could have something to do with reward methods. He's aware of Dr. Hackner's study that showed the problem with dogs who can't get rewarded in a screening scenario. He isn't the dog expert, so he hadn't been working closely with Sato-san on the dog side on detection methods, but they've now developed a more consistent reward system.

He and the local doctors will continue following the people whose samples the dogs marked as positive. "CT and endoscopy, blood and urine tests were all done for positive cases, but only one of those was found to have cervical cancer that was missed through the routine cervical checkup," he explains. "CT scans successfully visualized the tumor. Among other positives, they may have the latent tumors that may include thyroid tumor, prostate tumor. These are less malignant cancer and sometimes are carried lifelong. These are extremely hard to diagnose."

In the second year, the dogs will be screening fewer people—about six hundred—so Sato-san and his assistant can take more time with the dogs and run them through in a more careful manner, with the new and inspiring rewards system.

"I know that most scientific action begins with the failure," says Dr. Miyashita. "We are now set to do better, and hope others can learn from our mistakes and, I hope, from our future successes."

———

With all the work that's going into dogs detecting cancer, it may come as a surprise that most researchers don't envision dogs as the final stop on the road to better cancer detection.

As good as the dogs appear to be at sniffing cancer, they are not predictable machines. That's part of the joy of working with them, but for something as serious as cancer detection, reliability trumps fur appeal.

Dogs are happy and willing to do the job, but researchers are aware of their limitations. After the poor results of his lung cancer screening-style study, Dr. Hackner wrote in the *Journal of Breath Research* about how dog personalities play into achieving accurate and reproducible effects. "Dogs can only be trained for a limited set of applications and get tired, thus requiring a high turnover. In contrast to analytical instruments, dogs are subject to boredom, limited attention span, hunger, fatigue and external distractions."

Even if researchers figure out how to accurately screen for cancer using dogs, there would probably never be as many dogs as would be needed.

One day, dogs may be entirely out of the cancer-sniffing picture—replaced by analytical instruments that will be able to detect cancer easily, painlessly, inexpensively, and reliably. This type of device is commonly known as an electronic nose, or e-nose. It also goes by nanonose, electronic olfactory, or artificial nose. (I think it should be called Dog-e-nose—a little play on words that gives credit where it's due.)

The work dogs are doing now may help make e-noses for cancer viable. Many of the researchers you've read about here, including Claire, Dr. Otto, Dr. Hackner, and Dr. Miyashita, are collaborating with other scientists and cancer-sniffing dogs to create e-noses.

Since e-noses detect patterns in complex mixtures of VOCs, the scientists are trying to isolate and identify the components of cancer a dog might be smelling as that cancer's olfactory signature. They typically use a chemical-analysis technique called gas chromatography–mass spectrometry, or GC-MS. Cancer-sniffing dogs are given parts of a cancer odorant that have been isolated using GC-MS. If the dogs alert to those components, scientists will try to isolate them further and give them back to the dogs to see what they think. The process goes back and forth, with dogs informing the scientists and scientists checking back in with the dogs.

The amount of odor pulled from the GC-MS is much lower than what the dogs typically detect, Dr. Essler explains. That's why researchers at the Working Dog Center and some other cancer-sniffing venues are trying to find the lowest threshold for the dogs' detection abilities, and why dogs like Bobbie, detecting more diluted samples, cause their trainers to cheer when they show they have what it takes. The hope is that dogs will help researchers find out exactly what part of the scent makes a cancer smell like cancer.

There's much optimism about this partnership of dogs and researchers.

"If nature can do it, we can do it. It's just a matter of time," says physicist Andreas Mershin, PhD, research scientist and director of the Label Free Research Group at Massachusetts Institute of Technology. His group is part of MIT's Center for Bits and Atoms, described on its website as "an interdisciplinary initiative exploring the boundary between computer science and physical science. CBA studies how to turn data into things, and things into data."

In keeping with that mission, the MIT team has entered a collaboration with Medical Detection Dogs, Johns Hopkins University, and the Prostate Cancer Foundation. They're working on a pilot project in part to determine whether the e-nose technology MIT is developing can be used to detect urological cancer.

Most researchers considering the e-nose envision it as a relatively small device doctors could use in their offices. This kind of advance in the war on cancer would be revolutionary.

The MIT team's goal is bigger than some others. Or, really, smaller. An e-nose for specific cancers at the doctor's office is great, Dr. Mershin says, but he calls that a "conservative" look at the future. He wants this cancer detection available to anyone, anytime, anyplace, for any cancer. How to do that?

"We want this to be part of your cell phone," he says. "It smells you day in and day out, all the time, it learns what your normal scent is, and at the first instance of something amiss, sends you a notification to get checked out."*

Dr. Mershin is confident there is an overall cancer "fingerprint" dogs can recognize, and thinks that as more researchers work with dogs and technology, it will be found.

He's hoping such a device will be intriguing to a company like Apple, Amazon, or Google, and one will want to work with MIT to get the technology into the phones of tens of thousands of people who want to participate in a pilot study. (Fifty thousand people is his dream number.) Users would need to track their activities while having the phone with them at all times. And they'd need to skew older. The younger population may be more willing to do this, but it's rarer for them to get cancer, and cancer is what's going to teach this phone-e-nose and the researchers what they need to know.

---

*The technology may not be that far off. In spring of 2019 there was conjecture on tech websites that Apple Watch and iPhone models could soon come with "smell recognition capabilities."

If someone in the pilot finds out he or she has cancer, the researchers can go back and look for any signs of minute odor changes. As data accumulate, the researchers can fine-tune. The dogs will still be doing their part behind the scenes until this is perfected.

What about the e-noses that could be used in doctors' offices? Could they be a reality more quickly? Most scientists won't guess about the timeline of these e-noses either. There are too many variables.

For a brief moment, I had hope that e-noses might be around the corner. I was in an olfaction laboratory at Monell Chemical Senses Center in Philadelphia, speaking with George Preti, PhD, an analytical organic chemist who has been studying human odors at the company for forty-five years. He's working with Dr. Otto's group to find the unique odor signature for ovarian cancer—an essential step to developing an e-nose.

He is seventy-two. He told me he hopes there will be an e-nose for ovarian cancer before he retires. That seemed like great news. At his age, retirement can't be too far down the pike.

But then I took a good look at him. The Brooklyn native stoops slightly, but he also has a wiry runner's body and seems to be in excellent shape. He told me he can still bench-press 165 pounds if his arm joints aren't acting up. He wears a Fitbit.

"So, do you know when you might be retiring?" I asked, my hope waning.

"Oh, I have no intention of retiring in the near future."

It's likely to be several years before even larger versions of e-noses are introduced for limited clinical use.

Until then, our faithful companions will be at the forefront of the research, sniffing out cancer in exchange for a bounced ball and happy praise.

"When it comes to the least invasive, the earliest, and most precise cancer detection," Dr. Mershin says, "the ability of the humblest trained dog still far surpasses our best analytical laboratory tests."

CHAPTER 4

DOG, MD

Multitalented, Multipurpose Medical Dogs

Oscar the beagle looks like a stuffed-toy version of a beagle puppy. When I met him, I had the urge to look for a cloth tag attached to his hindquarters that tells what age child should have him, if he is machine washable, and where he was made.

Beagles are usually cute; let's just get that out of the way. They're even adorable when they're surrounding your suitcase when you're coming back to the US after visiting your relatives in Italy, and the authorities at customs confiscate your treasured hunk of Parmigiano-Reggiano cheese. It's hard to get mad at these smiling dogs just because they snitched and robbed you of the best cheese in Italy.

But there's something especially appealing about Oscar. He's seven years old, but he retains his youthful looks, partly because that's what beagles do. He's also a little more jowly than the average beagle. I'm a sucker for drooping jowls, at least on dogs. They make a dog seem stalwart and relaxed at the same time. Maybe even noble. Oscar's large brown eyes, each surrounded by a circle of soft white fur, help him look perpetually inquisitive and kindly.

The red cape on his back doesn't so much announce as whisper—in a small font on the edge—that he is a SERVICE DOG ON DUTY. The cape usually comes off when he's not in public, but Oscar is always on. He received formal training in diabetic-alert work, but he's broadened his practice to include ferreting out other serious medical troubles.

Oscar, like Brody the seizure/cancer/diabetes/heart dog, is a doctor dog of many trades. He was trained in one specialty and has branched out to a few others of interest to his nose and—not to anthropomorphize—maybe even his heart.

It's not just Oscar and Brody. I've run across a surprising number of dogs who have gone from one specialization to others. In the military, the dogs who have the most varied skill sets are called multi-purpose canines (MPCs). Cairo, the dog who accompanied Navy SEAL Team 6 on the Osama bin Laden raid, was an MPC.

Multipurpose canines, used by Special Operations forces, can sniff out bombs, track people, and apprehend bad guys really well. Because the units they work with have a wide range of missions, they need to be able to "adapt to multiple situations at a moment's notice," explains an article on the DVIDS (Defense Visual Information Distribution Service) website.

So in homage to those canine heroes, "multipurpose medical dogs," or "multipurpose MDs," is how I refer to Oscar and other dogs like him.

Oscar shares a four-thousand-square-foot home with Deanne (DeeDee) Kramer, on Catawba Island, Ohio, about an hour west of Cleveland. Catawba Island is actually a peninsula, but it's popular with boaters, and there are enough real islands around that it's easy to get away with calling it an island.

Since I had flown halfway across the country to meet Oscar, and since there are two vast and empty guest rooms at their house, DeeDee had insisted I stay with them during my visit. "Oscar and I would love the company," she told me when we were discussing trip dates. "And I make a really good breakfast."

When I arrived, Oscar wagged over to me with his ever-present smile and sat on my foot for an ear rub. DoubleTree's welcome cookies have nothing on this dog.

A couple of hours into interviewing DeeDee at the dining room table, my audio recorder ran out of juice. I dashed upstairs to my room to get new batteries. As I entered, I was surprised to see Oscar standing with his front paws on my bed, his nose near my leather laptop briefcase. He seemed surprised to see me as well. He jerked his head in my direction. His ears whipped around horizontally before flopping down to where gravity wanted them. Oscar stared at me for two seconds, then galloped out of the room without slowing down for so much as a pat.

In his gusto to exit, something had flown out of his mouth or off his fur. A sliver of red paper lay on the white rug. Not really paper but more like a wrapper. Like a candy wrapper.

Oh no. Please no.

I ran over to my bag. Reporter's notebooks, batteries, cash, my backup drive, an extra camera, pens, gum, and a spare recorder were all in their compartments. But one tight external pocket on the back felt wet. I slid my hand in and extracted the contents: about two-thirds of a Krackel bar with slobber at the top and most of the wrapper intact. I knew Oscar hadn't gotten more than a bite or two, because I'd had at least a couple of bites myself the day before.

It could have been much worse, but I was still concerned. I'm used to big dogs, and if they get part of a Krackel bar, it's probably not going to hurt them. Despite the warning to never give our dogs chocolate, dogs like Gus can handle a little, especially milk chocolate. But Oscar was a little dog, and he could have scarfed a couple of big bites. Was this enough to hurt him? Was I going to be responsible for the demise of this caped crusader?

I ran downstairs to confess to DeeDee so we could take him to the vet's or do whatever one does when a dog his size gets chocolate.

She laughed. Apparently this was not Oscar's first chocolate rodeo.

"He'll be fine, don't worry! Oscar gets into things. His nose takes him places."

Yeah, you could say that. The dining room is on the first floor on one end of the large house, and my room for the night was on the second floor on the opposite end, with the door partly shut. Oscar had not gone up with me when I dropped off my bags. But somehow he must have picked up on the scent of the crunchy chocolate bar. Maybe it left an odor trail, enticing him to follow when no one was looking.

Heeeere, doggy doggy! Come eat me! You know you want to, and you know where to find me . . .

Luckily, DeeDee was right. Oscar suffered no ill effects.

I should have known better than to bring chocolate into the home of a dog who uses his nose for a living. Especially a supersniffer multi-purpose medical dog like Oscar.

This is the same dog who detected some serious health conditions on DeeDee's friend Tina Brassel. One afternoon while Tina was over for a visit, Oscar kept nudging Tina's side, by her breast. DeeDee couldn't get him to relax.

"I'm sorry, Tina, he never does that. I don't know what's going on with him."

Tina was already scheduled for a mammogram. Doctors confirmed Oscar's apparent suspicions: She had a small, malignant breast tumor—right where Oscar had been poking at her. She underwent a lumpectomy, but they'd caught it early enough that she didn't need chemo or radiation.

A year later, in 2017, Tina was talking with DeeDee at the dining room table one evening when Oscar wouldn't leave her alone. He was sitting at her feet, staring at the back of her leg, sometimes bumping it with his nose. He'd whimper and run to DeeDee and back to Tina's leg, as if to say, *Something's wrong back here! Tell Tina!* DeeDee tried to get him to go lie down in his bed, but he kept coming back, sitting, and whining at Tina's leg.

Shortly after, Tina went in for some knee imaging to see if she was a good knee-surgery candidate. That's when the doctor found a blood clot behind her knee, right where Oscar had been bumping her.

In mid-2018, I got a call from Tina.

"I'm at Cleveland Clinic. Oscar sent me here."

She had been having dinner at DeeDee's when Oscar put his paws up on her chair and relentlessly pushed her side with his nose. He'd whine, walk over to DeeDee, walk back to Tina, and push some more.

Tina didn't want to say anything to DeeDee, but she'd been having strange pain in her side for a few days. Oscar's actions forced her to confess.

"You need to get that seen," DeeDee told her.

"You're right. But why can't he just lie on his bed during dinner like a normal dog?"

Doctors found kidney stones. Months later I learned that after numerous additional tests, Tina was diagnosed with chronic myeloid leukemia. She will probably be on oral chemotherapy drugs for the rest of her life.

"Oscar skunked me out again," she said. "But I'm grateful. Who'd have guessed a beagle could save my life? A German shepherd maybe, but a beagle?"

Oscar wasn't always a walking health screen. In late 2013, DeeDee's husband, Bill, convinced DeeDee to get checked for the usual ailments that come with age. It had been two decades since her last in-depth health checks, so she indulged him.

Doctors discovered she had both colon cancer and breast cancer. Three surgeries and radiation followed.

DeeDee thinks her cancers may have primed Oscar to detect Tina's health problems. She shrugs off the fact that Oscar didn't alert her about her condition.

"He had his hands full with Bill."

Oscar started life with a family in a wealthy suburb of Cleveland. The wife had never wanted a dog. After a couple of years, despite protests from her husband and child, she booted out the beagle. He was taken in by a dog trainer DeeDee and Bill had used for their previous dog.

Around this time, Bill had been making two to three trips a week to the emergency room because of his diabetes. His sugar was going to extreme lows and highs. Then he had a heart attack—his second. Bill had already had a quadruple bypass. His doctor suggested he consider getting a dog. "It might be good for you. Get you out and active."

On July 6, 2013, the Kramers met Oscar, fell in love, and brought him home.

Two weeks later, Bill had another heart attack. When he got back from the hospital, Oscar wouldn't let Bill out of his sight. He followed him everywhere, including the bathroom.

About a month after Bill's return, DeeDee was sitting on the couch in the living room watching TV. Oscar dashed in and barked at her once, ran down the hall to the bathroom, barked again, ran back into the living room and barked again. She realized what he was doing and raced to the bathroom, where she found Bill collapsed, although conscious. It was his heart again, and this time he was in the hospital for a couple of weeks.

During Bill's absence, Oscar didn't want to eat. The pep in his step disappeared. He didn't care about going outside. DeeDee knew he was depressed. Bill couldn't get back soon enough for either of them.

This time when Bill returned, Oscar stayed even closer to Bill. "It's like Bill is Oscar's patient, and he's always watching for any sign of a problem," DeeDee told a friend. The dog never left his side except to go out for a quick bathroom break. As soon as he was done with business, he'd hurry back to Bill.

Bill's heart held relatively steady. But his blood sugar didn't. He had developed insulin-dependent diabetes in 1989 as a result of chronic pancreatitis,* and it was challenging to keep up with the highs and lows of his blood glucose. He wondered if Oscar could give him an early warning if it went too far in either direction.

In their search for good, affordable training, the Kramers ran across Service Dog Academy. They purchased access to the online

---

*This form of diabetes is known as type 3c. It is often misdiagnosed as type 2 diabetes.

videos, paid for private phone consultations, and enlisted their own trainer to help them make sure they were doing everything right.

Within a few months, Oscar had become a star service dog, alerting Bill to his highs and lows in time for him to do something about them. Bill went from frequently being rushed to the hospital to never seeing the ER.

"It was the best training," says DeeDee. "And we end up with the cutest lifesaver in the world."

Oscar was happy to share his diagnostic talents with others. During visits to the VA, he trotted over to diabetic veterans and gave them a high five on their knee. This was no idle greeting. He was telling them they had high blood sugar. For low sugar, he'd get close to their face and paw at their chest and whine.

DeeDee, Bill, and Oscar had more than two great years together before the day Bill coughed up blood in October 2016. Multiple medical tests followed, but they wouldn't know anything conclusive until a biopsy.

At 4 a.m. a few days after Thanksgiving, DeeDee awoke to Oscar standing on her chest and barking. She knew the drill from before and, with her heart pounding, followed him into the bathroom. She found Bill collapsed on the floor. The ambulance raced him to the hospital, with DeeDee and Oscar right behind.

As Bill's service dog, Oscar was by Bill's side in the ICU with DeeDee every day. They'd get there at 8 a.m. and stay until 10 p.m. Oscar kept working—alerting promptly when he sensed Bill's blood sugar was off. DeeDee felt it gave Oscar a sense of purpose that he could still help Bill.

Bill Kramer was sleeping when his heart stopped at 9:03 a.m. on December 3. Oscar wailed even before the nurses burst into the room.* It was a haunting cry, a primal baying. As medical staff poured

---

*How did Oscar know this moment of transition? Did he sense DeeDee's emotion, or was it something more? His reaction reminds me of a poignant scene in an enchanting old film called *On Borrowed Time*. In it, Mr. Brink, the personification of

in to try to resuscitate Bill, there was no room for a mournfully howling dog. A nurse moved DeeDee and Oscar to a room a couple of doors down. Oscar continued, more high-pitched. DeeDee and Oscar were escorted to a conference room far from Bill's room.

Oscar fell silent.

A week later, Oscar attended Bill's funeral service at St. Joseph Church in Marblehead, Ohio. DeeDee and Oscar followed the pallbearers to the hearse. Oscar tried to jump into the hearse to go on Bill's last ride. Those who watched this act of loyalty say they will never forget it.

At the grave site, Oscar wailed as he had at the hospital. His cries drowned out the words of the priest. Several times he pulled toward Bill's coffin. At one point he managed to stand with his front paws on the edge of the coffin, but after a few seconds, DeeDee pulled him back.

"He would have stayed with him. He did not want him to go."

Three days later she took Oscar—without his cape, since he was no longer a service dog—to the cemetery. His wailing picked up where it left off. Then, to her horror, he put his head down and dug into the dirt that covered her husband. He flung several paws of earth behind him before DeeDee was able to pull him off the grave.

She called Oscar's trainer when she got home. "Keep him away for a month because he can still smell him," he told her.

About a year and a half later, I visited Bill's grave with Oscar and

death, comes to take a sweet old grandmother. Her cocker spaniel sees Death before she does, and he cries. When she takes Mr. Brink's hand and peacefully dies, the dog cries again. He knew what was happening, just like Oscar seemed to with Bill.

There's a long history and much mythology around dogs howling before or during the death of a human. Stanley Coren, PhD, psychology professor emeritus and author of a dozen or so popular books on dogs, wrote an enlightening article on this phenomenon in *Modern Dog* magazine. One of my favorite "explanations" for this behavior was his description of an ancient Norse legend: "It speaks of Freyja, the goddess of love, fertility, and magic, but also death. When she is acting as the goddess of death, she rides the crest of a storm on her chariot pulled by giant cats. Because cats are dogs' natural enemies, it is said that dogs would start to howl when they sensed the approach of Freyja and her mystical felines." If there are giant cats in the sky when it's my time, Gus is not going to howl. He's going to bark and chase them until they find a suitable hiding place, from which they will skulk away, never to trifle with me again as long as he's near.

DeeDee. It's near a grand oak tree at the Catawba Island Cemetery. Oscar seemed to have come to terms with his loss. He sat and looked at the gravestone for a while, and then he stretched, lay down, and fell asleep.

Bill's name and dates of birth and death are engraved on the left of the shiny black stone. DeeDee's name and birthdate are on the right. She will be with Bill when her time comes, and the last day of her life will be added.

Etched between their names is Bill's favorite photo. He and DeeDee are sitting on a bench. Bill is wearing a Hawaiian shirt and a baseball cap, with his back to the camera. DeeDee's hair is in a ponytail, and she's wearing a plaid shirt. Her back is also to the camera, but she is in profile, looking at Bill lovingly and leaning into him. They're holding hands. Oscar is sitting on the ground next to Bill, looking right into the camera.

Since Bill's death, DeeDee hasn't been eating much. She doesn't have anyone to cook for except when company comes. Her appetite seems to have been buried with Bill. Eating so little has worsened the symptoms of her nondiabetic hypoglycemia, a condition that often causes shakiness, sweating, dizziness, and rapid heartbeat. DeeDee's hypoglycemia tends to skew toward the more serious symptoms. Her vision blurs, she gets dizzy and weak, and she can't concentrate. If she doesn't eat something to elevate her blood sugar—she normally carries glucose, candy, and a sugary drink in the car for these occasions—she may pass out.

While Bill was alive, Oscar didn't seem to notice DeeDee's low blood sugar. She rarely had episodes because she was eating normally. But a few months after his death, while DeeDee was driving their GMC Yukon, Oscar scrambled up to the front seat and pawed at her. He kept pawing until she pulled into a parking lot. That's when she noticed a slight weakness and rapid heartbeat. She ate some of her candy and waited to feel better.

Since then, Oscar has been DeeDee's service dog, usually alerting to her condition before she notices the symptoms. He's also volunteering as a therapy dog at the VA.

Oscar has his cape back. DeeDee beams when she looks at her dog. "He looks good in red, don't you think?"

———

Oscar knew when Bill needed help after his heart attacks, but he never alerted to Bill's heart attacks. If he could team up with a dog named Penny, they'd have a well-rounded cardiac care practice.

Penny had a rough start in life. The boxer–Jack Russell mix had been surrendered to a Central Florida shelter three times by the same family within a few months. Whenever she'd go back to a cage, she seemed defeated, forlorn, hopeless. When her family came to get her again, she was over the moon. But they always brought her back.

It was during one of her stays that Kevin Turner* and his wife visited the shelter. They'd lost their old dog not long before and weren't sure they were ready for another. They were just looking. But as soon as Kevin saw Penny, he knew he couldn't leave without her.

"It's not something you can put into words. I just felt it in my gut," he says. "Penny and I both knew." It's a sentiment shared by many who have chosen a dog and feel the dog has chosen *them* at the same time.

Penny fit right into life with the Turners. She was a fast learner, friendly to people and dogs, relaxed, and a bit of a clown. The only downside: "She was an unguided missile of separation anxiety," Kevin says. The Turners lived on a thirty-foot sailboat, so they were with Penny almost all the time. But when they had to go out and leave her in a kennel on the boat, "she'd go psycho." She shredded her bed and even bent some of the wires of the kennel. Leaving her loose inside the boat didn't make separation any easier. She was only eighteen months old, but she had big abandonment issues.

Kevin could relate. He'd had a hellish start in life himself. His father was an alcoholic with a volcanic temper. He and his four

---

*Not his real name. He asked that his name not appear in the book because of family issues.

siblings and mother bore the scars from brutal beatings with fists and boots. His mother frequently had to put makeup on the children so their bruises and cuts wouldn't be obvious, especially during school.

Kevin started drinking at age nine and says he was a "roaring alcoholic" by his teens. He eventually straightened up enough to join the Air Force. It was around that time that he realized he had PTSD. Not from his military experiences—he never left US soil during his Cold War service—but from his childhood.

Two of his siblings committed suicide. He realized he had to face his PTSD so he wouldn't meet a similar end. Over the years, he's gotten help, but he still has nightmares and triggers that send him right back to his father's maulings.

One night when he was trapped in a dream about not being able to escape the wrath of his father, he woke up. This didn't usually happen. Usually these dreams seemed tortuously long. Then he realized why he'd woken up. Penny was licking him on the face.

He hugged her and praised her and nuzzled into her. She was a good girl. She was a good, gooooood girl. Since then, she has caught him during most of his nightmares and brought him back safely.

She was a special dog. He'd soon find out just how special.

While walking up some stairs on a larger vessel they'd moved to, Kevin felt out of breath. Much more so than he'd ever experienced. He stopped to catch his breath at the top. He tried to continue but was too winded.

Penny was with him, as always. When he stopped again, she took great interest in his right forearm. She licked at a small spot so intensely that he looked to see if there was food on it. There wasn't. It looked just like the rest of his skin. She licked it for a long time, occasionally stopping and gazing into his eyes. He didn't know what to make of it.

This happened a couple more times. He'd get exhausted after a minimum of effort, and she'd go right for the same spot and lick it as if it had peanut butter on it and she wanted to remove every molecule. As she was licking, she'd stare into his eyes.

He realized she might be onto something. But he wasn't sure what.

One morning he got to the top of the stairs and felt so out of sorts he sat in a chair. There was a little pressure in his chest and a nagging pinprick of pain in his heart area. Penny started in on his forearm again and looked at him. He knew what she was telling him.

Things are wrong. You need to get help.

Just then he felt a pain radiating down his left arm and realized Penny might be right. Their docked boat is only a five-minute drive to the closest hospital. Rather than wait for an ambulance, he drove himself to the emergency room.

After an EKG and some other tests, he learned he'd had a heart attack. Further tests revealed a 98 percent blockage in a coronary artery. Doctors told him it was a miracle he'd walked in with this level of blockage. It's often a widow-maker, they said. They inserted two stents to keep the artery open and put him on anticoagulants.

During the first several months after the procedure, Kevin had a few angina episodes. But unlike most people, he had an early-warning system. Penny would go right for his forearm with her usual intensity, and within fifteen to thirty minutes, the angina came on. Because of Penny, he always had his nitroglycerine ready, and at the first sign of angina, he'd take it and feel better.

She was right every time.

His last angina episode was a couple of years ago. She hasn't gone for his forearm since.

But Penny isn't letting her skills get too rusty. While they were out recently, a man asked if he could pet Penny. He knelt down and she poked her nose into his forearm and licked at it just like she used to with Kevin.

"I don't mean to intrude, but do you have heart issues?" Kevin asked.

"Funny you should mention that," the man said. "I was just diagnosed with congestive heart failure."

"You might want to go see your doctor or get to an ER," Kevin told him. "What I'm about to tell you is going to sound crazy, but please hear me out . . ."

The ability of dogs to sense impending heart attacks is purely anecdotal at this point. And the dogs who seem to have alerted their people to heart attacks weren't trained to do so. They've been pet dogs, or service dogs trained for other issues.

Dogs are sometimes trained as cardiac-alert dogs for other conditions that involve heart symptoms, such as a syndrome where people get a rapid increase in heartbeat as well as light-headedness or fainting when they go from reclining to standing up. But I searched for people training dogs to alert to heart attacks, and asked around the service dog world, and didn't find anyone doing this.

Heart disease is the number one killer in the United States and the world. Wouldn't it be great if dogs could tell us if our arteries are getting clogged, or if we're going to experience a heart attack or cardiac arrest? Dogs already help our heart health by getting us out for walks and reducing stress. If dogs could be trained to recognize some forms of serious heart conditions, chances of surviving a cardiac event could dramatically increase.

One of my favorite stories of dogs alerting to heart attacks is from a segment on *Arthur C. Clarke's Mysterious Universe*, a TV series in the mid-1990s. I ran across the story because it happened to come right after a little story about Baby Boo (named just Baby in her segment) and her discovery of Bonita Whitfield's melanoma.

The piece featured a Southern California firefighter named Lorenzo Abundiz who went hiking in a desolate hilly area with his two rottweilers. Usually one of them, Cinder, liked to hike out in front on the trail, but on this day she kept turning around and trying to walk back down the trail. She'd never acted like this before.

The hilly hike usually takes about four hours, but Lorenzo thought Cinder might be sick and turned around after a half hour. Cinder didn't lag on the way back. "She immediately became the leader," he said.

When Lorenzo got home, she was staring at him, and he was worried about her. He didn't want to take any chances, so he got up to call the veterinary office. "Immediately I felt like something just grabbed my lungs with all their might and just like two hands squeezing everything." He fell to the ground.

Then he felt Cinder nudging his hand, and he felt the phone. He barely managed to dial 9-1-1. The paramedic was interviewed for the show and said Lorenzo's blood pressure was dangerously high and he was in "great danger of having a massive heart attack. I think he was on his way to that."

If Cinder hadn't coaxed him down the trail, both Lorenzo and the paramedic believe he would have died on the hike. There was no doubt in Lorenzo's mind that Cinder knew what she was doing. "We just need to take time to listen to our animals," Lorenzo said.

What was it that Cinder, Penny, and other dogs might have been sensing? (I'm going to assume that at least some of these dogs I've learned about were really sensing heart trouble and it wasn't just co-incidence.) Could it be heart rhythms? Blood pressure? Scent?

Maybe it's all of these, or something else, but chances are that scent is key.

Researchers are studying the volatile organic compounds associated with cardiovascular disease. (Unlike the scientists looking into cancer VOCs, the heart researchers haven't used dogs so far.) A 2018 paper in the *Journal of Breath Research* describes how the authors were able to discriminate older patients with congestive heart failure from healthy people, and even from those with chronic obstructive pulmonary disease (COPD), by their VOCs. Other studies examine cardiovascular disease biomarkers in exhaled breath.

If any doctor dogs are looking for a specialty, canine cardiologists may soon be in high demand.

———

Dogs alert to diseases, but they don't need to know the name of what they're finding. You don't tell a dog, "Please sniff out the urine that has prostate cancer" or "Buddy, be a good chap and tell us if this is hypoglycemia." With dogs, it's about odors, not names of diagnoses. As long as motivated, focused dogs get good training linking a scent with a reward, they'll have a decent chance of being able to sniff out the scent. Just ask any self-respecting explosives-detection or narcotics-detection dog.

Or you can ask Koira, a multipurpose MD who saved the life of her young man on hundreds of occasions—even when doctors had misdiagnosed him.

When he was a child, Paul Willis loved to entertain his friends with demonstrations of his flexibility. He would twist his arms and legs in bizarre ways that made them squeamish. He'd easily put his feet behind his head. He could fit himself into the tiniest spaces—the overhead compartment of the bus, inside school lockers—by folding himself like some high-tech gizmo.

On a couple of occasions he walked by a classroom window pretending his leg was broken by facing it in the opposite direction. When the kids ran to the window in alarm, he twisted it back around, smiled, waved, and walked off.

He figured he was just flexible—like his mother, only more so. But after a while, his joints and bones and muscles and skin began to hurt. If he was awake, he was in pain. His parents sought help, but no one could figure out what was wrong.

Shortly after his seventeenth birthday, he was diagnosed with hypermobile Ehlers-Danlos syndrome, an inherited connective-tissue disorder caused by defects in the protein collagen. His mother, Vivian, would turn out to have it as well, but her physical problems were minor compared with Paul's. Besides the pain, his joints would dislocate with ridiculously little pressure. It got to the point where he couldn't hold a pen without some of his finger joints coming undone.

Just as debilitating were the gastrointestinal symptoms, especially severe nausea and digestive problems—common issues with this form of Ehlers-Danlos syndrome. He missed nearly all of the last two years of high school because of the effects of the illness, and had to go through a special program to get his high school diploma.

By the time he was eighteen, he was in a wheelchair most of the time.

When he was nineteen, he was hit by another cruel condition. He had been having a good day, so he accompanied his mother to get a gift for a friend at Toys R Us. While there, he developed a debilitating headache. Vivian found him a seat just in time for half of his body to go limp with paralysis. He drooled on the side that had lost all muscle tone, and one eye swiveled off at a disturbing angle, out of sync with the other one.

She asked him to smile, and only half of his face moved. Her first thought was that Paul was having a stroke. They were only one highway exit away from their favorite emergency room—they'd gone there for multiple dislocations—so rather than wait for an ambulance, she had the store employees help him onto a flat-platform shopping cart and wheel him to her car.

At the emergency room, the doctor immediately called a Code Stroke, and the room filled with ten medical staffers, with everyone hurriedly working on Paul. Vivian couldn't keep track of what was going on; it was all happening so fast. All she knew was that her son's life could be in danger. She couldn't believe this poor kid who'd already had such a rough go of it might now have suffered a major stroke.

But MRIs and CT scans of his brain showed no evidence of a stroke or any other brain damage. By the time Paul got back to the emergency room, he was able to move his pinkie finger. Within a couple of hours, the episode had ended. The on-call ER doctor diagnosed him with a hemiplegic migraine and discharged him.

Hemiplegic migraines are rare. Their hallmark symptom, besides a headache, is extreme muscle weakness, usually on one side of the body. It's often mistaken for a stroke. Paul's parents hoped it would be an isolated incident, but less than a week after his first attack, he had another episode. This time there was no headache, just sudden paralysis of half his body.

Local specialists confirmed the migraine diagnosis and sent Paul to the Mayo Clinic, where it was reconfirmed.

But soon the paralysis stopped playing by the rules and started involving his whole body. Paul would get no warning of an impending paralysis. No headache, no weakness, no aura.

If he was standing up or walking, he'd drop hard to the floor. It was as if he were a marionette whose strings have been instantly severed. If he was sitting, he would slump over. He'd usually dislocate something, often multiple joints.

He remained conscious, aware of everything going on around him. But he didn't panic. He was logical about it. He knew he wasn't having a stroke, so he figured there was nothing to worry about except getting his dislocated joints back in place once he could move again.

His parents were not surprised that he handled these episodes with a certain amount of serenity. He'd always been a calm kid. And now, with the average paralysis lasting an hour, he was just as level-headed.

The worst paralyses lingered for eight hours. When Paul came out of the longer ones, he would tell his parents how boring it was to be stuck in a body that wouldn't move. The family tried to keep him entertained. Someone might put on a movie for him. Or they'd joke with him.

When an episode ended, they'd get to the work of putting him back together again. Depending on how he fell, he could look like the Scarecrow in *The Wizard of Oz* after the Witch's minions got through with him—body parts all helter-skelter, twisted in ways that would be impossible for most people.

Since Vivian, a geologist, had left her environmental-consulting job to be at home with Paul full-time, she was usually the one to start repairing him. If he dislocated both shoulders, she would pop one back in. It made her feel queasy, but once his shoulder was back and he had a hand free, Paul took care of the rest of his joints.

It was an awful way to live, but the family tried to make the best of it, keeping their sense of humor alive for Paul. After a trip to Los Angeles for an upright MRI, he became paralyzed while his parents were pushing his wheelchair along a sidewalk. They wheeled him into a tourist shop and put ridiculous hat after ridiculous hat on his head, asking if he liked or wanted each of them. One blink meant yes, two meant no. Even though he was trapped inside his body, he enjoyed the diversion.

Then one day during a paralysis, Paul stopped breathing. He could handle everything else, but not this. The inability to breathe was the start of a new and frightening turn in the disorder. Someone always had to be nearby, ready to use a manual bag-mask ventilator or race to get his bilevel positive airway pressure (BiPAP) machine, which he used at night to make sure he breathed when he was sleeping.

The only way he could communicate during paralysis was by blinking. As usual, one blink meant yes, two meant no, and now the new blink code—rapid blinks—meant he could not breathe.

It was too much. If someone wasn't always near him in time to ventilate him until he started breathing, he could die.

While desperately researching alternative ways to help her son, Vivian found out about dogs who can alert to migraines. They already had a couple of dogs, and while they were sweet, they were not medical dog material. Vivian thought if Paul could get a migraine-alert dog, they could have some warning about the paralyses. Even a few minutes would be enough time to prepare. She knew it was a long shot, but they had to try everything.

As Oscar the beagle's folks did when they were looking to train their dog to be a diabetic-alert dog, the Willis family ended up finding dog trainer Mary McNeight. Mary ran the then-Seattle-based Service Dog Academy that focused on training diabetic-alert dogs.

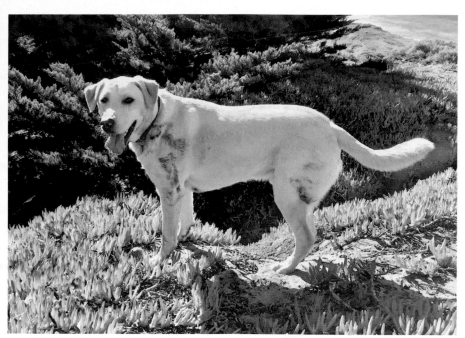

Like most dogs, the author's dog, Gus, revels in a world of scent. When Gus becomes transfixed by a favorite smell, he may blissfully cover his body in it, as he did on this walk near their home in San Francisco. The author wonders if—with the right training—Gus could channel his love of scent to become a doctor dog. *(Maria Goodavage)*

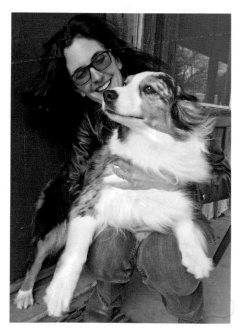

Stewie, an Australian shepherd who has been trained to detect cancer in laboratory samples, occasionally seems compelled to alert to people—despite her trainer discouraging this unscientific moonlighting. When the author, who has a family history of ovarian cancer, met Stewie, she steeled herself. *(Maria Goodavage)*

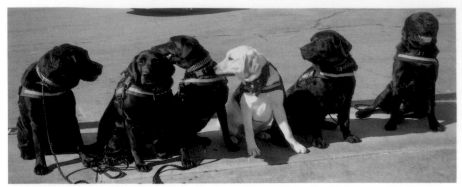

Diabetic-alert dogs, like these dogs trained by Canine Hope for Diabetics in Southern California, can outperform sophisticated technology for detecting diabetic lows and highs. But when it comes to lining them up for a photo, they can be just like any other dogs. *(Maria Goodavage)*

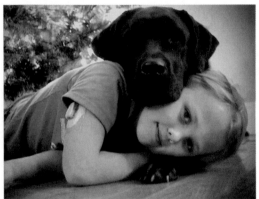

Luke Nuttall's diabetic-alert dog, Jedi, has alerted to thousands of his diabetic highs and lows, rarely missing anything. "He's not just another tool against diabetes," says Luke's mother, Dorrie. "He's an extremely special part of our family." *(Dorrie Nuttall)*

Dogs trained at Dogs4Diabetics undergo rigorous, fun training to achieve a minimum of 80 percent reliability before being placed with diabetics. *(Maria Goodavage)*

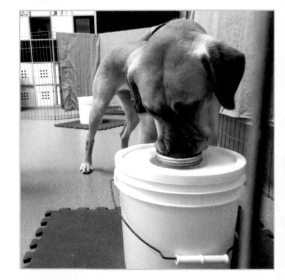

Clay Ronk's diabetic-alert dog, Whitley, was a campus favorite during Clay's high school years. She went to most of his classes, keeping an eye (and nose) on him throughout the day. *(Maria Goodavage)*

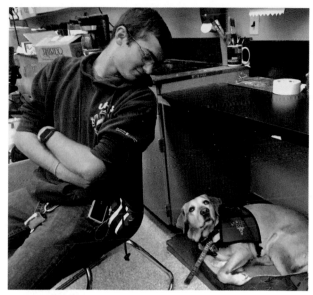

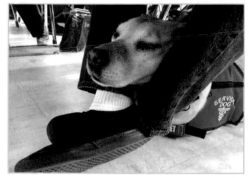

Whitley often dozed in class but would wake up and alert Clay when she sensed his blood sugar was off. *(Maria Goodavage)*

When Whitley strode on stage with Clay at graduation, the audience went wild with cheers. She is now attending college with him. *(Lori Barnes Speas)*

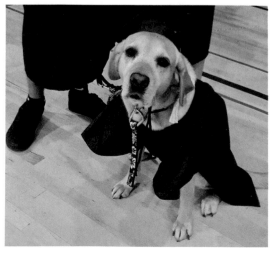

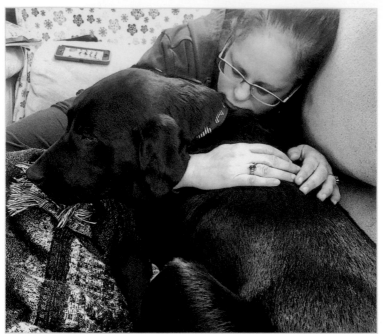

Seizure-alert dog Bud stays close to Leslie Fong before, during, and after her seizures. Shortly before this photo was taken, he had alerted her to an oncoming tonic-clonic seizure, so she was able to hunker down in a safe spot. *(Brandon Fong)*

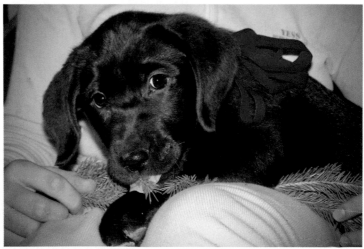

Even as a puppy, future seizure-alert dog Frida, of Zagreb, Croatia, would run to Davor Kobešćak and lick his face when he was felled by a seizure. To the family's amazement, Davor would often become aware again. "She loved him from the beginning. She could sense he needed her, and she knew what to do," says Davor's mother. *(Sanja Kobešćak)*

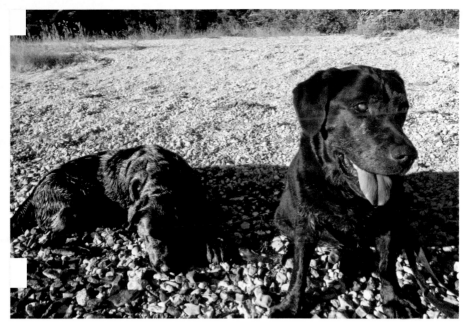

Frida devoted her life to helping Davor with his seizures. When she got older, the family brought in Nina to learn the job and take on the responsibility so Frida could rest. The water-loving Labs enjoyed many fun outings to beaches near the family's summer home. In this photo, Frida is ten and a half and Nina is two. *(Sanja Kobešćak)*

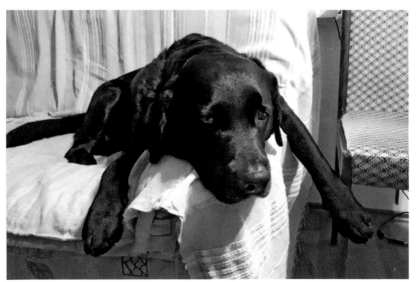

Nina is anything but a couch potato. But since she can sense impending seizures from a distance, she sometimes takes advantage of a comfy couch while on the job. *(Sanja Kobešćak)*

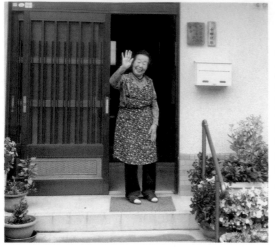

The residents of the bucolic Japanese town of Kaneyama have some of the highest stomach-cancer mortality rates in the country. Residents like Tsuruko Chigahara are putting their hopes in a pilot screening program that uses dogs to rapidly and noninvasively detect cancer in urine samples. *(Maria Goodavage)*

Kaneyama mayor Hiroshi Suzuki discusses the cancer screening with other city officials before a town meeting to update residents. The town council voted earlier to spend 11 million yen ($98,000) annually to conduct a screening study of up to 1,000 of its 5,600 residents. *(Maria Goodavage)*

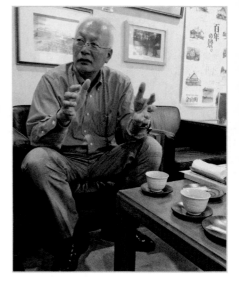

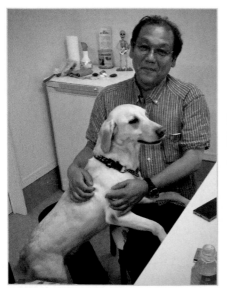

Cancer-detection dog Bea affectionately greets Masao Miyashita, MD, PhD, the Tokyo-based doctor in charge of the screening pilot. *(Maria Goodavage)*

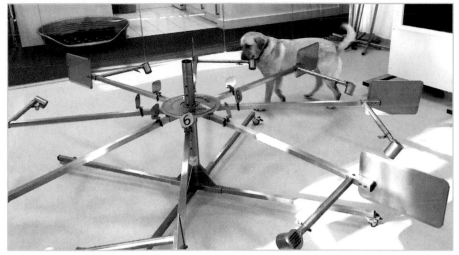

A dog in a prostate cancer study walks around a scent carousel at Medical Detection Dogs in the English village of Great Horwood. The organization is involved in a variety of groundbreaking medical studies around the world. The studies have one unifying element: They use dogs to detect the scent of illness. *(Maria Goodavage)*

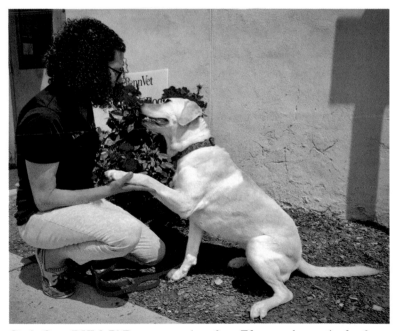

Cindy Otto, DVM, PhD, gets some love from Ffoster, a dog on the forefront of ovarian cancer research. "If there's an odor, we can train [dogs] on it," says Dr. Otto, founder and executive director of the Penn Vet Working Dog Center at the University of Pennsylvania. "They're heroes without knowing how important they are." *(Maria Goodavage)*

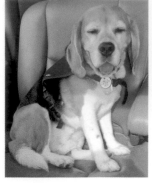

Oscar the beagle is a doctor dog of many trades. He trained as a diabetic-alert dog but appears to have branched off into a variety of other medical specialties on his own. *(Maria Goodavage)*

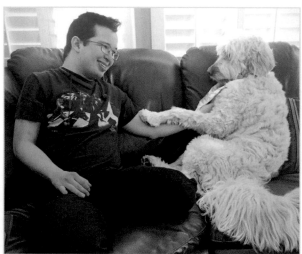

Like Oscar, Koira is also proficient in a few medical specialties—among them, being able to tell her best friend, Paul Willis, when he is about to experience full-body paralysis or agonizing dystonia. *(Maria Goodavage)*

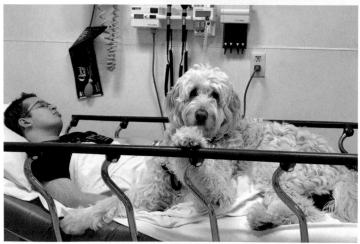

When Paul has to go to the hospital, Koira stays with him, offering comfort and also medical assistance. Paul says that when she lies on his legs, it seems to help the blood flow better to his brain and makes him improve more quickly. *(Vivian Willis)*

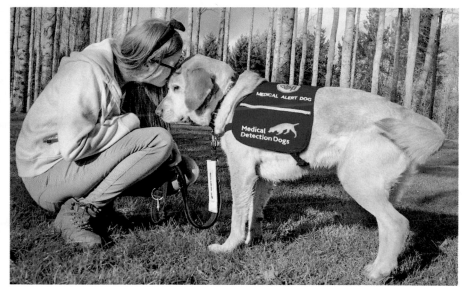

Nimbus is so good at his job warning Jodie Griffin of impending losses of consciousness that he got to meet Queen Elizabeth II. Not only did he meet the monarch, but he took a good sniff of her black leather handbag, which was hanging from her arm at dog-nose level. *(Jodie Griffin)*

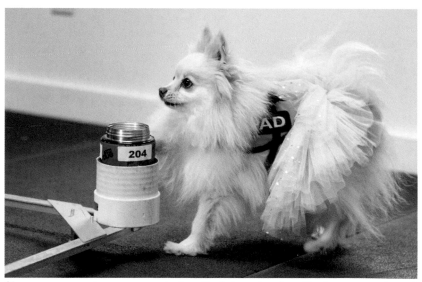

Shugga, a rescue, is not your typical medical-detection dog. She has a reputation of being a bit of a diva, but that doesn't get in the way of being a stellar detector of Parkinson's disease. *(Amber Chenoweth Photography)*

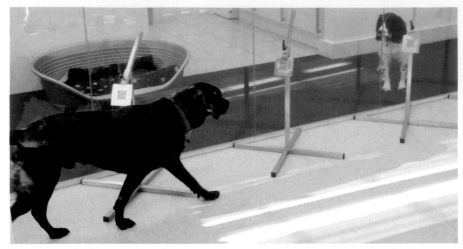

Future malaria-detection dog Freya watches star *Pseudomonas*-detection dog Oakley as he nails his task time after time at Medical Detection Dogs. During the author's visit, Freya appeared smitten with the calm, regal Oakley, even running to greet him as he exited the detection room. *(Maria Goodavage)*

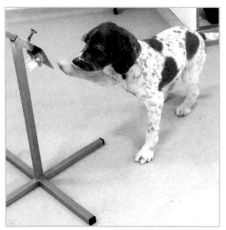

Not all the canines at Medical Detection Dogs are as laid back as Oakley. Lizzie, also a *Pseudomonas*-detection dog, has a far more frenetic style, but she's nearly as good as Oakley when put to the test. *(Maria Goodavage)*

Angus, an English springer spaniel, has every dog's dream job. He gets to sniff for poop for a living. But not just any poop—poop that contains the superbug *Clostridium difficile*. He is a star at the Vancouver hospital where he helps keep the highly contagious and sometimes deadly bacteria in check. *(Maria Goodavage)*

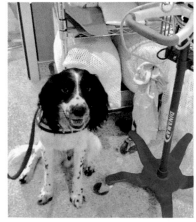

Until Matthew LaMott got his service dog, Lloyd, he was unable to cope with most outings because of his autism spectrum disorder. His family had given up on restaurants, and haircuts and visits to the dentist were nightmares for everyone. But Lloyd has opened their world. Here the pair walk through Muir Woods, north of San Francisco, during one of many vacations the family has taken since acquiring Lloyd. *(Christine LaMott)*

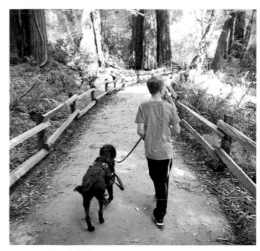

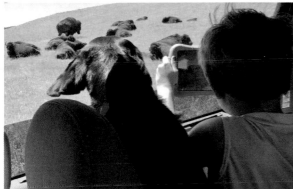

Matthew cried tears of happiness for the first time in his life when he met Lloyd. The two clicked immediately. "It was as if they were made for each other," his mother, Christine, says. "Matthew became a whole different kid." *(Christine LaMott)*

Matthew's parents say Lloyd's actions calm Matthew better than any therapy they've tried. "Dogs love without prejudice. They don't expect any verbal interaction, like people do," Christine says. "I think that takes the pressure off. Autism is a skyrocket. Lloyd brings him back down safely." *(Christine LaMott)*

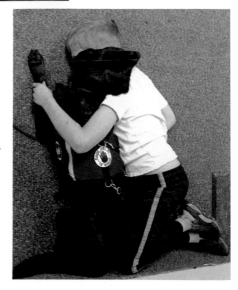

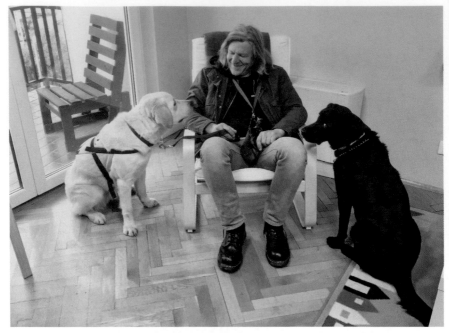

Damir Vučić, head service-dog trainer at the Croatian Guide Dog and Mobility Association, relaxes at the organization's Zagreb headquarters with a couple of favorite trainees. Within a few minutes of this photo, he would be bringing Bob, the dog on the left, to live with a young girl with autism spectrum disorder. "We chose a gentle, sweet, sensitive girl for him. Today is the big day for everyone." *(Maria Goodavage)*

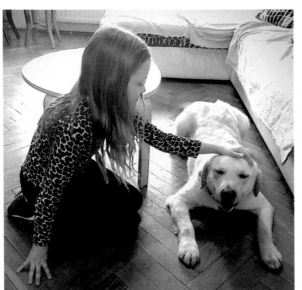

Ira Petek had been joyfully counting the days until Bob arrived. After Bob explored his new home for a few minutes, he settled in next to Ira, and their bonding began. Bob would go on to change Ira's life. *(Maria Goodavage)*

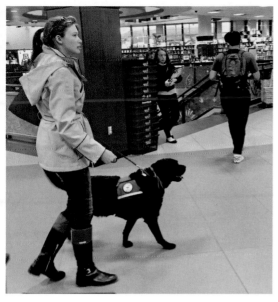

Psychiatric service dogs are trained to mitigate a wide range of mental illnesses. Here, University of Arizona student Kit Heyser, who suffers from debilitating anxiety, demonstrates how her dog, Angus, can lead her out of a store on his own if she becomes overwhelmed. *(Maria Goodavage)*

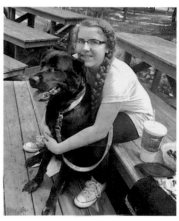

Molly Wilson was diagnosed in her teens with schizoaffective disorder and severe depression. Her dog, Hank, is trained to prevent her from cutting herself and helps her manage some of the worst aspects of the illness, including hallucinations. *(Melanie Wilson)*

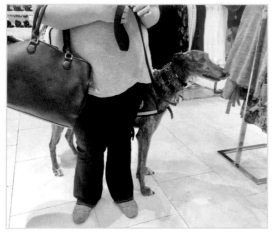

Pippin, the psychiatric service dog of Elizabeth Horner, is a retired racing greyhound with a less-than-stellar track career. But Elizabeth, who has bipolar disorder, says Pippin is a winner when it comes to helping her function comfortably in public and in her home. *(Maria Goodavage)*

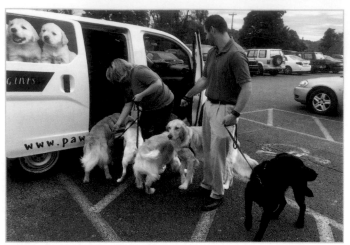

A few times a year, dogs trained by inmates in prisons in West Virginia make a ten-hour drive through the Appalachians to Wilmington, North Carolina, where they get further training and move on to a variety of jobs, including psychiatric service dogs for people with PTSD. Saying good-bye to the dogs can be emotional for inmates, but they take comfort knowing their work could change—or even save—lives. *(Maria Goodavage)*

Army veteran Wil Nobles deployed to Iraq twice. He returned from his second deployment with PTSD. Doctors prescribed a variety of medications, but it took a dog to give him his life back. "I've hardly had any angry outbursts since Harnett. He's brought out the real me. Medicine only hid it." *(Maria Goodavage)*

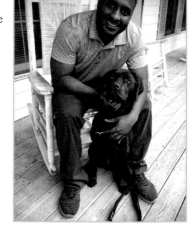

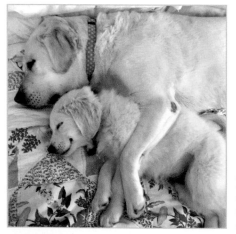

In a heart-melting moment, Daisy, a psychiatric service dog for PTSD, snuggles with future PTSD service dog Oprah. *(Judy McDonald)*

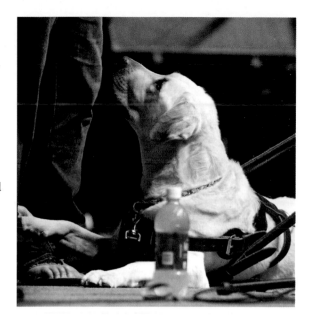

Daisy frequently accompanied her person, Judy McDonald, on stage during Judy's comedy performances. Daisy was a calm, stable presence whose companionship and training helped Judy cope with the PTSD from years of childhood sexual abuse. *(Judy McDonald)*

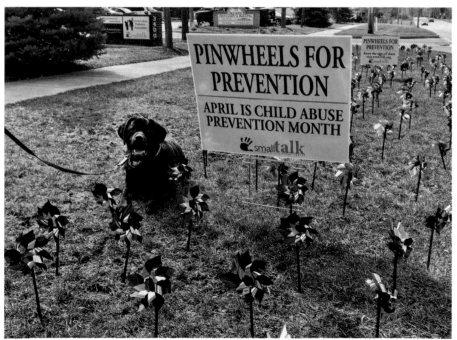

The sentencing of former USA Gymnastics and Michigan State University doctor Larry Nassar was an emotionally fraught time for the dozens of victims who testified as he stood just feet away. Preston, who works as an advocate for abused children, was at the courthouse for anyone who needed a little extra comforting. *(Thomas Grieb)*

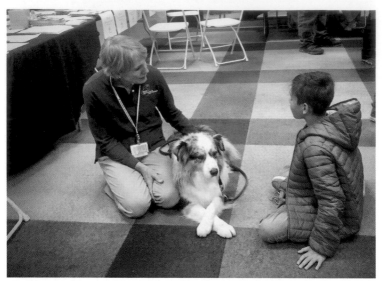

Cody is one of a growing number of dogs who specialize in helping people in the aftermath of crises such as hurricanes, floods, mass shootings, and fires. Here he and his handler help comfort a boy who lost his home during one of the worst wildfires in California history. *(Maria Goodavage)*

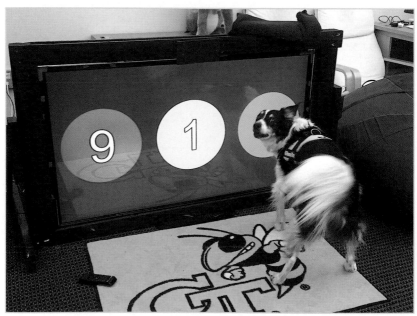

Researchers at Georgia Tech are studying ways to help dogs communicate better with people. Talking vests and touchscreen technology may one day lead to dogs being able to "tell" researchers the strength of a cancer scent or to help someone take action that will avert a mental or physical health crisis. *(Maria Goodavage)*

Her own service dog had gone from helping her with her hypoglycemia to spontaneously alerting to her migraines with no training.*

Once Mary realized dogs could alert to migraines, she decided to try to help people train their dogs using the scent of their saliva before or during a migraine. She used a similar technique to help people train their dogs for diabetes.

She knew it wasn't scientific, and that some might scoff at her techniques. But she says with the right dog—usually a puppy who can be trained early on scent—and rigorous, reward-based training by highly dedicated owners, it has worked most of the time.

"I was so surprised at first," says Mary. "But if trained dogs can find whale poo in the ocean, it shouldn't be a shock that trained dogs can find something right beside them. We won't ever explore what dogs are capable of unless people like me say, 'Hey, let's just try this and see if it works.'"

She says that in her experience, as long as there's some kind of biochemical change, there's a chance a dog could alert to it. "We're not talking trick knees," she says. "But there's a lot of potential for dogs to be able to alert to illnesses in areas we haven't thought of yet. We just have to try."

Paul's migraines were different from those of any of her other students, but Mary was fairly confident there was hope, although she couldn't guarantee success. She directed the family to a breeder that was about to have a litter of goldendoodles. This breeder was known for producing high-quality, successful service dogs, and Mary felt one of these pups would give Paul the best chance.

Paul's family was able to secure a puppy. When Koira was seven

---

*The ability of dogs to sense an oncoming migraine is hopeful news to the more than thirty-eight million Americans who suffer from migraines. This skill isn't just the purview of trained dogs. A neurologist at the University of Pittsburgh surveyed more than a thousand migraine sufferers who have dogs. She reported in a paper in the *Journal of Alternative and Complementary Medicine* in 2013 that one-fourth of those surveyed recognized changes in their dogs' behavior before a migraine. Self-reporting may skew the figures, and more research is needed, but it's worth exploring.

weeks old, the breeders hand-delivered Koira from Idaho to the Willises' Southern California home. They were driving Koira's brother and a couple of Great Danes to the area, so the Willises' house was on the way.

Koira's name was originally going to be Dog. Paul had always wanted a dog with the name Dog. But she wouldn't respond no matter what they tried. He eventually gave up and decided to name her Dog in another language. He settled on the Finnish word for "dog," and Dog became Koira.

She was the size of the family's little bunny when she arrived. They all fell in love with her immediately. She was sweet, affectionate, and calm, even as a newly arrived puppy.

Training began the next day, using homework Mary had given them.

Every half hour, Paul would chew on a cotton ball. Unless he had a paralysis within a certain window of chewing on the cotton ball, he would throw away the sample. Mary felt this would give the puppy the best chance of smelling a change in Paul. She had taught the family a special technique to create many samples from one. This was important since they wanted to give Koira fresh, new samples, not ones she had alerted to before.

They trained her to associate the smell of the scent with good things—just as Luke's pup, Jedi, had been trained for his diabetes. Vivian punched a hole in a paper bowl and set it inside another paper bowl that had a cotton ball with Paul's preparalysis scent. They fed Koira a little kibble at a time in the top bowl so she could pay attention. Each new meal got new bowls and a new sample. Food was always paired with Paul's "pre-paralysis."

After a couple of weeks, the family began training Koira to paw at the sample as someone held it. They hoped this would eventually become her alert. It was a work in progress when they packed up and headed to Seattle, for classes with Mary. Koira was three months old.

Koira gave her first alert at the rental car counter at the Sea-Tac Airport. She had been calm, as always, but became a jumping bean, bouncing all over Vivian and then Paul, and licking Paul's face rapidly while he was sitting. They'd never seen her like this before. Within a few minutes of getting into the rental car, Paul slumped over in paralysis. It was a relatively brief attack, and he could still breathe.

"Afterward, we're thinking *noooo*, that was just coincidence," says Vivian.

They settled into the hotel, and Koira began the same oddly energetic behavior again, jumping around and licking Paul's face.

"By that time we're like we *know* what she's doing. We gave her a whole bunch of treats," says Vivian. A few minutes later, Paul became paralyzed.

When Mary heard that Koira was trying to tell Paul and Vivian about an upcoming paralysis, she was thrilled. She decided it was time to refine the alerts, and by the end of the four-day course, Koira had learned a more proper alert. She would paw at Paul, gently but insistently, and stare at him as she did so, as if searching his soul.

In a matter of months, Koira was solid with her alerts. She could warn Paul thirty minutes ahead of an impending episode. If Paul wasn't paying attention, she automatically sought out someone else. And if he collapsed and no one was around, she'd make it her job to find someone.

"She is a wonder dog," says Paul. "She saved my life so many times. Besides that, I was relieved not to have to crash to the floor anymore."

But there was no rest for Paul. Shortly after Koira was able to alert to his episodes, he developed a disorder that was equally dangerous and far more painful. Instead of his muscles completely losing tone and being unable to move, they did the opposite. They gripped and contracted all over his body. Imagine the most agonizing charley horses or foot cramps, only in every muscle.

He had the worst form of dystonia. It took over his body, including his throat and mouth, twisting him out of control. About a quarter of the time, he was unable to breathe. With paralysis, emergency ventilation was straightforward. With dystonia, it was difficult to get air into him without strength and determination.

As if all this wasn't bad enough, because of his Ehlers-Danlos, these muscle contractions caused numerous dislocations, with multiple bones often being thrust out of their sockets. Like his paralysis, his dystonia attacks came on with no warning. Sometimes an attack would start in one large muscle, but there was no time to do anything before it snaked its chokehold around his body.

A neurologist at the University of California, Irvine, thought it was impossible that he was getting these dystonia attacks because of a physical problem. "You can't have these seizures concurrent with a paralysis disorder," she told them. "It doesn't work that way."

She thought he had a condition called conversion disorder, where anxiety or trauma causes psychological symptoms to "convert" to physical ones. She didn't want to treat him further until he got psychiatric care. He and his parents were livid. "Just because standard testing couldn't find something, the experts shouldn't assume it's a mental illness," says Vivian.

A psychiatrist saw him twice. For his second (and what would turn out to be his final) visit—when she decided he didn't have conversion disorder—Paul purposely wore a T-shirt imprinted with the caption "I'd love to stay and chat, but you're a total idiot."

He never went back. His parents supported the decision. But they despaired that Paul had to face another strange and life-threatening rare disorder with so little help. He'd been through so much. Why him? And what could they do?

One day when Koira was alerting to a paralysis, Vivian had a thought.

"Wouldn't it be nice if she could alert to dystonia?"

"Maybe she can!" Paul said before paralysis struck.

They consulted with Mary. She told them it shouldn't be a problem to train Koira on a second alert and encouraged them to try.

They did the training much the same way, only with a different alert. They chose "sit pretty," where she would sit on her haunches with her two front paws resting in front. At first she would fall over, but after she strengthened her core muscles, she was a rock.

A couple of months after they started training, Koira sat pretty on her own for the first time. Five minutes later, Paul was in full-body dystonia.

They didn't dare to get excited. They thought it could be a coincidence. But when it happened again a week later, Vivian had Paul's alprazolam ready, and it significantly diminished the episode. Shortly after, they trained her to fetch his medicine pouch when she detected the scent, so Paul would be able to self-administer the medicine.

Paul was having about three to six dystonia episodes a month, and ten to thirteen paralyses. Koira never missed a paralysis alert. Paul could be showering behind a closed bathroom door, and she would scratch at the door until she got his attention. Sure enough, a half hour later, he was down. She rarely missed a dystonia alert either—only if she was too far away or sleeping.

Even with Koira's help, the attacks—on top of the Ehlers-Danlos—were taking a toll. The medicine for dystonia was slowly losing its effectiveness. And his paralysis could be brought on by something as simple as turning his head.

The family decided to consult with a New York neurosurgeon known for his work with Ehlers-Danlos to see if he could offer any ideas on how to help Paul. During a videoconference with him, he suggested they try traction the next time Paul was paralyzed.

He asked them to take hold of Paul's head and pull it up and off his neck.

They thought it was ridiculous. None of them wanted to try it. How could pulling his head up stop his paralysis? They ignored his advice until just before their next video appointment, when they realized they hadn't done their homework.

The next time Koira alerted to Paul, he sat on the couch in the living room and waited for the paralysis. He sat in a position where he wouldn't slump over and fall onto the ground.

When the paralysis descended, his mom got behind him and carefully lifted his head up toward the ceiling. At first nothing happened, but then she hit the sweet spot, and Paul could talk and move again. She was so shocked she almost dropped his head back down.

"You can move?"

"Yes!" Paul said, and wiggled his arms and kicked his legs to show her.

"And everything feels normal?"

"Yes, totally normal!"

"This is amazing!"

"I know!"

"Is it OK if I put your head back down? It's getting heavy."

"Yes."

When she lowered his head back down—it was like holding a bowling ball and she couldn't keep it up for long—he became paralyzed again. She felt terrible that his ability to move was in her hands in such a literal way.

"Can you move now?"

He blinked twice—their signal for no.

"Do you want to try again?"

One blink.

They repeated the success. A few days later, when Paul's dad was home, they were able to take a video of another paralysis and demonstrate the wonders of manual traction. They sent it to the neurosurgeon, who was as delighted as his parents were to see such clear evidence of what he thought the problem could be.

After more MRIs, CT scans, and a test traction system complete with pulleys, the neurosurgeon determined that Paul's paralysis was not caused by any kind of a migraine after all—and that it was, in fact, related to the dystonia. Even if his scans had not showed anything clearly—he said they often don't in cases like his—the doctor would have been confident in his diagnosis because of Paul's symptoms, and his improvement with the traction.

The cause of both disorders seemed to be a pathological instability of his craniocervical junction—where the skull and the upper spine connect. People with Paul's type of Ehlers-Danlos syndrome often have troubling spinal instability. The craniocervical junction tends to be where the most severe symptoms appear.

His mother explained the root of the problem to his sister in the simplest way:

"Basically his brain stem is being squashed."

They marveled that Koira, trained to alert to what they thought were hemiplegic migraines, had been able to sniff out the chemicals associated with something completely different. Human doctors usually need to know a diagnosis to treat a disorder. Doctor dogs just need the scent.

"It turns out it doesn't matter that we didn't know what Paul really had, as long as the scent was consistent, and it was," Vivian says. "We are so amazed by Koira, so grateful. Without her, Paul would not be here now."

During the next year, Paul would undergo two surgeries to fuse his spine from his skull to his C6 vertebrae, with his skull held in the correct position by bars and other hardware. The paralysis and dystonia initially disappeared after the first surgery. Koira didn't have much to do other than keep him company. She seemed depressed. She didn't want to play as much and stopped listening to commands.

"It was like she felt she lost her purpose. She couldn't help him anymore," says Vivian. They started training her to do things like turn on and off lights, and fetch certain objects. Having a job seemed to help pick up her spirits.

But six weeks after the surgery, the paralysis and dystonia came back. Even though it had been so long since Koira had needed to alert, she was on it, pawing at him and giving him warning. His first paralysis was fierce, sending him to the emergency room because he passed out, had a seizure, and stopped breathing. Even with the alert, he dislocated four fingers and a collarbone. Doctors implanted a breathing pacemaker so his diaphragm would keep working during paralysis.

Since the second surgery, in June 2017, he hasn't had an episode of dystonia or a paralysis related to his craniocervical instability. But Koira is still gainfully employed.

For a few years, Paul had been having less-troublesome episodes of paralysis—different from the ones that had come without warning. This had been diagnosed as hypokalemic periodic paralysis (HKPP), which would start as weakness he often dismissed as regular fatigue, but would render him a rag doll if he didn't get potassium into his system stat.

Koira had never picked up on those, probably because they had a different odor. Not long after Paul's second fusion, a couple of dog-loving friends were visiting and suggested the family train Koira on the HKPP episodes. It would give her something to do, and would help Paul know he needed to take immediate action. These paralyses didn't happen often and seemed to be triggered by physical exertion. But the family decided to do what they'd always done. They gave it a try.

They trained her for a few sessions with cotton balls infused with Paul's saliva taken a few minutes before an HKPP episode. The next time he had one of these paralyses, she alerted. The family was thrilled.

Her alert for HKPP is different from her other two alerts. She stands on all fours and hops her front legs up and down a couple of inches, like an excited dog inviting another dog to play. You can't miss it.

Besides helping with his HKPP, Koira has also become a mobility-assistance dog for him. The worst complications from his Ehlers-Danlos may be gone, but it's still a serious condition, making it difficult for him to change positions or pick things up.

Now that she's down to just one detection job, and an intermittent one at that, Koira has taken quickly to her new responsibility. She helps brace Paul when he gets out of bed, or when he needs to go from sitting to standing, or when he needs help with balance. She also picks up objects for him.

He started school again that fall, taking a couple of classes at community college to see how it would go. Just three years earlier, it had seemed impossible he'd ever be able to do anything without a wheelchair, or even hold a pen again without dislocating several joints in his fingers. His life was a series of unpredictable brushes with death, and the worst pain he'd ever experienced. And here he was, walking into classes like most of the other students, only with a canine companion. He could write again, thanks to intensive physical therapy for his hands. And he didn't have to worry about death lurking around every corner.

This dog had been there for the worst of it, helping him survive against the odds. Now she was at his side for this next adventure. She has proved to be a great social lubricant, helping Paul meet several new friends.

He has now gone back to school full-time, with a goal of getting a degree in economics. Koira goes to all his classes with him. He's hoping that in addition to everything Koira still does for him, she might be able to help get him a girlfriend.

"Look at everything she's managed. If she knows I'd like a girlfriend, she might do something about it—right, Koira?"

Koira, who had been sitting next to him on the couch, leaned against him and licked his cheek.

PART II

RARE BREEDS

CHAPTER 5

FAINTING IN FRONT OF
THE QUEEN

And Other Problems Tackled by Doctor Dog Specialists

I know a dog who met Queen Elizabeth II. Not only do I know this dog, but when I was visiting his home in the charming town of Cannock, England, he ran up to me and took great interest in my reporter's notebook, looking as if he were trying to read it. While I was laughing (no one but me can read my writing, not even a dog), he took the opportunity to give me a kiss. By this I mean that he gave a big wet lick to my wide-open mouth. This made me laugh more, and he seized the moment and went in for another smooch, but I closed my mouth in time and he just got my cheek.

At the time, Nimbus hadn't yet met the queen. But when I heard that months later Nimbus, a Lab–golden retriever mix, had been in her company, I felt as though *I* had made her acquaintance. As an American about 1,053 degrees of separation from the queen, this is probably the closest I will ever come to meeting her. Not only did Nimbus meet Her Majesty, but she beamed at him and Jodie Griffin, the twenty-seven-year-old woman he watches over. While this was going on, he had a good sniff of the queen's black leather handbag, which was hanging from her arm at dog-nose level.

You may be wondering what he smelled in her purse. With the queen's love for her corgis, I'd like to think there were several perfect royal dog biscuits tucked away inside a gloriously silky compartment. Jodie jokes that she asked Nimbus, but he didn't remember.

She can't blame him because she doesn't remember the conversation she had when she met the queen and Camilla, Duchess of Cornwall, a.k.a. Camilla Parker Bowles, wife of Charles, Prince of Wales, and a longtime supporter of the organization that provided Nimbus to Jodie. She knows they had a lovely chat, both warm and genuine, that they were intrigued by Nimbus, and that the duchess stroked his head and he snortled the queen's purse. But the conversation is a blur. Even right after, when reporters asked her what they talked about, she couldn't recall.

Sometimes when people are caught up in the moment and the moment is big, they may forget what happened—thus the odd condition of wedding-day memory loss. But in Jodie's case, the more likely reason was that she had fainted several minutes earlier. Thanks to Nimbus's expertise in alerting to Jodie's fainting disorder, she didn't slump out of her chair and onto the floor in front of the queen.

Nimbus told Jodie she was going to pass out while she was sitting in a circle of about thirty people with the queen and duchess. They were in Buckingham Palace's Royal Mews, watching a demonstration by two biodetection canines from Medical Detection Dogs and learning about what they do.

A brown cocker spaniel named Kizzy nailed the cancer detection on the scent carousel time after time. The queen and duchess looked focused and serious as they watched her every step, and applauded enthusiastically when Kizzy was done. Next up was Peanut, a black Lab. As Peanut launched into his own successful round of sniffing for the scent of Parkinson's disease, Nimbus abruptly stood up and began wagging and wiggling at Jodie. He sniffed the air and licked her arm. Jodie realized what might be going on.

Nooo. Please don't tell me I'm going to faint. Not here, not now.

She tried to settle him, but if he's alerting, he won't settle. Nimbus sniffed again and stared at her, his eyes glistening with excitement. Then *boom*. The front half of his body plopped onto Jodie's lap. His legs wrapped around Jodie's sides, and he licked and nudged her. There is no clearer signal. Jodie knew she had just a few minutes to lie down before she collapsed.

Jodie hoped they didn't think her dog was misbehaving. She walked to the back of the room, sat on the floor, and took some medicine. She felt weak and shaky. Time to lie down. Nimbus tucked into her chest and leaned against her as she lay on her side with her knees toward her chin. She draped her arm over him and waited.

Doctors haven't been able to figure out the cause of Jodie's syncope. They've trotted out a variety of diagnoses since her first collapse at age six. Most doctors agree she has POTS (postural orthostatic tachycardia syndrome). One of its main features is a rapid heartbeat and a loss of consciousness, usually when going from sitting or lying down to standing. But Jodie can faint while she's sitting or even lying down, and she has other troubling symptoms, so experts have come up with several disorders with alphabet soup acronyms.

It's a dangerous malady, whatever it is. She was nine when she collapsed face-first onto a hard floor. Her upper front teeth jammed into her lower lip and shattered. She still has fragments of teeth in her lip. When she was nineteen, she collapsed while crossing a busy street. When she came to, cars were veering around her and pedestrians were watching her with no offers of help.

For a while she was fainting up to ten times per day. By taking medicine and paying attention to her triggers—like standing up and most physical activity—she's down to fainting two to four times a day. The less activity, the less chance she'll faint.

Until she got Nimbus in 2015 from Medical Detection Dogs, she rarely ventured out without a wheelchair. But now her wheelchair, like Paul's, collects dust most weeks because Nimbus can give her warning a few minutes ahead of her syncope, allowing her enough time to get into a safe spot.

As Queen Elizabeth sat watching Peanut's demonstration that day in the Royal Mews, Jodie's episode began. She describes it: "I often feel a strange pulling sensation, like gravity dragging me straight down through the floor. My vision goes all gray at the edges and then it's suddenly black. I can't see. My hearing is very distant, like somebody turned the volume down and made voices sound all distorted or bubbly, like we're underneath water. My arms and legs start to feel very heavy and I can't move them or lift them.

"If I were still seated in a chair or in a standing position, I would have just fallen straight to the floor in a heap, unable to speak or move."

Jodie doesn't know if she fully lost consciousness at Buckingham Palace. If so, it was for only a few seconds. As she started to feel better, she was able to move her hand. She felt Nimbus's soft fur. His tongue licked her hand. Her legs were shaking hard, as often happens. She thinks it's her body trying to get enough blood back to her brain so her body can function again.

She sat up and gathered herself. It had been a short episode, just a few minutes. Sometimes she can be out for an hour or more. She realized where she was and stood up carefully. She felt weak and unbalanced, and one leg was still shaking. She looked over and saw that the demonstration was done, and the queen and duchess were meeting with the dogs and their people.

"Are you OK?" someone with Medical Detection Dogs asked.

"I'm fine," Jodie said, and smiled convincingly.

Before she got Nimbus, her illness had kept her from so much. She was not going to add this to a bucket list of regrets.

Jodie focused on the queen's white gloves and, with Nimbus flanking her, made her way toward the smiling ninety-one-year-old monarch.*

Nimbus is one of a growing number of dogs trained to do a medical job outside the norm. He's a specialist, as most doctor dogs are, but

---

*I received an email from Jodie just as I was wrapping up writing the book. The latest Medical Detection Dogs magazine had come out, and she was happy to read what she said to the queen. She isn't sure if someone had taken a video and transcribed it or if someone there had a great memory and reported her words, but she was glad to finally know what she had said. "Nimbus is my best friend . . . Having him has just transformed my life. I can be affected up to two or three times a day and had been too scared to go out in case I hurt myself. He has changed everything . . ."

with an unusual gig. Service dogs for people with POTS are becoming more popular, but Jodie doesn't have a clear-cut diagnosis. So Nimbus is just going by his nose.

He was trained on skin swabs and breath Jodie collected while she was feeling "unwell," as she puts it. When his trainer felt he was ready, Jodie and her mother drove down to the organization's headquarters to train with Nimbus. They took him back to their hotel on the first night.

"We were fast asleep. Nimbus woke up and was crying and pacing around the room. He kept licking my face, then walking around to Mom's bed crying. He did it a few times, so I woke myself up and had tried to sit up to call him over to settle him to stop him wandering up and down. That's when my symptoms hit, and I got really hot and dizzy and realized I couldn't speak to tell him to settle down and the room was all spinning. I lay back down quick before my arms went all weak. He came over and was still just licking at me. I assume I blacked out and that's all I remember.

"Luckily I hadn't got out of bed, so I didn't faint or hit the floor. But we literally didn't think any more of it. I just fell back to sleep because I was completely exhausted from the training day and I assume Nimbus did, too. The next day when Helen the trainer asked about alerting, I said I thought that he had in the night but I really wasn't sure and I asked if it could be a coincidence. And Helen asked if he got up in the night at any other time. We both said no, he was perfectly settled and completely quiet, didn't get up or make a single sound all night. Even in the morning he didn't wake me up for breakfast. He was just curled up in his bed.

"And it was only then when I realized properly what had happened and why he had woken us up and it started to sink in and I suddenly believed it was all possible. I tried not to get my hopes up too much, but I really believed it from that morning and I was already so proud of him and genuinely amazed."

Since then his record is almost perfect. He missed only a couple of times, toward the beginning. Within a few of weeks of their partnership, Nimbus had alerted in shops, at her college art class, and on walks. He's been with her for hikes in the countryside and trips to Disneyland Paris. She is a huge Disneyland fan, and Nimbus, ever the sport, is game for any ride she wants to go on—not that she can go on the more intense ones. And he seems to get a kick out of wearing Mickey Mouse ears.

"His detection of my illness has changed my life," says Jodie. "But the fact that he does it with such goofy joy and fun and happiness is the best part."

———

And then there are diva doctor dogs like Shugga—a fluffy Pomeranian with attitude (and occasionally a pink tutu). When she reports for her unusual volunteer job as a Parkinson's disease–detection dog on Washington State's San Juan Island, she doesn't let anyone get in her way. She barks at the training-area gate steward to open the gate *now*. She yips with dissatisfaction when a dog detecting Parkinson's ahead of her in the next room is taking too long.

It's almost as if Shugga knows that her work is important, and the sooner she gets on with it, the better for humanity. Then again, she probably just wants to have fun playing the game where she gets a delectable treat and praise when she does well.

Shugga is one of fourteen dogs on the Parkinson's-detection team at PADs for Parkinson's. She's joined by Hudson, Buster, Ella, Dez, Ajax, Rudi, Quil, Topper, Levi, Sasha, Russell, Rowan, and Mia. Most of the dogs are giants compared to her, but there are a couple of scrappy little terriers in the mix. They all live at home and train two to four days a week, depending on their level.

These dogs have it made. They get to smell T-shirts—sometimes even ones with underarm odor strong enough for humans to smell—in exchange for little pieces of home-cooked turkey. The T-shirts are tucked into metal canisters, and one dog at a time walks around the canisters and alerts if the scent of Parkinson's is present. The dogs don't see one another, and samples are always switched out, as they are in any kind of biodetection in a controlled setting.

PADs cofounder and program director Lisa Holt says it takes about four hundred exposures on dozens of Parkinson's T-shirts for the dogs to show the first signs of recognition.

"We know it is a complex signature, and of course, they're sorting this from a huge canvas of background noise," she says.

The dogs are doing an impressive job. Overall they've got 94 percent sensitivity and 86 percent specificity. (In case you skipped the cancer chapter, this means they detect 94 percent of the Parkinson's samples and recognize 86 percent of controls as being controls—or, on the flip side, they miss only 6 percent of Parkinson's and misidentify 14 percent of controls as positive.)

At this point, PADs is not involved in a study, although data are collected carefully. The organization's goal is not to become a screening facility for anyone who wonders about their Parkinson's status. As helpful as that would be since there are no tests that can help diagnose Parkinson's in its early stages, Lisa realizes how difficult it is to do screenings using dogs—a lesson some cancer researchers have been learning. Since no one would know if the T-shirt wearer has signs of Parkinson's, it's tricky to figure out a reward system that keeps a dog confident and accurate. She says one way around this would be to run just one or two unknown samples per dog per week. It could work for screening small numbers of people.

But for Lisa, the work is more about dogs' noses helping science identify and isolate the VOCs from Parkinson's—just as researchers are doing with cancer-sniffing dogs. When she was putting the organization together, an analytical chemist and professor at the University of Washington happened to be bringing his dog in to one of her puppy classes. Jack Bell, PhD, lives on the island and volunteered to join the team. He's working in tandem with the dogs to identify and isolate VOCs. At the time of my most recent correspondence with Lisa, Dr. Bell was providing her with the compounds acrolein and

4-hydroxynonenal (HNE) to see if there was anything about them that the dogs recognized.

"A biomarker is like a fingerprint at a crime scene," she says. "I believe the noses of the dogs can help to uncover important clues left on the path of PD disease progression. By working together, we may find clues left at the beginning of the path.

"The dogs, once they know what odorant molecules to look for, can be used to fast-track this step by saying 'Yes, that's it' or 'No, that's not it' when introduced to a lab sample. Jack was so excited when he figured this piece out."

If the dogs and Dr. Bell can find a biomarker for Parkinson's, this could one day lead to early detection for a disease that's usually diagnosed only once symptoms appear. Researchers say early diagnosis would mean fewer dopamine neurons being lost and might result in new ways of treating the disease.

In England, Medical Detection Dogs is working with Manchester University on a two-year study funded by Parkinson's UK and the Michael J. Fox Foundation for Parkinson's Research. Four dogs there are hot on the trail of the scent: Peanut and Rumba, both black Labs; Bumper, a golden retriever; and Zen, a large rescued black cocker spaniel.

"Zen is also nicknamed What-a-Mess, as he comes in from a walk bringing half the field with him," says Jenny Corish, biodetection coordinator at the organization. "He is the loveliest, sweetest boy."

A total of eighteen dogs are rooting out Parkinson's in the US and the UK. That's a lot of nose power coming at the disease. Maybe one day, with the help of dogs, a diagnosis of Parkinson's will be far less devastating than it is today.

But dogs won't get all the nose credit this time around. The first nose that made headlines for sniffing out Parkinson's belonged not to a dog, but to Joy Milne, a retired nurse from Scotland.

In the mid-1980s, Joy smelled a strange scent emanating from her husband, Les. Joy described it as a musky odor, and not necessarily an appealing one. She often asked her husband, a busy anesthesiologist, to shower and brush his teeth without realizing he had just done so. Eventually she stopped talking about this odor since it upset him. About a decade later, he was diagnosed with Parkinson's disease.

Whenever Joy attended Parkinson's support group meetings, she noticed that same smell all around her. Years later, at a lecture about Parkinson's, she asked the speaker why people with Parkinson's smell different. The doctor didn't know what she was talking about, and got in touch with her after speaking with colleagues about her question. They put her to the test and had her smell twelve T-shirts—six worn by people with Parkinson's, six without. She identified seven T-shirts as having the Parkinson's smell, the rest as normal. The researchers were impressed that she got eleven out of twelve.

Within a year, the person who had worn the T-shirt she had "misidentified" was diagnosed with Parkinson's. Make that twelve for twelve.

When Joy's story came out in 2015, it led to the MDD study and inspired Lisa to put her extensive canine background to use in a meaningful way.

"It would be the greatest honor of our existence to participate in a journey to help point research in the direction of a biomarker," Lisa says.

It's a heavy responsibility for Shugga and her baker's dozen friends (and frenemies—every diva has them). But they are blissfully unaware as they wag around the scent wheel in hopes of a roast-turkey reward for their efforts.

———

As trainers come to realize how willing and able dogs are to learn skills that can help our health, they're getting more creative with what they ask them to do. In my search for doctor dogs with uncommon jobs, I found a dog who had been trained to help with a serious sleep condition. He's one of only a handful of dogs around the world who have had this job.

Rollo is going to wait for his introduction until after you get to know his young woman, Danielle Brooks. Waiting is something he does well.

Anything that abruptly changes Danielle's emotions can cause her muscles to go slack: It could be a cockroach skittering across the floor. A funny friend. Pain or fear. An adorable frog showing up at a swim meet.

Sometimes these emotional changes cause only a minor facial droop, especially if it's just a slight shift of emotion. But too often Danielle experiences a frightening and sudden loss of muscle tone. She can go from a heartily laughing young woman to what looks like a limp rag doll in a matter of seconds.

At first her speech slurs as if she's drunk, and her jaw goes slack. Her head starts nodding, and everything becomes blurry as her eyes close. Then her knees buckle. If she's standing or walking, she'll slump to the ground. If she's lucky, she can grab onto something to break the fall.

When people see her collapse, they think she has fainted or passed out. But she's fully conscious—trapped in an unresponsive body, unable to move, barely able to talk, sometimes struggling to breathe. She can be down for ten seconds to ten minutes.

Danielle has cataplexy, a rare neurological disorder where the muscle paralysis normally experienced during REM sleep bubbles up into waking life. Our muscles need to lose tone during REM (rapid eye movement) sleep so we don't act on our dreams.

What's helpful while sleeping is a nightmare while awake. During high school in Buford, Georgia, Danielle was a champion swimmer. One day while poised on the starting block during a competition, she felt the cataplexy overwhelm her. She couldn't say a word, couldn't move to save herself from what she knew was next—landing either in the pool or on the hard concrete of the pool deck. She went limp and dropped into the pool. It wasn't a severe episode, and she managed to pull herself out of the pool, even though she couldn't feel her legs. (She was disqualified.)

Some people with cataplexy end up trying to live life as a flat line—no ups, no downs, and as emotionless as possible. The consequences for laughter, anger, surprise, or excitement are not worth it.

Danielle has suffered scrapes, bumps, and a concussion. Cataplexy feels like it's lurking close to the surface most of the time—especially when she's tired. Yet when she was diagnosed during her freshman year of high school, she made a promise to herself:

"This disease won't change who I am but will hopefully make me a better, stronger person. I still choose to laugh, even if I look like I am drunk or slump to the floor in front of my friends. I will never let my illness define who I am."

Cataplexy rarely exists on its own. It's usually always bedfellows with narcolepsy, a chronic neurological disorder that causes extreme daytime sleepiness. Like cataplexy, the condition is a breach in the brain's ability to regulate the sleep-wake cycle. Narcoleptics are often extremely tired and can fall asleep with little warning. It can feel as though they haven't slept for twenty-four hours even if they've recently napped.

About 70 percent of people with narcolepsy have cataplexy. This double whammy of sleep disorders is called narcolepsy type 1. It's relatively rare, afflicting between one in two thousand and one in five thousand. Narcolepsy type 1 is an autoimmune disease caused by the destruction or death of brain cells in the hypothalamus that produce the neuropeptide hormone hypocretin (also known as orexin). One of hypocretin's main jobs is to promote wakefulness. Without it, staying awake can be a losing battle. Narcolepsy type 1 often starts during adolescence, but it can take years to diagnose, with symptoms being confused with laziness, lack of sleep from schoolwork or social life, or depression.

Danielle was one of the lucky ones. It took only a year from the onset of her symptoms to her diagnosis.

She had always been athletic, and began swimming competitively at a young age. She swam almost every day, and by age fourteen she had top age-group time standards. She was swimming five thousand to seven thousand yards per day, five days a week. She loved the sport, but during her freshman year, no matter how hard she tried, she was getting slower. Practice became exhausting, and she came to dread it because it took so much out of her. Her parents thought she had lost interest—something normal at that age. But she hadn't. Her passion for the sport still drove her, but she couldn't get her body or mind to cooperate.

During that year, her life spiraled down. She was sleeping more, but couldn't stay awake longer than a few hours. School became a struggle. She had always been an A student, but she was so tired that she had a hard time focusing and often fell asleep in class. Her algebra teacher called her parents and described her sleeping as "disrespectful." Her friends joked that she was a bobblehead as they watched her head jerk up and fall back down as she tried to stay awake in class.

She could fall asleep anywhere, at any time: riding home from school, watching a movie, doing homework, eating dinner, even leaning over to pet one of their dogs. Her parents took her to several doctors, who tested for numerous physical problems, including low iron and mononucleosis, but they never found anything. They said she was healthy.

If her younger sister, Gianna, hadn't been a natural comedian, her diagnosis might have taken much longer. Gianna thought it was hilarious that she could make her sister laugh so hard that she would collapse to the ground. So did Danielle. When she pointed out this amusing observation to her parents, they finally had the missing piece of the puzzle. Her mom did an internet search for "buckling knees laughter" and there it was: Cataplexy. Narcolepsy. The likely answer to this mystery that had so abruptly robbed their daughter of the life she had known.

After a visit to a pediatric sleep specialist and an all-night sleep study, Danielle was relieved to finally have the answer. There is no cure for her narcolepsy, but medications and regimented naps can help. She adjusted her life to make room for the diagnosis. Her life improved, but she felt imprisoned by the disease.

Narcoleptics typically drop almost immediately into REM sleep. Their dreams are often frightening, vivid, and realistic. They rarely get the restorative sleep they need. Doctors prescribed Danielle a new and expensive drug that improves her sleep and diminishes the nightmares. It's been a godsend, but it's short-acting. She has to wake up at 3 a.m. for a second dose every night. Getting up at a normal hour in the morning is enough of a challenge for Danielle, much less at 3 a.m. Even when she set two alarm clocks, her parents usually had to wake her up.

Danielle worked hard at being a normal, involved teenager. She kept going to school, studying as diligently as possible, hanging out with friends, doing volunteer work, and swimming two to three hours a day—changing from a mid-distance swimmer to a sprinter. (Her friends gave her the nickname "the nautical narcoleptic," and it's still in her email address. Many photos of her at swim meets show her sleeping on the sidelines before or after her competitions.)

At the same time, she was cautious and guarded while performing everyday tasks like taking stairs, standing near windows, riding in elevators, or even walking alone to a friend's house. She would worry and think *What if I fall?*, and the twinge of anxiety would cause her cataplexy to rear up and she would fall.

The idea of going away to college in three years concerned her and terrified her parents. She began to question if she could ever be truly independent. She wouldn't be able to drive. But if she took a bus, she could easily fall asleep and miss her stop and end up who knows where. Anything could happen. How would she wake up without her parents there to help her?

One day while laughing with a friend in front of her house, she felt the cataplexy take her over. Her face drooped, her words slurred, her vision blurred, and her head bobbed. She collapsed onto her driveway and slammed the back of her head on the concrete. The fall resulted in a concussion and some bruising. Because of the concussion she had to remain in a dark room with no stimulation for a week and wasn't allowed to take her medications. She couldn't go to school and fell behind on her homework. Keeping up was hard enough. Catching up was daunting.

It was the turning point for Danielle. She realized she needed help beyond what her parents and medications could offer. Her father is a veterinarian, so she had grown up knowing about the benefits of service dogs. She wondered if there were service dogs for narcoleptics. She imagined what it would be like to have a constant companion who would give her back her independence. A friend of her father's suggested they check an organization about an hour west of Philadelphia. They got in touch and she was encouraged to apply. The organization had never trained a dog for a narcoleptic, but trainers thought they might be able to make it work.

Danielle wrote a long, clear, heartfelt essay as part of her application. Here's how it ended:

> Narcolepsy and cataplexy cause you to be scared and question who you are. You fight the urge everyday to just stay home and shrink away. Everything is different for you, but I have a choice. My choice is to fight this head on and to be smarter, stronger, and more resilient than I ever have been before. However, I thought it would be easier than it is proving to be and while I can try to go it alone, I would deeply love and appreciate the help, confidence and companionship, a service dog would provide in reaching my dreams and future. WE will do great things together and he or she will be a part of it all. Thank you for considering my request. I will love and respect him forever, I promise!

After the people at Canine Partners for Life reviewed her application and interviewed her, they knew they had to try to get this girl a dog. She got a call a few months later that they had a match for her.

His name was Rollo, a smiling, handsome, sturdy yellow Lab with a coal-black nose and a big, wide head. Like most of the organization's other service dogs, Rollo had spent four months with a foster family, eight months getting basic training in a prison program, and another year training at the organization's headquarters in Cochranville, Pennsylvania.

Rollo had a friendly, outgoing temperament, was energetic, and had passed an important and unusual test: Trainers had placed him for a few days with the client who has several seizures every day and tests dogs to determine if they have a natural ability to detect seizures. (You met him briefly in Chapter 2.) Rollo seemed to be able to tell that the man was about to have a seizure, though that didn't mean he would alert to Danielle's impending sleep attacks or cataplexy. Still, even if he couldn't, there was so much he could do to make her life better.

He had spent his life training for this role.

It's a bright spring morning, and Danielle's alarm is going off. She doesn't stir. She'll be late for classes at the University of Georgia if she doesn't rise and shine soon. Rollo has been sleeping right next to her, with his head on her stomach, but now it's time for him to be her alarm clock. He stands up over her and licks her face. He takes a moment and watches to see if she wakes up. She stirs, opens her eyes, blinks a few times, and smiles back at the happy face above her. She loves how delighted he is to start a new day.

She tells him, "Good boy!" He jumps off the bed and stretches a full, languid downward-dog.

It wasn't the first time that morning that Rollo had woken Danielle. A few hours earlier, at 3 a.m., he heard the alarm that wasn't waking her up and licked her face until she sat up and took her medication.

He might wake her later in the day, too. Rollo knows their bus stop, so every time the bus driver announces it, Rollo stands up. This has helped Danielle several times when she's been too exhausted to notice. When Rollo gets up, she'll feel him on the other end of the leash or harness and usually awakens. As a backup, she also sets an alarm for a few minutes before she's supposed to arrive at her destination. If that doesn't wake her up, Rollo licks her and prods her with his nose until she's awake.

Danielle and Rollo have been together four years. They spend nearly every waking and sleeping moment next to each other. Her friends can't picture one without the other. Wherever Danielle goes, there's Rollo: on buses, in classes, at restaurants, at the movies, in bathrooms, on planes, and recently even on a semester abroad in Scotland.

Rollo has gotten rid of the ominous "what if" factor that used to haunt Danielle under her confident exterior. Her friends say he's a knight in shining armor. You could also see him as a trusty steed, outfitted daily in his mobility harness and service dog vest.

When Danielle falls, Rollo catches her; he'll stand steady and strong, and she can lean against his harness handle as her knees buckle. He'll watch over her when she can't move. When she's ready to get up, he gets into position and she can use him to help steady herself. When she walks, he pulls her along with the harness. This helps her use less energy. Less energy use means less fatigue, which means less chance of cataplexy. In fact, since she's had him, she's had only a handful of falls. Before Rollo, she was falling a couple of times a month.

If she needs a nap, he will lie with her and wait for her as long as it takes. Minutes or hours, he won't leave her side.

He doesn't alert to her cataplexy. Danielle thinks it's because her cataplexy is always just a laugh or surprise or headache away. It happens so quickly. There is no time for him to slip an alert between when someone says something funny and when she drops.

But Rollo does have other alerts. He often lets Danielle know she's going to have a sleep attack—when she falls asleep in places she shouldn't. Danielle suspects he may sense a level of fatigue she's not aware of. It tends to happen if she has pushed off her nap too long. "He gets in my face," she says. Typically, if she's about to crash during homework, he'll stare at her and paw and lick her.

She was surprised to find that Rollo also alerts when she's going to have a headache. Headaches are common in people with narcolepsy, and if Danielle gets a warning, she can do something to try to prevent it or diminish it. She may need water, or a nap, or medicine, or to get to a cooler place. Rollo has a distinct alert for headaches: He licks her palm. She had to learn to read his signals, and together they worked out their own special language. Once he knows she's taking action to mitigate a problem, he relaxes.

Rollo has been trained to do dozens of other tasks. These help keep Danielle from getting too tired and let her rest if she's exhausted. He does them with his usual verve. He turns on lights; picks items like phones, coins, keys, and socks off the ground; carries grocery bags; opens the refrigerator and gets her a drink; picks up his food bowl; loads and unloads laundry; tugs off her socks, jackets, and other clothing items; and pays cashiers.

And he does something else Danielle loves. Maybe the most important task of all. He makes her laugh.

"He's so expressive, and when he's out of harness, he's so silly. He makes the funniest noises," she says.

Danielle has stayed true to the promise she made to herself when she was diagnosed. She will never stop laughing. She laughs until she drops. But now, with Rollo at her side, she doesn't have to worry so much about the consequences.

———

Clinical psychologist and behavioral sleep medicine specialist Mary Rose, PsyD, would like to see many dogs like Rollo in the future. At the moment, dogs who help people with sleep problems are rare.

"That needs to change," says Dr. Rose, a clinical associate professor at Baylor College of Medicine and a staff psychologist at TIRR Memorial Hermann. "Dogs are a valuable and underappreciated option in sleep disorders."

The Centers for Disease Control estimates that about seventy million Americans suffer from sleep disorders. And it's not just the

United States. Sleep medicine is a growing field around the world. Dr. Rose hopes that as scientists continue to learn about the importance of sleep for health and well-being, some will want to focus on what dogs can do to help people with sleep disorders.

"Research into the vital roles dogs can play should be a top priority," she says. She points to some common sleep disorders (besides narcolepsy) where dogs have already proven helpful:

Obstructive sleep apnea. CPAP (continuous positive airway pressure) masks aren't a lot of fun. They strap around your head and can cover your nose, your mouth, your nose *and* mouth, or your entire face. A long, flexible tube attaches the mask to a CPAP machine, which applies mild air pressure to keep your airway(s) open and unobstructed. Or, as a good friend who uses CPAP explains: "It blows air into my orifices all night, and I look like an elephant, but it's good for me, so I do it."

Masks can fall off, and sometimes wearers unconsciously pull them off in their sleep. (Go figure.) Many CPAP users have woken up in the morning wondering where their mask went. Dr. Rose wrote in an article in the journal *Sleep Review* about a dog who had been trained to put "a paw on the patient's CPAP mask if she attempted to remove it at night." (I would guess that not all dogs would be good candidates for this job. If I had to wear a CPAP mask and it came off, I'd probably wake up to a mass of mangled plastic covered in Gus drool.)

A reader left an interesting comment at the end of the *Sleep Review* article. She has apnea but can't use CPAP because of a damaged sinus wall. She wrote that her dog Teddy has been trained to nudge her when she stops breathing. It's usually enough to get her breathing again without waking her up, but if her blood oxygen levels go below 85 percent, Teddy barks and wakes her up.

Wow, well done, Teddy! I asked Dr. Rose what she thinks about this setup with this clever little fellow. She thought the dog was great but had concerns about the woman.

"The problem is her oxygen levels are continuously fluctuating, so this certainly isn't ideal," she wrote me. "Keep in mind apnea is basically suffocation, so just being warned that one is suffocating is a poor substitute for preventing it from happening in the first place. In this case I'd suggest she review options with her sleep doc for a possible oral appliance to manage her apnea. But kudos to her dog for his sensitivity and talent in being able to decipher these events, and thus to be useful once she is treated in warning her if her treatment may be suboptimal."

Nightmares. I find this one fascinating. Dr. Rose has young patients incorporate their pets into their nightmares to help manipulate the course of troubling dreams. The dog should be sleeping close to the child, preferably right next to the bed so the child can see her and reach out and touch her.

Say a boy has been having a recurring dream involving a monster chasing him and trying to hurt him. Dr. Rose asks him what kind of superpower he'd like for combatting the monster. He says he'd be a great swordsman. She asks what his dog's superpower would be. He says his dog could fly.

They devise a scenario where the next time he has this dream, he goes after the monster with his sword, knowing his dog is right beside him, and when it's time, he can grab hold of his dog and they chase the monster away, from a safe distance. She has the boy rehearse this in his head and write it down until it's engrained. If the boy wakes up afterward, the dog is right there in real life. "Even just having the dog there before sleep is grounding and reassuring for children with nightmares," she says.

It's a more creative version of a technique called imagery rehearsal therapy (IRT). She often uses IRT with adults who have nightmares related to post-traumatic stress disorder, although she doesn't use dogs as partners. It's a way of breaking into lucid dreaming so the dreamer has an element of control and can help shape his or her actions in the dream.

Sleepwalking. One of Dr. Rose's patients has multiple sleep disorders, including sleepwalking and obstructive sleep apnea. Even with medication, she used to leave home several times a night. Sometimes she'd get hurt. If a roommate tried to intervene, she'd become aggressive. She was tired of being tired all the time, and scared that she might end up under a truck one night.

Not knowing where else to turn, the woman turned to dogs. She found an organization that agreed to try to train a dog to help with her sleep disorders. It was a gamble because this is pretty much uncharted territory. But it worked. Her dog is like an all-in-one sleep solution: He blocks her if she tries to leave her room or the house when she's sleepwalking. He helps keep her from tearing off her CPAP mask by pawing at her or bumping her face with his nose. (She has to wear a full face mask and is claustrophobic—bad combination.) He's there for her nightmares as well. He doesn't wake her up, but if she awakens on her own, he's by her side, and she calms down and goes back to sleep more easily.

Insomnia. If your dog has ever shared your bed, you will probably have one of two types of reactions to the suggestion that dogs can help with insomnia:

"Yes, I love to feel my dog beside me when I go to sleep. I feel safe, and it's comforting to have her right there." Or:

"Are you crazy? I can't move with my dog on my bed. She fidgets, and she scratches, and she runs in her sleep. Oh, and don't get me started on her gas. I'm lucky to sleep at all if she's on the bed!"

I recently dreamed I was lying on the beach near my house, reveling in some rare San Francisco summer sunshine. I heard a far-off bulldozer. The sound sped closer—so close it sounded like it was going to run me over. And then, I regret to say, it did run me over. Not only did it run me over, but it decided to stop on my chest. It was heavy, as bulldozers tend to be. I couldn't open my eyes and couldn't breathe, and I felt a wave of panic.

Why is this bulldozer on me?! Why won't it move? If I'd used my sense of smell in my dream, the next question would have been, *And why does it smell like dog breath?*

I finally managed to lift my eyelids, and instead of a bulldozer on my chest, I found Gus. At some point during the night he had jumped on the bed and draped himself across me—all eighty-five pounds of him. His head drooped over my shoulder at an angle, and he was snoring. I jostled him awake and somehow twisted myself up high enough that he plopped onto his cushy dog bed on the floor. Less than a minute later, he resumed snoring. I never got back to sleep.

An oft-cited survey by the industry trade group American Pet Products Association found that 50 percent of Americans let their dogs sleep on their beds. (This is not a surprise since the same group recently found that 60 percent of us think of our dogs as family members or children.)

But co-sleeping with a dog is not for everyone. It depends on the dog and the person. Sleeping next to a dog can leave you feeling groggy in the morning if your dog is large and/or mobile and you're a light sleeper. A small study published in *Mayo Clinic Proceedings* concluded that dogs on beds can be disruptive, but a dog simply in a bedroom doesn't interfere with sleep.

If you sniff around the internet, you'll run into all kinds of warnings against sleeping with your dog on your bed beyond lack of sleep—everything from fleas to hygiene to creating dominant or clingy dogs. There's a simple solution to most issues: Keep your dog flea-free and relatively clean. If you think your dog has dominance issues, consult a behaviorist if you're concerned about sharing your bed. Same for dogs with separation anxiety.

As for insomnia, some swear by the relaxing effects of sharing their bed with a dog. They say minor sleep interruptions are a small price for the joy of spending the night next to their best pals.

"We found that many people actually find comfort and a sense of security from sleeping with their pets," Lois Krahn, MD, a sleep medicine specialist, stated in an article about the Mayo study, which she co-authored.

Dr. Rose has run across this with many of her patients. She says the benefit can come just from having a dog in the room, but it appears to be greatest when the dog is within arm's reach.

"Having your dog next to you can be deeply reassuring and comforting. If you have worries or feel anxious and can't sleep, feeling your dog's respirations under your hand, feeling their warmth, their chest go up and down, can really help. There's nothing like a dog to ground you when you've got troubles, day or night."

CHAPTER 6

HIDDEN ENEMIES

Super Dogs for Superbugs

I t's a busy Monday morning at Medical Detection Dogs. Most of the dogs have filed in for their day of work, dropped off by their doting foster parents. They wag around, greeting one another, sniffing fore and aft in slow circles as if catching up after the weekend.

Mornin', Marlowe.

Mornin', Bumper.

Have a good weekend, did ya? From the aroma back here I'd say you had steak last night!

Oh ho ho, don't tell the folks! I grabbed a bit of gristle from the bin when the missus wasn't looking.

Good dog! Looking forward to another week of sniffing urine and getting treats for it?

You bet! How could I not? It's like taking candy from a baby. Not that I've done that—recently.

Excuse me, here comes Karry. She smells like dog shampoo, poor girl. See you round the scent room?

Not if I see you first!

The watercooler communications die down as the dogs are called to practice their skills or wait their turn or go for walks. On this brisk November day, the prostate-cancer-detection dogs are the first to get to work in the large detection room. They pad around the scent wheel, alerting correctly almost every time to the urine samples from men with prostate cancer. Just as important, they don't alert if there is no prostate cancer sample. Marlowe, Karry, Florin, Midas, and Jobi seem to have this down to a science, which is good, because that's what it's supposed to be.

Next up are the dogs I'm here to see. They're part of a proof-of-principle study to determine if dogs can detect the bacteria *Pseudomonas aeruginosa*. These organisms are fairly ubiquitous in the environment. They're usually found in moist places like sinks and soil and vegetation. For healthy people, *P. aeruginosa* (which we will refer to simply as *Pseudomonas* from now on) doesn't usually present much risk.

But for people with weakened immune systems, *Pseudomonas* can be deadly. It's easily spread in hospitals and long-term health care facilities, which are full of people with compromised immune systems.

Infection with *Pseudomonas* can be a lifelong struggle for those with cystic fibrosis, a serious genetic disease affecting at least seventy thousand people worldwide. It causes fluids like mucus, sweat, and digestive enzymes, which are normally smooth and thin, to be thick and sticky. The thickened mucus can trap microorganisms in the lungs, which can lead to chronic infections and impede lung function. It also can cause severe damage to the digestive system, liver, and other organs.

By adolescence or young adulthood, the majority of cystic fibrosis patients are infected with *Pseudomonas*. Normally people with wet coughs can produce sputum to be tested for the bacteria, but it's harder for people with cystic fibrosis. Testing on babies and young children usually involves using a cough swab, but it's not a reliable technique. Even if sputum is produced, culturing it and identifying it can take several days, which can lead to delays in treatment and possible cross-infection.

Jane Davies, MD, professor of pediatric respirology and experimental medicine at Imperial College London and honorary consultant in pediatric respiratory medicine at Royal Brompton & Harefield NHS Foundation Trust, specializes in cystic fibrosis in children. She'd like to see monitoring for *Pseudomonas* infections that can be done frequently and rapidly, and doesn't necessarily rely on sputum, so infections can be caught in the early stages.

She and her colleagues are working on several high-tech ways to detect *Pseudomonas*, including mass spectrometry, cell-free biosensors, and optoelectronics. "But this machinery stuff is quite difficult," she said at a talk at Imperial College. (She regretfully declined speaking with me for the book because she was nervous about doing anything that could jeopardize publication of the study you'll read about shortly. That's why I'm quoting her from videos and getting background information from other sources.)

While waiting for technology, they decided to see if there was a less high-tech approach for reliably and quickly detecting *Pseudomonas*. "We have begged the question, 'Is nature already able to help us in a way that this technology is trying to reinvent?'"

Cue the dogs.

Pseudomonas produces volatile organic compounds that some say have distinctive odors. In small samples provided by patients, humans can't smell it. But when grown on bacteriological media where the bugs can proliferate, it has been described as smelling like everything from flowers to grape juice to fresh tortillas. The idea is that if people can smell it in concentration, maybe dogs can smell it at normal levels.

If the dogs at Medical Detection Dogs can easily identify the bacteria, this could lead to rapid screening for *Pseudomonas* in the patients who need fast diagnoses. Patients, especially those who have a hard time producing sputum, could send in coughed-on tissues and breath samples on a fairly regular basis for inspection by bacteria-sniffer dogs. Dr. Davies told the audience it could be an inexpensive way to keep on top of infections.

Working with dogs has been a refreshing change for Dr. Davies and her staff. "It's a bit of a laugh. We're having a good time doing it, and it may come to something."

A short black Lab named Mason is the first in the *Pseudomonas*-detection lineup today. Although Mason is only two years old, he's already on his third career. He was trained to be a guide dog, but that didn't work out. When he came to Medical Detection Dogs, he was trained as an assistance dog, but that didn't work out either. He is drooling a lot today. Maybe that has something to do with it. But he seems to have found his calling as a medical detection dog.

He's the new guy on the team and is just getting familiar with the scent of *Pseudomonas*. A trainer wearing latex gloves kneels at dog level and holds out a vial containing a sterile sample of the bacteria. All Mason has to do is approach it and give it a nice, close sniff. As soon as he does, she presses the clicker and tells him "Good!" in a high and happy voice. That's only part of his paycheck, though. Being a Lab, he likely prefers the other part, where she skitters a few tiny treats a couple of feet across the floor. He chases after them and gives them a couple of chomps before he notices she's holding out the magic vial again. A string of drool hangs from a jowl.

Sniff. Click. "Good!" *Skitter. Chomp.*

He's got this. As he aces it time after time, I spot a black-and-white springer spaniel–ish dog lying down on the other side of a glass observation wall, watching Mason. I learn that her name is Freya, and she's in training to be a malaria-detection dog. She doesn't have anything to do today. Her detection happens on other days, but she's here anyway because she lives with one of the trainers.

Even though she could be hanging with other dogs during their downtime, or meandering around the offices and being adored, she's chosen to repose on the burgundy carpet on the other side of the glass. She lies in a splash of striped sunlight shining through the blinds of a window in the training lab. Her eyes are fixed on Mason, a good fifteen feet away.

Sniff. Click. "Good!" *Skitter. Chomp.*

Freya is riveted, moving her head only if the skittering kibble goes farther than normal. She's like a music teacher watching her student from afar during an audition, urging him on psychically, hoping he'll perform as well as she knows he can.

Mason approaches the vial again, but this time he dips in for a whiff when he's at least a foot away. He stands expectantly, waiting for his praise and his kibble. Not receiving it, he sits and takes on a serious demeanor. He looks at the trainer. She holds out the vial to give him another chance, but he just sits and stares at her.

Excuse me, ma'am, I believe you're forgetting something?

She smiles and hides the vial under her arm. When she brings it back out, he's on top of his game again, touching his nose to the rim and giving a sniff.

Click. "Good!" *Skitter. Chomp.*

A few more rounds and he's done.

"Good job, Mason! Gooooood boy!" she tells him.

Freya watches him leave the room. She rests her head on the carpet and closes her eyes.

Lizzie is next on the roster. She's part bearded collie, part springer spaniel, and today she is also part Ping-Pong ball. She runs into the detection room and skids to a stop at the feet of her trainer. She sits and looks up at him, squeaking some excited barks. The trainer stands calmly and looks back at her. She squeaks some more, then canters to one side of the room and back.

"She's always like this at the start of the day," he says. "Plus it's Monday, so she's raring to go. I just let her get it out of her system. She needs to know that she doesn't always have to get right to work in this room."

Lizzie runs toward the observation wall and glances at Freya, who is now standing up, staring at her, her mouth slightly agape.

Lizzie is six years old, so this isn't puppy energy. She was trained as a bedbug-detection dog elsewhere, but as with Mason's previous gigs, it didn't work out. "She's impulsive," says the trainer. "We're working on focusing her. She's got a great nose once she settles in."

Her training today is a little more advanced than Mason's. Whereas he just had to head a few feet over to a trainer who was holding a vial, Lizzie is supposed to enter the room and walk about seven feet to a short metal stand containing a vial with the *Pseudomonas*. Once there, she should sniff it and alert calmly. That's the idea, anyway.

The first few times she does it, she runs in, smells the sample, and slams the device so hard with her paw that it moves a few feet.

"Try to work on that paw action not happening," another trainer advises Lizzie's trainer *du jour* from the other side of the room.

Freya is still standing and watching through the observation window. Her upper lip has somehow gotten caught up on her gum and is stuck in a curled position. She's looking pretty judgy.

Lizzie tries again. This time she whacks at the sample with both paws and it moves farther toward the center of the room.

"Lizzie, no," the trainer says, and points for her to leave the room. The next time she enters, she runs to the device, sniffs, and sits. *Click.* "Good girl!"

Treat. Wag!

After a couple of successes, she's on a roll. She sits and stares at the vial. She looks like Nipper, the dog listening intently to the gramophone in the famous painting *His Master's Voice*. Only instead of hearing a gramophone, she's smelling a Gram-negative bacteria.

After a few perfect rounds, Lizzie takes to vigorously licking the vial each time, as if it's an ice cream cone.

"That's probably enough for now," the other trainer says.

Out jogs Lizzie, and in saunters Oakley, a large black Lab with a red collar. Compared to normal dogs, he is calm. Compared to Lizzie, you have to resist the urge to check his pulse.

Oakley is regal. Oakley is confident. Oakley is da bomb.

He walks over to a row of four detection stands. Three contain controls (different bacteria common to cystic fibrosis and an uninfected sample); one contains the *Pseudomonas*. Or maybe they're all controls with no *Pseudomonas*. Oakley doesn't know. But he knows if he alerts to the right one, or if he doesn't alert if there's no *Pseudomonas*, he'll get a reward.

The detection stands are next to the observation wall, where Freya is now lying with her head on her paws, facing the glass. She looks like a fangirl.

Oakley walks calmly to the first stand, sniffs, then on to the second stand, sniffs, then the third stand, sniffs, keeps his nose there, and slowly wags his tail.

Even his alert is calm.

Click. "Yesssss! Good boy!" *Treat. Chomp.*

Without taking her eyes off him, Freya stands up to watch the master at work.

He is perfect every time.

When he's done, Freya stretches. She leaves her post and walks toward the entrance to the detection room, where she waits for Oakley.

There's another dog on the team, but I'm told he doesn't like working in front of someone he doesn't know. His name is Flint, and apparently he's got the biodetection-dog equivalent of stage fright.

These four unique canine characters could make a significant difference in health outcomes for a vulnerable population.

Months after my visit to Medical Detection Dogs, the first phase of the study had been completed. Dr. Davies couldn't talk about the results, but I learned what I could from a poster abstract that was presented at a conference.

Mason was too new to the project to be part of this trial, but he'll be in on the next phase. The other three dogs each did extremely well in the double-blind trial.

Even Lizzie.

They each sniffed out two hundred samples in a double-blind externally supervised trial. A bar graph indicates that Oakley correctly detected 100 percent of the bacteria. (Freya is surely even more smitten now.) Flint the Shy wasn't far behind. Lizzie the Hyper dragged down the success rate of the team a little with a detection rate just under 90 percent. But still, quite impressive.

The next phase of the research will involve exhaled breath and coughed-on tissues. Gus, who is an aficionado of used tissues, would be a natural for this job. Alas, he lives too far away, so he'll sit this one out and let Lizzie and her friends handle it.

———

Researchers have only recently begun to explore the role of dogs as rapid, inexpensive, noninvasive means of detecting some of the most dangerous microscopic bad boys—pathogens and parasites. The science is in its infancy. Most of the research has focused on whether dogs can even detect these invisible dangers. Proof-of-principle studies so far have been demonstrating they can.

The research doesn't usually make headlines the way studies about cancer-detection dogs do. But the potential benefits could be even more far-reaching: Rapid discovery of a virus or harmful bacteria could stop an infectious disease from spreading to a wide population, or dramatically reduce the waiting time for test results, leading to timely and possibly lifesaving treatment.

Researchers with the Canine Performance Sciences program at Auburn University recently showed that the odor of a virus is detectable by dogs. Not only did dogs recognize the virus among uninfected cell cultures, but they could discriminate between the target virus and two other viruses. This is pretty big news in the world of dogs and science. But maybe because the dogs were sniffing bovine viral diarrhea virus (BVDV) instead of something more dramatic that infects us—like the flu—reporters weren't clamoring for interviews.*

Surely research showing that dogs can detect a notorious antibiotic-resistant superbug wouldn't go without notice. It would be a pretty big deal if dogs could find something as harmful as methicillin-resistant *Staphylococcus aureus* (MRSA). MRSA is a highly contagious pathogen that's often picked up during stays in hospitals and long-term

---

*For those who have an insatiable curiosity about bovine woes, the viruses the dogs learned to ignore while seeking BVDV were bovine herpes virus 1 (BHV-1) (you don't want to read the symptoms if you are eating) and bovine parainfluenza virus 3 (BPIV-3).

health care facilities. The bacteria are resistant to many common anti-biotics, and if the infection spreads to the heart, bloodstream, lungs, and bones, it can be deadly.

A couple of research teams have been investigating the possibility that dogs can detect MRSA's volatile organic compound scents. Yet when Toronto researchers reported the results of a study showing that dogs *can* detect MRSA, and can even distinguish it from similar strains, the news didn't go much further than the *Journal of Hospital Infection*.*

Fortunately, publicity is not what drives most researchers—or dogs. If other doctor dog discoveries inspire TV segments while the pathogen-pursuing pups only end up in a published paper, they don't mind.

A study with exciting potential for practical application in the near future is also a study with one of the best understatements ever: "Sniffing urine is an innate behavior in dogs," write the authors of a paper on canine detection of urinary tract infections, in the journal *Open Forum Infectious Diseases*.

Anyone who endures daily walks with a dog who stops frequently to read "pee-mail" can attest to this. Yes, sniffing urine is indeed innate. The paper discusses the reasons dogs do this, and amazingly, "to vex the person on the other end of the leash" is not among them. The main reason the authors give for dogs sniffing urine is identifying other dogs and their notable characteristics, including their fertility and health status.

It turns out that the canine fascination with urine may be a boon for humans. The authors write that dogs are predisposed to "exceptional accuracy in identifying disease in humans by sniffing urine samples."

The study's dogs, who were trained to identify urine samples for *E. coli* and three other types of bacteria (*S. aureus*, *Enterococcus*, and

---

*The dogs were tested monthly for potential colonization of MSRA in their noses. Safeguarding the dogs who detect disease is essential for this kind of research.

Klebsiella) in double-blinded conditions, correctly detected nearly 100 percent of the positive samples. Even when the samples were diluted with distilled water and contained very low bacterial counts, the dogs could sniff out the troubled waters. The authors suggest that dogs could provide early detection of urinary tract infections (UTIs).

UTIs are a common health problem, accounting for ten million visits to physicians every year in the United States. For most patients, they're easily treated. But for some, especially the elderly and people with limited mobility because of neurological conditions, UTIs can lead to complications. If left untreated, they can rapidly become lethal.

The study suggests that highly trained future service dogs for those with, say, spinal cord injuries could do double duty. They could help their people with mobility, and they could also serve as UTI monitors. Early detection from a best friend who also steadies you out of bed, picks up your dropped phone, and helps you get up if you take a tumble? It doesn't get much better than that.

Research continues.

Meanwhile, in Canada, a dog is already hard at work detecting another nasty bug. This bug isn't in urine, but in another form of bodily waste that's a real crowd pleaser in the canine world.

———

A black-and-white English springer spaniel named Angus may consider himself the luckiest doctor dog in the world. While other medical detection dogs busy themselves sniffing out cancer and diabetes and all manner of disorders, Angus spends his days sniffing for something close to the heart and soul of any self-respecting dog: feces. Or, as we'll call it here because we are all friends: poop.

When Angus is working, it's clear that this is a dog who would not trade his job for all the tennis balls at Wimbledon. With handler Teresa Zurberg on the other end of his bright orange leash, he zips and clips and wags and zags up and down the halls of Vancouver General Hospital. His quarry is poop, but not just any poop. It's poop that contains the superbug *Clostridium difficile*, otherwise known as *C. difficile*, or more commonly (and more cool-sounding) *C. diff*.

My favorite description of *C. diff* comes from a museum dedicated to microbes, in Amsterdam.

> *Clostridium difficile* is the black sheep in the Clostridia class. The other members are mostly useful intestinal bacteria which break down fibres in the gut, producing important nutrients for the cells in the intestine . . . The other intestinal bacteria usually keep *C. difficile* under their thumb but antibiotic use can get rid of these "good" bacteria. The *Clostridium difficile* spores are able to survive the antibiotic attack and can reproduce unchecked.

C. diff is a highly contagious and sometimes deadly bacteria. Its most common victims are people whose beneficial gut bacteria have been compromised by antibiotics. The main symptom of a *C. diff* infection is diarrhea—in severe cases, it's miserably uncontrollable. If that's not bad enough, it's often accompanied by fever, abdominal pain, and rapid heartbeat—"immense suffering," in the words of a former CDC director.* In the United States, *C. diff* causes half a million infections a year, and fifteen thousand to thirty thousand deaths.

Hospitals are a delectable environment for *C. diff*. They're filled with sick people on antibiotics, and if a patient is infected and has diarrhea, the spores can easily be transferred from one person to another, or to objects common to hospitals—anything from bed rails to stethoscopes to remote controls. The rugged bug can live for months on surfaces and will happily travel from the hand of someone

---

*You might think that the "*difficile*" part of the bacteria's name came about because it makes life so difficult for those who have it. But that's not the case. If it were, other nasty bacteria should follow suit, with specific epithets (not swear words, in this case, but the second "name" of a species in binomial nomenclature system) like "*miserabile*" or "*payamillionbuckstogetridofthiswretchedthing*" becoming standard. *C. difficile* actually comes by its name because when it was first identified in 1935, it was hard to isolate, and it grew slowly in culture. In other words, it was difficult.

who touches the contaminated surface to its next victim, where the whole cycle of misery starts anew.

Angus's job is to sniff out *C. diff* in the hospital environment before it has a chance to go on its next joyride from hand to mouth to gut. The *C. diff* he seeks has already traveled to places it shouldn't be. His aim is to make it a one-way trip.

A photo badge identifying him as a hospital volunteer dangles from his blue harness emblazoned with the words "WORKING DOG." As far as the hospital is concerned, he's a volunteer. But anyone who sees Angus at work knows he is well compensated for plying his trade. Treats, a ball, praise—the paycheck varies, but he's always happy and has never asked for a raise.

He whisks his way down the corridor of the fourteenth-floor medical unit, directed partly by Teresa but mostly following his own nose. You don't realize how many devices have wheels in a hospital until you're with a dog who smells all of them. A wheeled cart here, a wheeled contraption there, a wheelchair, a wheeled stool under a sink, a shelf on wheels, wheeled drawers known as isolation carts. He sniffs the wall, inhales at a plastic garbage can, inspects a laundry bag. He is trained to avoid contacting surfaces with his nose so he doesn't end up with *C. diff* or other goodies on his snout.

Everyone wants to say hi to him, but he's a dog on a mission. Visitors stop and watch. Staff members smile as he passes their stations. "Hi, Angus!" He looks up and wags but gets right back to it. He is vigilant and focused. Nothing will distract him.

Almost nothing. He spots a stuffed toy bear at one of the nurses' stations. His eyes fix on it. He looks at Teresa, then the toy, then Teresa. His eyes seem wider than they were before, and there's a pleading quality to them. His message is clear:

Can I have that please?

"No, that's not yours, Angus."

They move on. She gives him a "Good boy!" every time he sniffs something. They come to a metal cart with three shelves. It's stationed between two patient rooms. The top shelf holds several boxes of disposable gloves. The next shelf down has a couple of folded patient gowns and something medical-looking in a plastic bag with white wires coming out of it. The lowest shelf contains two white mesh bags stuffed with yellow isolation gowns.

Angus sniffs the bags, sniffs under the cart, sniffs the side of the cart. His tail wags faster. He stares at Teresa. Then he sits. Hard. He stares at Teresa more. He wags harder. The floor is so smooth and shiny that his hind legs drift apart until they're so far away from each other he can't sit anymore. He stands and stares at Teresa and wags some more.

She leads him away. He looks incredulous. He stops and sits and stares at her. She pets him, tells him he's a good boy, and explains to me that there's a glove on the ground under the cart, and he probably just wants to get the glove. He follows her for a step, then sits again and stares at her. She pets him more and tells him they'll come back.

They walk on and he jumps up on her legs. He really wants to tell her something. But they continue on their rounds.

As promised, in a couple of minutes they're back at the cart. Angus sits and wags and stares again. He doesn't stick his nose under the cart, where the crumpled glove hides. Teresa realizes it's probably not the glove after all.

"GOOD boyyy!" she says with the enthusiasm of someone whose dog may have just thwarted a deadly outbreak.

Happy to have his discovery acknowledged, Angus trots away with her.

Teresa tells a couple of nurses about the location of the possible *C. diff*, and we head back to her office. She plays a little tug-of-war with him and gives him a couple of dog cookies.

When he's done with his snack, I ask Angus a question while I pet his soft coat, which has the pattern and color scheme of Oreos crumbled in milk.

"What does *C. diff* smell like, Angus?"

He stretches and walks into his soft-sided kennel, where he curls up and promptly falls asleep. My question doesn't seem to interest him, but Teresa jumps at the chance to describe it.

"It smells kind of like boiled bamboo shoots."

I have no idea what boiled bamboo shoots smell like. They could smell like cotton candy for all I know.

"Be right back!"

She returns a minute later with a sealed jar. It contains a two-inch square of gauze. She explains that this gauze had been exposed in a different jar to the poop of someone with *C. diff.* The poop and the gauze coexisted, though didn't touch, for twenty-four hours. So the gauze should have the odor—and only the odor—of *C. diff.* It's what Angus trains on, partly because it's not dangerous since it contains just the odor, not the spores, and partly because poop has so many variables.*

She unscrews the lid, and I lean in to take a whiff of *C. diff.*

I can say with confidence that it does *not* smell like cotton candy. I can also say with confidence that it's one of the worst things I have ever smelled. I have a dog who rolls in seriously decayed animals when he gets the opportunity, so that's really saying something. I have smelled ugly, and this is ugly.

It's a nasty, sharp, acrid odor that jolts you to the depths of your sinuses. It creates almost a burning sensation, but that's not quite it either. It's impossible to describe the smell of true *C. diff,* but when you smell it, you know it's something you want to avoid.

Many health care professionals say they can sniff out *C. diff* in a patient even before the lab tests come back. Here are a couple of colorful descriptions from an online forum for nurses:

> It smells like using an outhouse or J-John during 3 months of 110+ degree temperature days. It does not smell like normal poop; it smells like something that has

---

*We won't go into the obvious and discomfiting details about poop's variables. But if you've become a fan of VOCs by this point of the book, you will be excited to know that the poop of healthy humans has been found to contain 381 volatile organic compounds. That's a lot compared to, say, blood, which has 154, but way less than breath, which has 872. The lesson here is that just because something smells bad to us doesn't mean it has more VOCs.

been dead and laying in the hot sun with just a slight tang
of poop smell . . .

To me it is like that rotten chicken meat smell, (like when
you smell that chicken and go . . . "no way . . . can't make
this tonight! PUEWWWWWW") mixed with baby dia-
per sweet smell (like when they are very young!), mixed
with old blood smell. Once you smell it . . . you won't forget!

And yet Angus is happy to find it. Ecstatic, actually.

As Teresa and I discuss the smelly superbug, I realize I'd just been
petting a dog who sniffed possible *C. diff* in a hospital unit. Could he
have rubbed against it? Probably not. Just in case, I fish out the bottle of Purell in my bag and squirt it onto my hands.

"Oh, sorry," Teresa says, in the endearing way many Canadians
say "*sorry*." "Purell doesn't really protect against *C. diff.*"

What?! Purell and other alcohol-based hand sanitizers boast that
they kill 99.99 percent of common germs that cause illness. That's a
really large percentage. Like pretty much everything. When you see
"99.99 percent," you don't think there's going to be anything harmful
in the remaining 0.01 percent. You don't even think of that 0.01 percent. Maybe these sanitizers should say something like "Kills 99.99
percent of common germs that cause illness but NOT the superbug
C. diff, which can make you really REALLY sick. Go wash your
hands with soap and water—*now!*"

The journal *Infection Control & Hospital Epidemiology* confirms
Teresa's warning: "Alcohol is not effective against *Clostridium difficile*
spores," it states, and adds an example to drive home the point: "Re-
sidual spores are readily transferred by a handshake after use of
ABHR." (Alcohol-based hand rubs have their own acronym in certain circles.) The paper goes on to state that thorough hand washing
is far more effective.

I excuse myself and wash my hands twice as long as usual. When

I return, Teresa tells me, "Better safe than sorry. Believe me. You do NOT want *C. diff.*"

This sounds personal. Turns out it is. In 2013, Teresa had a leg wound that became septic, and the antibiotics she had to take depleted her beneficial bacteria. This left *C. diff* to colonize and proliferate.

She had it bad, with diarrhea four to five times an hour, necessitating diapers, much to her embarrassment. The infection also brought fever, pain, and chills. She spent five days in the hospital, and in the course of one week with *C. diff* lost twenty pounds.

"I almost died," she says.

She finally got better—thanks, ironically, to antibiotics.

During her recovery her husband, Markus, ran across an article about a beagle in the Netherlands who was trained to sniff patients for *C. diff.* Teresa was a dog handler and trainer at the time, working with bomb- and drug-detection dogs in the private sector.

"Do you think you could train a dog to find *C. diff* in the environment?" he asked. Markus, a nurse working in Quality and Patient Safety for Vancouver Coastal Health, knew there were no fast, accurate ways to detect *C. diff* lurking in hospital settings.

"If it has a smell, I can train a dog to find it," Teresa told him with conviction. Based on her bout with the bug, she was pretty sure that *C. diff* stinks in more ways than one.

She had recently acquired a pup named Angus and was planning to train him as a detection dog for a security job. He was in the right place at the right time. Markus and Teresa approached the health authority that oversees the Vancouver General Hospital with their idea.

"We thought they'd laugh us out of the room," she says.

But the hospital liked their proposal of a pilot program. If it could help make the hospital environment safer, they were all for it. Teresa began training Angus. It took about a year because she was also working full-time as a cardiology technician. After double-blind validation/certification testing, the team became fully operational in the fall of 2016.

Angus has had a wildly successful early career. A study done in-house and published in 2017 in the *Journal of Hospital Infection* reported that his recognition of *C. diff* in containers was 100 percent (this is called sensitivity, you may remember from the cancer chapter), and he alerted to only 3 percent of negative samples as if they were positive (in other words, the specificity was 97 percent). During searches, his sensitivity was 80 percent (it has greatly improved since then, Teresa says) and specificity was 93 percent. And during clinical sweeps in a five-month period he was 100 percent on *C. diff* samples hidden for quality control.

The study concluded that "a dog can be trained to accurately and reliably detect *C. difficile* odour from environmental sources to guide the best deployment of adjunctive cleaning measures and can be successfully integrated into a quality infection control programme."*

Angus has had more than five hundred alerts in his career. He's been asked to assess several other hospitals either for outbreaks or to do baseline assessments. His finds have resulted in units and whole hospitals changing their protocols and procedures.

He used to frequently alert to staff lockers, for instance. It didn't take long to figure out what was going on. Staff would put their work shoes in their lockers at the end of a shift. The shoes sometimes had *C. diff* contamination. When they arrived for their next shift, they'd take out their work shoes and put their personal effects—jackets, purses, lunch bags—into their lockers, setting up a scenario for cross-contamination.

---

*A study published the following year in *Open Forum Infectious Diseases* looked at two Toronto dogs trained to detect *C. diff*. The authors came to a different conclusion. The study found poor agreement between the dogs, and the authors wrote that "this finding limits the practical value of using dogs as a point-of-care CDI test" and suggested that future research focus on strategies that speed up current molecular diagnostic testing process.

Teresa thinks there was a problem with the dogs used in the study: "Basically the study shows not all dogs have what it takes to be working detection dogs."

The Vancouver program has proven so successful that Vancouver Coastal Health has hired one more handler and at press time was looking to hire two more. It's also added four more dogs for a total of five detection dogs (three in training, by Teresa).

The solution was simple; the units provided shoe racks for staff. No more shoes in the locker means no more locker alerts from Angus.

Occasionally Teresa comes across nurses telling her they don't need a dog to tell them there's *C. diff*—that they already can smell it. Her response: "I know you can smell *C. diff*, but can you tell me where exactly the spores are, and are you willing to crawl on your hands and knees to find it?"

End of discussion.

Some of Angus's biggest fans are in the infection-control department at Vancouver General Hospital. Doctors there say there has been a "significant decrease" in *C. diff* since Angus started. A recent study found that *C. diff* rates have decreased in hospitals across Canada in the last several years thanks to better testing and more careful use of antibiotics. But there's only one Angus, and he's getting lots of credit for his hospital's decrease.

When he detects *C. diff*, staffers clean the area using an ultraviolet light disinfection robot. But Angus has helped reduce *C. diff* in less tangible ways as well.

Just having him scour the hospital for *C. diff* seems to make staff more aware of the bacteria, explains Diane Roscoe, MD, head of the Division of Medical Microbiology and Infection Control at the hospital. They're more careful because there's a four-legged inspector who randomly sniffs his way through the hospital.

"Angus raises the bar," Dr. Roscoe says. "The crew is so much more aware because of him. And the beauty is there's no finger-pointing. He's good in so many ways."

As we sit discussing the virtues of Angus, Dr. Roscoe's phone rings.

"Good news!" she tells Teresa. "They found a brown stain where Angus alerted this afternoon. They're taking care of it."

Teresa does a happy dance in her chair.

"Yes, I get excited about poop!" she tells me.

She's in good company. She can't wait to go tell Angus when we go back to her office.

———

In the Gambia, local health care workers recently collected urine, breath, and fingerpick blood samples from six hundred children in two schools and gave the children a pair of beige nylon ankle socks to wear for twenty-four hours. The socks were then cut lengthwise into four pieces that were packaged neatly into tiny plastic bags and shipped *en masse* to Medical Detection Dogs.

The baggies of sock pieces waited in drawers of a deep freezer as the organization assembled a team of dogs whose job would be sniffing the socks for a scent well-known to mosquitoes: the scent of someone infected with malaria.

A Labrador retriever named Sally and a Lab–golden retriever mix named Lexi were chosen for the initial team. If successful, the duo could help usher in a new way of preventing the spread of a scourge the Centers for Disease Control calls "one of the most severe public health problems worldwide."

(Freya, the spaniel you may remember as the not-so-neutral observer during the *Pseudomonas* study, was to be on the original team, but it was decided she'd be trained for another phase of the study.)

Malaria is an infectious mosquito-borne disease that cuts a swath of illness and death in a wide band around the equator, but especially in Africa, which accounts for 90 percent of malaria victims. In 2016, the most recent year for which statistics were available, there were 216 million cases of malaria worldwide. To put it in perspective, that's the population of the fifteen most populous US states. We're talking everyone in Massachusetts, Arizona, Washington, Virginia, New Jersey, Michigan, North Carolina, Georgia, Ohio, Illinois, Pennsylvania, New York, Florida, Texas, and California.

Malaria claimed the lives of 445,000 people that year. The disease affects mostly young children and pregnant women. It's a leading cause of illness and death in many developing countries.

As daunting as these figures are, they're greatly improved from the previous decade. The CDC reports that malaria mortality has decreased by 45 percent, "leading to hopes and plans for elimination and ultimately eradication." Governments and organizations around the world have been scaling up malaria-control interventions, including widespread distribution of bed nets and application of insecticides, as well as increased testing and treatment.

The Gambia is one of the countries that has seen a substantial decline in the disease, but a cross-sectional survey published in the *Malaria Journal* concluded that "current interventions are not sufficient to interrupt transmission . . . and new approaches need to be urgently evaluated . . . The Gambia offers an ideal setting to test new interventions aiming at interrupting malaria transmission."

In 2016, the Bill & Melinda Gates Foundation—which has made eradicating malaria one of its top priorities—awarded a $100,000 grant for a joint collaboration of the canine kind.*

The initial study is simple in concept: to see if dogs can smell malaria. If this proves successful, dogs could one day be used for screening travelers entering malaria-free areas, much as airport dogs screen travelers for drugs or explosives or certain foods.

The dogs could also be used to sniff out malaria within communities in a much faster and less invasive way than current methods. Right now, malaria detection usually involves a finger-prick blood test that has to be evaluated in a laboratory.

Steve Lindsay, PhD, a public health entomologist at Durham University in northeast England, is the study's lead investigator. He has worked in the Gambia regularly since the 1980s, devoting much of his career to developing malaria-control measures. He has high hopes for these doctor dogs without borders.

---

*And yes, when this was announced, there were predictable comments suggesting Microsoft eradicate its own bugs first.

"Dogs could hugely accelerate efforts to completely wipe out this terrible disease once and for all," says Dr. Lindsay.

When he learned that the Gates Foundation was looking for researchers to develop a noninvasive malaria diagnostic tool, he immediately thought of dogs. He has had dogs most of his life, although he is "now in the awful time between dogs" since the death of his Labrador retriever. And he's been aware of the power of a dog's nose for a long time. As a young man, he wanted to be a veterinarian and found a weekend job working with bloodhounds and taking them to shows to compete. Thanks to his travels, he's also been screened by plenty of dogs at airports.

He invited fellow dog-lover and colleague James Logan, PhD, head of the Department of Disease Control at the London School of Hygiene & Tropical Medicine, to collaborate on the study. One of Dr. Logan's fields of research is the potential odor change of people with malaria.

"Infection with malaria creates a human perfume that seems to make people more attractive to mosquitoes," Dr. Logan says.

A brief lesson in malaria transmission might be handy to make sense of why this would be. When a mosquito infected with a parasite that causes malaria bites someone, the mosquito's saliva transmits the parasite in a spore-like form directly into the person's bloodstream. The parasites first invade the liver and grow and multiply there until they leave in a more mature stage of life to grow and multiply again, this time in red blood cells.

When a mosquito takes a blood meal from someone infected with the parasite, she'll pick up some of these parasites, and they'll also grow and multiply inside her. In ten to eighteen days, the parasites are in the sporozoite stage in the mosquito's saliva. With her next blood meal, she'll start the cycle again, infecting a new person (unless she happens to bite someone who already has malaria).

The parasite's chances of spreading increase if mosquitoes are drawn to people who harbor the parasite. While earlier studies showed that those with malaria have a different smell and are more attractive to mosquitoes, a study co-led by Dr. Logan and published in 2018 zeroed in on chemicals that seem to attract mosquitoes.*

They found the main attractants were compounds called aldehydes, including heptanal, octanal, and nonanal, which easily evaporate and are used in perfume making. Perfumes using aldehydes—and some of the most popular perfumes do—are described as floral or fruity.

"The malaria parasite is very clever, manipulating the systems of the mosquito host and the human host," Dr. Logan says. We can only hope the dogs will also be clever, using their noses to help manipulate the parasites into oblivion.

In the early phase of training, Sally and Lexi were alerting to something, but it wasn't malaria: it was the difference between the odors of the two schools where the socks were worn and collected. The scent of the schools turned out to be stronger than the smell of the malaria. Once the researchers and the Medical Detection Dogs trainers realized this, they were more careful about how the samples were presented until the dogs got the hang of what they were supposed to be sniffing.

The dogs ended up with only 175 pair of socks out of the initial 600, so the sample size was far lower than the researchers and MDD had wanted, especially since only thirty pairs were positive for malaria. But Dr. Lindsay said they decided to be "über-careful" with the samples. "We needed to make sure the negatives were negative and the positive samples were positive. For this reason the positive samples were those where we could see malaria parasites down a microscope (not detected by PCR) and the negatives were those that were PCR-negative. PCR detects much lower parasite densities than does microscopy." (PCR stands for "polymerase chain reaction." It's a technique for finding incredibly small pieces of DNA, and is frequently used for diagnosing infectious diseases, including malaria.)

---

*This involved placing microelectrodes on the antennae of mosquitoes. "It is tricky putting electrodes on mosquitoes," Dr. Logan says.

The preliminary results were announced in late 2018. They made headlines around the world. Sally and Lexi detected 70 percent of the positive socks and 90 percent of the negative socks. Dr. Lindsay believes that if the sample size had been larger, the dogs would have done even better, but he says he considers these "excellent results" for the limited samples.

They're now seeking funding for more research. They hope to eventually test dogs at ports of entry in sub-Saharan Africa. If the dogs chosen for the mission prove to be good at what they do, doctor dogs will enter a new stage in helping keep humans safe from hidden enemies: the world stage.

PART III

OUT OF THE DARKNESS

CHAPTER 7

THE DOG WHISPERERS

From Freud's Dog to the Trombones and Hills on the Autism Spectrum

Matthew LaMott had always been a fussy baby. He had to be swaddled tightly to go to sleep, and even then, he would cry for hours, no matter what his parents tried. Bassinet, arms, rocking, singing, silence, lying with him in bed, white noise, lavender—nothing worked. When his mother, Christine, brought him into the shower with her to see if the gentle warmth of the water would help calm him, he screamed in what seemed to be physical pain. She never tried that again.

His temperament took her by surprise. His sister and stepsister hadn't been like this. But Christine knew plenty of babies were sensitive and not so good at falling asleep. She figured he'd grow out of it by the time he was old enough for day care.

But day care was a disaster. He wouldn't play with the other children, and if he engaged, it would usually end badly. It seemed to his parents that he couldn't "read" people. He'd get angry and frustrated, and would have frequent meltdowns. Sometimes he bit other children. If someone took his toy or accidentally bumped him, or even if someone was too close—anything that threatened his environment—he would lash out. Once he drew blood.

"I thought it was a stage. But it lasted far too long and was too severe," says Christine, who got her share of hard bites when she had to restrain him during a meltdown.

The best word she could think of for him was "intense." When he was about two and a half, Matthew became obsessed with the color blue. Everything had to be blue, from his underwear to his clothes to his cup and plate. If something wasn't blue, he had meltdowns of "epic proportions," sometimes lasting more than an hour.

He couldn't run through the sprinkler like the other kids because he said it hurt when the water touched him. He couldn't stand fluorescent lights, loud noises, strong smells. Brushing his teeth, brushing his hair, trimming his nails, or any personal grooming was a two-person job.

An occupational therapist diagnosed Matthew with sensory processing disorder. She and his parents worked to expose Matthew to sensory skills in fun ways, like jumping in a ball pit, swinging, playing with shaving cream as paint, blowing bubbles, making noises.

But it seemed to Christine that there was something wrong beyond this sensory diagnosis. She felt it in her gut but relied on the experts.

She took him to see a psychologist and was glad when Matthew had a meltdown in front of him. She thought this would help the psychologist come up with a more accurate diagnosis. But he said it was just normal two-year-old behavior. Christine wanted this to be true, but she couldn't really believe it. "So many things were just off," she says.

It would be another year before Matthew was diagnosed with autism spectrum disorder. Everything finally made sense to Christine and to Matthew's dad, Jon. As they navigated the treacherous waters of the fresh diagnosis, they tried to continue life as normal— although they could barely remember what normal was.

That Christmas, the relatives came to their house. It didn't take long for Matthew to crash. Christine doesn't remember what set him off, but she was embarrassed by his screaming and yelling and biting and head-butting. She didn't want this to be happening at all, much less on Christmas and in front of the relatives. She whisked him into the closest room—the bathroom—and hoped he would calm down. If nothing else, the relatives would have a break from his storm.

There was a knock at the door. Christine could barely hear it through the screams. It was Christine's sister, who had brought her two Doberman pinschers to the festivities.

"Let Dior in. She's a mama," she told Christine.

The Doberman walked into the bathroom. Matthew immediately fell silent. Dior walked over to Matthew. He reached out his arm and stroked her fur. He rubbed her side. He hugged her.

Christine had never seen anything like this. *What just happened?* she asked herself as she emerged from the room with a transformed child a few minutes later.

She looked for information about the benefits of dogs for children with autism. She learned that Can Do Canines—the same organization that had trained Terri Krake's dog, Brody, from Chapter 2—also trained autism-assistance dogs. The organization was close, and the dogs were provided free of charge.

It seemed too good to be true. She applied for a dog.

Within a few days she learned there was a waiting list of 177 people.

It would turn out to be a four-year wait. But Christine didn't know that at the time. She's glad she didn't; just the idea of a dog who could help her son gave her hope and comfort during dark times.

In the interim, the LaMotts gave up going to restaurants because it was too much for Matthew. The family had a well-worn three-ring binder of takeout menus. It was the closest they could come to eating out. They never went on vacations. At home they had what they needed to survive—his familiar room, weighted blankets, noise-canceling headphones, a library of books they could read aloud. Reading usually calmed him. But only in the house.

Leaving the house was hell, especially when it came to appointments beyond Matthew's therapies.

Haircuts tormented him. He usually had long, shaggy hair because in the salon chair he screamed and writhed and had to be held by his mom. Christine and the stylist understood that haircuts were frightening to him, and that the little hairs that fell on his neck probably felt like needles. They tried to make it as soothing and gentle as possible, but no matter what, it was enervating for everyone.

The dentist was worse. They'd been only twice before he was seven years old. Christine had to lie on the chair with Matthew in her lap. He spent the appointment banging his head into her and screaming. The first time the hygienist tried to clean his teeth, he bit her. Doctor visits were just as traumatic. He was petrified of doctors and nurses. His parents usually had to hold him down for him to get even a basic exam. They hated taking him to the doctor almost as much as he hated going.

Christine grew weary, and sick of the looks people gave her when Matthew had meltdowns, especially in stores. Shopping was one activity they couldn't avoid. When she had to bring him with her, she used all her strategies to keep him calm—going late in the evening when it was less crowded, putting him in a stroller and letting him play with his iPad. Inevitably, at some point something would set him off.

If he wasn't in his stroller, he might bolt away. She'd have to leave everything and run after him. She'd hold him as he screamed, or she'd try to sing to him. The dirty looks from people with judgmental *MY child would never get away with that* expressions got to her. She had been one of those people before Matthew came along.

Usually the only solution was to rush home to a calmer environment.

Matthew often couldn't or wouldn't talk. He was considered high-functioning on the autism spectrum, yet words frequently wouldn't come to him, especially when he was overwhelmed.

But his parents noticed something intriguing: While he might not talk to people, he would readily talk to the neighbors' dogs. He would tell the dogs things he wouldn't tell anyone. He'd tell them about his day—often about problems with other kids. The dogs just listened. So he told them more.

His parents decided they'd waited long enough. It was time to get a dog, even if he or she was just a pet and not a service dog trained to help Matthew.

They settled on a golden retriever puppy. He was adorable, of course. Matthew named him Chase, after a dog in the animated children's series *Paw Patrol*. It was fun, but it was chaos. And unfortunately, as Chase grew up, he became scared of loud noises—just like Matthew. When Matthew had meltdowns, Chase ran away.

At least school was going OK. Sometimes. Matthew did well with the structure provided by school, especially since he could take "sensory breaks" in a special room with calming lighting and equipment like swings and fidget toys. But he would still sometimes lash out at the teacher. Even the principal wasn't immune.

Christine went to the principal's office one day and saw that he had bloody scratch marks all over the top of his hand from Matthew. "I was horrified and mortified that Matthew had done this, at the same time I felt terrible that Matthew had gotten to the point where he was that upset."

At home, his parents were following the advice of therapists and structuring his time there as much as they could, including giving him some chores. "He can't get a pass just because he has a disability," Christine says. "That's not how it works in the world."

It was still taking Matthew two hours to fall asleep. He had daily meltdowns, sometimes more. If someone tried to calm him with words or speak to him during meltdowns, it seemed to push him further over the edge. "Stop talking to me!" he'd yell.

Everyone was at a loss.

And then, just when the LaMotts were thinking they'd never get off the wait list for a service dog, they got the call. Can Do Canines had a dog they thought would be perfect for Matthew—a calm, good-natured, shiny black Lab named Lloyd.

The LaMotts had no idea of the changes that were in store, or that a dog could alter the course of a family's trajectory so profoundly.

Lloyd's first meeting with Matthew came at the end of a school day when Matthew was seven years old. Tears streamed down Matthew's cheeks as he greeted his new dog. He buried his face in Lloyd's fur.

It was the first time he had ever cried tears of happiness.

The two clicked immediately. "It was as if they were made for each other," Christine says. "Matthew became a whole different kid."

Lloyd's magic comes mostly from being a calm fellow, never ruffled, ever the unflappable and steady friend.

Matthew's meltdowns have dwindled to maybe one per month, usually lasting no more than fifteen minutes. When he starts getting to where he might boil over—raising his voice and becoming agitated—Lloyd nudges him.

What's going on? What are you doing? Let's just chill now. You'll feel so much better. Let me help you. Give me a hug!

Lloyd may also lick Matthew, and rather than run away, he stays by his boy's side. His parents are quick to tell people that Lloyd's actions calm Matthew better than any therapy they've tried.

"Dogs love without prejudice. They don't expect any verbal interaction, like people do," Christine says. "I think that takes the pressure off. Autism is a skyrocket. Lloyd brings him back down safely."

The takeout-food binder is forgotten in a drawer. As long as Lloyd is with them, the whole family can go out to restaurants. The overstimulating atmosphere doesn't upset him anymore. He usually hangs out under the table with his dog. Christine is aware that it's less than sanitary down there, but it's not a battle she's interested in fighting.

Recently, during a visit to Panda Express, Matthew asked to sit at his own table—just him and Lloyd. His mother watched in joyful shock as he took his food and settled at a two-person table. Lloyd lay at his feet as his boy ate his whole meal under the bright lights of the chain restaurant.

For the first year or so, Matthew was tethered to Lloyd during shopping trips since Matthew was still inclined to bolt.* Christine held Lloyd's leash so there was never a danger of him being dragged off with Matthew, and Matthew was never violent with Lloyd. She says the tether gave her son a chance to pause and rethink what he was doing. When he tried to escape, Lloyd sat and wouldn't budge.

Lloyd helped temper Matthew's sensory overload until he was able to express it in words instead of bolting. Now Matthew will tell his parents when he's about to go downhill.

"I'm feeling triggered," he'll say. Christine will get him to sit somewhere away from crowds—a quiet aisle, if they're shopping—and Lloyd immediately lies down across Matthew's lap. "This gives Matthew the weighted, warm, soft feeling that helps him regulate his senses," she explains. Then she'll ask her son what's going on, and he's usually able to put his frustration into words. They work it out.

Getting more sleep may be helping every aspect of Matthew's life. He no longer spends a couple of hours lying awake. At bedtime Lloyd zips tight against Matthew, who usually falls asleep within twenty minutes.

Everything is easier with Lloyd. Matthew gets through haircuts without a struggle as long as Lloyd is right next to him and within petting distance. The stylist can even use buzzing electric clippers. Lloyd's black fur ends up covered in little blond hair clippings, but he doesn't mind. Like everything else, he just shakes it off.

At the dentist, Lloyd lies across Matthew, almost like a blanket. Matthew sits quietly with his arms around Lloyd's neck. During their first dentist appointment together, the dentist was even able to apply sealants to Matthew's molars.

---

*Tethering a child to even a trained service dog is not recommended by many service dog organizations, although others maintain that if done the way Christine did it, with an adult maintaining control of the dog at all times, it's safe for the dog and the child. The website of the organization Autism Speaks explains the problem with the way the practice is often done: "Tethering a dog to a child can be extremely dangerous. Like any animal, a service dog can panic under stress, resulting in tragedy for both the child and dog. While some agencies claim they can train dogs to stop children from leaving a home or yard, dogs are not appropriate babysitters."

A few months after getting Lloyd, Matthew fell ill with a high fever. Christine took him to urgent care. Once she assured him that Lloyd could be on the gurney with him, he let her lift him onto it. Lloyd jumped up after him and lay down. Matthew cuddled him as he waited for the doctors and handled everything like a pro during the exam.

"It was like Lloyd had lifted this enormous weight off of me. I cried all the way home," Christine says.

The LaMotts have made up for lost vacation time, too. Since Lloyd, they've been to California (including a ride on San Francisco's clanging cable cars), Mount Rushmore, and Universal Studios Florida. With Lloyd at his side, Matthew can handle every aspect of travel, including cross-country plane trips.

Most important and heartwarming, Christine says, is that Matthew is making friends at school. He has blossomed since Lloyd arrived. He attends school functions (albeit sometimes with earplugs to muffle the noise) and has a confidence that wins over other kids, even if he still isn't as adept at interacting as most children. He gets invited to parties and sleepovers. The kids like his sense of humor— something he comes by naturally from being raised in a family of jokers.

Lloyd doesn't attend school because Matthew would have to take care of him there, and he's still young and unaware of his dog's needs. But sometimes Lloyd visits school—usually when Matthew is having a rough day. A few minutes of quiet time with his dog leaves Matthew in a better place.

To the amazement of his family, Matthew has joined the school band. He wanted to play trumpet, but the band teacher evaluated him and said that because he has excellent pitch sensitivity, he'd be a great trombone player. During the initial band practices Matthew tried to play the trombone and cover his ears at the same time because of the other instruments. That didn't work out so well. Christine bought him some earplugs that significantly reduce the noise. They seem to be helping.

Matthew brings the instrument home to practice on weekends. His parents realize beginners in any instrument will be rough on the ears, and they bear with the baying sounds and squawks. But Lloyd is another story. He was trained for only so much.

The trombone was not part of the job description.

When Matthew practices at home, Lloyd barks as if an intruder were in the house. He's never complained about *anything*, so Christine and Jon take the dog's protestations seriously. They have Matthew practice on one floor, and make sure Lloyd is far enough away on another floor where it doesn't bother him.

"It's the least we could do after what he has done for us," she says.

———

In the 1960s, child psychologist Boris Levinson, PhD, of Yeshiva University, broke new ground in a presentation to the American Psychological Association when he described how his dog Jingles affected therapy sessions with uncommunicative children. By chance he discovered that when Jingles was in the room, these children would open up and become significantly better at communicating.

Stanley Coren, PhD, professor emeritus in the Department of Psychology at the University of British Columbia, and author of many engaging and excellent books about dogs (you met him in a footnote in Chapter 4), was in the beginning stages of his career when he attended the talk. He recalled in a column in *Psychology Today* the reaction to Dr. Levinson's presentation.

"The reception of his talk was not positive, and the tone in the room did not do credit to the psychological profession," Dr. Coren wrote. "Levinson was distressed to find that many of his colleagues treated his work as a laughing matter. One even cat-called from the audience, 'What percentage of your therapy fees do you pay to the dog?'"

Dr. Coren lamented the response. He thought it might be the end for that line of "work" for dogs. But he wrote that around that same time, biographies of Sigmund Freud were being published. The books discussed the psychoanalyst's use of his own dogs in therapy sessions.

In the 1930s, Dr. Freud's dog, a fluffy red chow chow named Jofi, originally joined him in his sessions just as his cherished pet. She was there mainly to keep Freud company. He had been smitten with Jofi from the beginning. "She is a charming creature, so interesting in her feminine characteristics, too, wild, impulsive, intelligent and yet not so dependent as dogs often are," he wrote when Jofi came into his life. "One cannot help feeling respect for animals like this."

It didn't take Dr. Freud long to see Jofi's effect on patients. "This difference was most marked when Freud was dealing with children or adolescents," Dr. Coren wrote. "It seemed to him that the patients seemed more willing to talk openly when the dog was in the room. They were also more willing to talk about painful issues."

When Dr. Freud's findings appeared in these books, Dr. Levinson's work started being taken more seriously, according to Dr. Coren. Eventually this led to studies of dogs and their effect on children with autism spectrum disorder.

Considering that one in fifty-nine children in the United States has been identified as being on the spectrum, there's a surprising dearth of quality, peer-reviewed studies of this relationship. The authors of these studies tend to conclude they're encouraged by the results, but call for more research.

Some studies find that dogs in therapy settings can help children on the spectrum. One study of twenty-two children showed more improvement in language use and social interactions during occupational therapy sessions that incorporated animals (dogs, but also llamas and rabbits) than sessions without them. In a study of a dozen boys in sessions with therapy dogs, children showed less aggression and self-absorption, and more smiling, visual contact, and affectionate behaviors.

But it's not all unicorns and rainbows. An earlier study, published in the *Western Journal of Nursing Research,* found an increase in hand-flapping in a dog's presence and less eye contact with the therapist.

In addition, the children provided less-detailed answers to questions. Still, the authors leaned on the study's more positive results in their conclusion: "Children exhibited a more playful mood, were more focused, and were more aware of their social environments when in the presence of a therapy dog. These findings indicate that interaction with dogs may have specific benefits for this population and suggest that animal-assisted therapy (AAT) may be an appropriate form of therapy."

As for autism-assistance dogs like Lloyd, the little research that's been done points to the kind of positive outcomes the LaMotts have experienced: a calmer child who sleeps better and has fewer tantrums and other behavioral problems.*

Not all dogs are miracle workers like Lloyd. Sometimes these dogs aren't a good fit for families with autism. But when it's a strong match, autism-assistance dogs seem to be able to help across the spectrum. And around the world . . .

———

With his shoulder-length grizzled bob swept to one side, his leather bomber jacket, his faded jeans, and his ice-blue eyes, Damir Vučić looks like a rock star from another era. Even as he drives a Fiat Doblò that smells like dog food through the winding streets of Zagreb, Croatia, the fifty-two-year-old comes across as someone who belongs on a stage holding a guitar.

But a closer look reveals he's a rock star of a different sort. He wears a necklace that ends in a pouch. The pouch is full of dog kibble. Also around his neck are a couple of leashes. His jacket pockets brim with dog treats.

———

*What about the dogs? Most doctor dogs are not in situations where they could potentially be hurt. Stressed? Yes, sometimes, although their people usually do what it takes to mitigate stress. But physically hurt? No.

A study that looked into the welfare of autism-assistance dogs points out that depending on the child, these dogs can potentially be in harm's way. Children prone to aggression might unintentionally mistreat their dog. The study found that the dogs eventually learn to roll with the punches, so to speak, by figuring out when to move away and when to move in to distract the child.

Damir had spent plenty of time in the spotlight, but always with a dog at his side. He's a respected and popular dog trainer, and has devoted much of the last quarter century to raising and showing big, fluffy, light-cream golden retrievers, and being a show judge throughout Europe.

A couple of years ago he became the head trainer for the Croatian Guide Dog and Mobility Association. He loves the work, and finds it more rewarding than anything he's ever done. "To help improve someone's life by training a dog for them feels very good," says Damir. "Dog is my brother, so it's a natural fit for me to help them help people."

I ask him what he means about dog being his brother. I've heard "dog is my copilot," but the brother reference eluded me.

"It's my surname. 'Vučić' means 'little wolf,' like a wolf cub. So dogs and I get along very well." He adds that he was born in Dalmatia, so he is also a Dalmatian. "I am all about dogs."

I'd met Damir earlier that day when I was learning how the association uses dogs as educational aides for children with developmental disabilities. Psychologist and counselor Lea Devčić had been showing me some of the ways dogs have been helping children with their reading and numbers skills, days of the week, months, seasons, colors, and even coordination, empathy, recognizing emotions, and overcoming sensory issues.

Dogs are active parts of the lessons. At the office, Lea works with her dog Leo, a black Lab, to demonstrate skill-building exercises to parents and children. If a child has a service dog, that dog will be part of the lessons at home.

It's all a game for the dogs (as always), and learning becomes a game for the children. Let's say a child is struggling with months and seasons. The family has been given a big red cloth bag reminiscent of Santa's Christmas sack, filled with goodies for various lessons. The child or parent fishes out four big wooden numbers, each in a different color and with the name of a season, and sets them on the floor somewhere in the room. Near the child is a big circular calendar with all the months radiating out from the center, color-coded in sections to match the wooden numbers, which are inscribed with the seasons.

The parent or child asks the dog to "fetch" a number, and the dog brings the number to the child. The dog gets a treat. Children are usually happy to be working with a wagging and nonjudgmental educational facilitator. It seems to be able to make it easier to learn without frustration, and to participate in answering questions. Typical questions or requests from a parent doing this lesson go something like this:

"Which number did the dog bring you?"

"What is that season?"

"What months and color does that season go on? Can you read me the months?"

"Go ahead and set the number on the right season."

The dog is usually watching, even if from a corner of the room. Depending on the child's imagination, the dog is still participating in the lesson. Children often look at the dog during the activity, even when the dog isn't actively engaged. Some lessons are all about the dog—like matching a ball color to a dog's bandanna, which the parent changes. During the sessions the dog can bring different-colored balls to the child, or the child can choose a ball and bring it to the dog.

Balls and dogs and children are a winning combination.

"Dogs are great motivators for learning and skill development," Lea explained as she poured her sack of educational props onto the floor. "They're nonthreatening, nonjudgmental, and give unconditional love. There's no better teacher."

Just then, Damir walked in with a yellow Lab–golden retriever mix.

"This is Bob. He's going to go to a very nice girl with autism spectrum disorder today," Damir said after Lea had introduced him.

I'd never seen a service dog being placed with a child before.

"Is there any chance I could go with you?"

. . .

Bob is lying in a large kennel in the back of the van. For all he knows, he's going to the nearby grassy park—maybe the one with the big crunchy autumn leaves all over the ground. Or back to Damir's.

Bob had been staying with Damir and his wife for the last three months. He had come to them after spending most of his early life with a volunteer puppy-raiser family. And now Bob was ready for the next stage of his service dog career. Bob, who is eighteen months old, has had the time of his life at the Vučićs'. He shared the couple's large home and fenced meadow with their nine golden retrievers and a couple of other dogs Damir has been training for the organization.

He also shared the Vučićs' bed. There are dog beds scattered around the house, but most nights you can find several dogs piled into bed with the couple.

By day, Damir worked with Bob on basic obedience. Damir has known Bob since puppyhood. In fact, Damir was the one who named Bob. His full name is Bobby McGee. Damir shrugs and smiles when he tells me. This man clearly knows his Janis Joplin.

I'm fond of short human names for dogs, and to meet a dog named Bob in a country where I can't pronounce most names is a treat. I find myself saying "Hey, Bob!" in an idiotic voice every time I see him looking at me from his kennel. *Bang bang* goes his tail against the frame. "Bahhhhhb!" *Bang bang!*

Bob is a mellow, friendly dog. The organization, known for raising and training guide dogs, was hoping he'd be a guide dog. But after Damir and some other members of the staff tested him, they realized he didn't have the right stuff for guiding the blind. He was a little nervous in certain new situations. He would pant, with his ears back and tail down. Guide dog work can be high pressure, and they needed to see a more confident temperament. But all was not lost. They simply found a new career path for him.

"Bob is sweet and sensitive and gentle," Damir tells me. "We chose a gentle, sweet, sensitive girl for him. He met her and her family last week and they were all so happy. Today is the big day for everyone."

We pull up to a modest house and park along the street. Damir opens the back door of the van and out pops Bob, who stretches, yawns, and looks at Damir to find out what's next. Damir, flanked by Bob, starts up the exterior stairs of the house.

I glance at a window on the second floor and see a girl looking out. She has long straight blond hair and is smiling tenderly. Her hands are little fists of excitement under her chin.

When we get to the top of the stairs, Renato Petek opens the door. Bob runs up to him and his wife, Kosjenka. Bob is wagging and smiling, licking them on the face. He seems to recognize them from their first encounter last week with their daughter, Ira.

Ira scampers into the kitchen from the room where she'd been watching for Bob. Her eyes are wide and glittering with excitement. She doesn't say anything, but she seems to revel in Bob's presence.

"He's here, Bob is really here! We have a dog!" Kosjenka exclaims. Her eyes well up. "We have all been looking forward to this day for such a long time."

She invites me to the small kitchen table for a cup of coffee while Damir talks to Renato and Ira in the adjoining living room about Bob and the kind of training they will be doing with him. Bob knows basic obedience, and the family will have to learn how to work with him to keep up his skills. The training for Ira's needs will happen after Bob passes some obedience tests. Renato will be Bob's main adult handler since he's off work for a while because of an injury.

Ira sits on the couch, and Bob lies at her feet. She reaches down and strokes his fur, staring at him, rapt, silent, while she listens to Damir speak with her father. Bob licks her hands. She beams and looks at her mother, who is watching from the adjoining kitchen.

"This makes me so happy," Kosjenka says, setting a plate of buttery Croatian cookies on the table. "Ira has been talking about Bob nonstop. The idea of a dog has been a source of great happiness for a long time."

Ira is in second grade. She has been having a rough go of school the last couple of years, since leaving her Montessori kindergarten for public school. She hasn't been engaging with children well and feels uncomfortable in the classroom. At first they thought she was just shy, but it gradually got worse. She doesn't like to leave the house, preferring the comfort of familiar, calm surroundings to the outside world.

A year ago, she was diagnosed with autism spectrum disorder. Her autism looks much different from Matthew's. She may also have some learning issues. Ira is bright and attentive, but she's been having trouble with reading, math, and other school subjects. She's scheduled for evaluation in a few months to see if she has dyslexia or other learning disabilities. In the meantime her parents have been working with her so she won't fall far behind. Her mom is a primary school teacher, so Ira is in good hands.

In the months they've been waiting for a dog, they've been visiting Lea and Leo for learning enrichment. Ira has thrived during lessons with Leo. Kosjenka wishes it were the same at school.

It's been difficult for Kosjenka to watch her daughter struggle academically at such a young age. But far worse is seeing her longing for friends and having a hard time making them. She's at a stage where she still wants to play with dolls and stuffed animals, while some of her classmates have already moved on to talking about makeup and boys. Ira often comes home from school in tears. Or she has meltdowns because school and the outside world feel so overwhelming.

"I don't like seeing my daughter suffer," Kosjenka says. "She's a kid, she should be enjoying life. Every parent wants their child to be happy, and she's such a good girl."

They'd applied for a dog months earlier and were ecstatic when Lea told them their application was accepted. Once Bob had a career change, Lea knew just the place for him.

The Peteks have been gearing up for Bob for a while. Preparations included a trip to the pet store, where they bought him a bed, a collar, a leash, some toys, and food. Ira has a large Labrador retriever doll on her bed, in the room she shares with her parents. She has been sleeping next to the toy dog at night. Her parents will let Bob sleep in her bed, hoping his calmness, his warmth, and his affection will help Ira be more relaxed and sleep better.

As Kosjenka is showing me the "Bob doll" in the bedroom, Ira walks in, followed by the real Bob. Her smile is broad, her eyes alive with happiness. Bob's big tail wags as he snortles an inspection around the room.

Ira says something quietly to her mother.

"She wants me to show you her painting," Kosjenka says, looking at something behind me.

I turn around and see a square canvas painted with a couple of green hills. Above the right hill is a dark sky with stars and a giant moon. Above the left hill is a lighter sky with puffy clouds and sunshine. If you look closely, there is a little golden figure running to the left, from the hill on the dark side toward the hill on the lighter side.

Bob.

Without knowing it, Bob has already been helping Ira with something she finds difficult: understanding calendars, including days of the week. Once she and her parents knew Bob's arrival date, she made a little countdown calendar with her mother's help. It shows the days of the week, including the numeric order, and the big arrival date with an exclamation point and a heart and his name in ALL CAPS.

Ira had never taken to calendars, but at the end of each day she couldn't wait to cross off another square and say the day of the week and count how many more days until Bob Day.

We follow Bob and Ira back to the living room. Bob lies down on the parquet floor, and Ira tucks herself on the ground facing him. She holds his paws in her hands.

"She is so peaceful with him," her mother says. Tears well up again. "He is the perfect dog."

As we talk, Ira and Bob get up together and she starts skipping around the small apartment. Bob follows, with what seems to be a little smile. In that moment, Ira looks like any happy child, without a trouble in the world, flanked by her loyal, happy dog.

Kosjenka hopes it's just the beginning of a newfound confidence and joy for Ira, and a lighter load for her daughter to carry. Because now she can share it.

After three hours of talking with the family, Damir has to get going. He has a guide dog to train. He has left Renato with everything he'll need for continuing Bob's training until Damir's return in a few days.

Damir suggests Ira and her dad take Bob for a walk. Since Renato is the one who will be learning obedience with Bob, he takes the leash. We say our good-byes to Kosjenka, who hugs Damir extra hard and thanks him for bringing them the best gift they've ever had. (Dogs are placed free of charge.)

"It is my joy," Damir tells her.

We walk to the Fiat. Damir gives Renato a couple more training tips, and there are hugs all the way around. Damir and I stand and watch as father, daughter, and dog walk down the road. She is swinging her father's hand and checking in with Bob. Bob bounces along, wagging. He gives Ira's hand a lick. She giggles.

In a couple of blocks, they turn a corner and disappear from view.

A few months after my visit, I got the good news that Renato and Bob passed the equivalent of a public-access test for service dogs. About ten months after my visit, Kosjenka wrote me. Here's a portion of her note:

> Ira and I also started studying and writing homework with Bob, especially maths which she struggles with. He patiently sits by her side and takes part in our "classes" and learning activities at home.
>
> Her teacher says Bob made big difference and everything about Ira changed since she got him—she says Ira

finally opened up and started communicating both with her and with her classmates. At school she used to mask and pretend to understand everything, to be on top of everything and then when we would come home, she'd completely fall apart and it was hard to get on with the day for her. Things are better now because she looks forward coming home to him, taking him out, the whole environment is different. And she behaves more freely at school because many kids like to talk and listen about Bobby . . .

Greetings from Zagreb,
Kosi, Ira, Renato and Bob

CHAPTER 8

A HEARTBEAT AT MY FEET

The Difference Dogs Make in Mental Illness

Elizabeth Horner was four years old when she asked her mother to end her young life. They'd been playing on the living room floor, and she said it almost robotically, as if all the feeling had been sucked out of her.

"I want you to kill me." Just like that.

Sharon Horner felt her heart tighten. She couldn't have heard her right. This was her happy girl, the girl she'd just been tickling, the girl who makes friends easily with that winning smile.

She took a breath. *Stay calm.*

"What did you say, Elizabeth?"

"I want you to kill me." Same flat delivery.

Sharon was a registered nurse. She knew how to react calmly to emergencies. But nothing had prepared her for her daughter asking her to take her life.

"Oh my gosh, why would I do that? I *love* you! I want you to be happy!" She managed to say it without sounding like the bottom had dropped out of her world.

A psychiatrist diagnosed Elizabeth with anxiety and depression and prescribed Prozac. It was the beginning of an on-and-off battle with major depression, anxiety, agoraphobia, and what would eventually be diagnosed as bipolar disorder.

Medicine helped sometimes, but often her prescriptions made her feel worse, especially when she was on a few at the same time. During high school, Elizabeth grappled with panic attacks and crippling social anxiety. One time her mother dropped her off at a church event, and Elizabeth wouldn't let go of the handle of the van as she drove away. Her mother saw her and stopped. She told her she wasn't letting her back in and that she had to go to the event. By this point, several people were watching. Elizabeth peeled her hand off, her heart racing.

High school was hell. Agoraphobia often prevented her from being able to leave home, and frequent panic attacks prevented her from learning. She ended up homeschooling. By that point, she had eight younger siblings—most of them adopted, and all with special needs. Even with the chaos that could bring, she found it was a better learning atmosphere.

Her mental illness grew more severe as she became a young adult. She was feeling anxious and depressed most of the time, with little hope she would ever be able to live away from her family. She searched online for anything that could help. She was desperate for something good to happen. She wanted to live life, not hide from it. She wanted to be somebody.

It was around this time that a racing greyhound named Gable Sandstorm was having his own difficulties. The sleek seventy-pound brindle was pushing four years old. He had raced 120 times during his career at Tucson Greyhound Park. It wasn't where the best dogs raced. The really fast dogs usually went to parks with bigger earnings.

Gable Sandstorm had been able to keep his career going for nearly a couple of years. But a look at his racing record showed he was no track star.

"The dog was maybe mediocre. It wasn't the worst career I've seen, but it was far from stellar," a career greyhound-racing expert we will call Henry told me when he saw Gable Sandstorm's track record. (Henry didn't want to go on the record because he was only supposed to be helping me decipher the dog's racing records, not passing judgment on some poor retiree.)

Greyhounds get an official comment for each race. It's kind of like a greyhound report card. Here are some comments the track's chart writers gave Gable during his career. The comments in brackets are mine. (Unlike the report cards of most humans, his charts are available in perpetuity on the internet. Yes, Gable is a sight hound, but it's probably good that he can't read.)

> *Stumbled backstretch*
> *Collided 1st turn*
> *In it Briefly* [yes!]
> *Never in It*
> *No Threat*
> *Held Gamely* [good job!]
> *Not in It*
> *Not a Contender*
> *Couldn't Keep Up*
> *Always Back*
> *Stmbld Badly Far Tn*
> *Furious Finish, Inside* [sweet!]
> *Not a Factor*
> *Failed to Threaten* [who writes these things?]
> *Faded Off*
> *Not in It*
> *Never Improved*
> *Not in It*

"Dogs know when they don't win," Henry said. "They see the other dogs running ahead of them. They know they're not getting that extra biscuit some of the others got, or the huge praise the winner gets. They'll get an encouraging pat. You've got to keep the dog motivated. But it's not winning."

Gable Sandstorm had viewed plenty of greyhound heinies in his career. Bringing up the rear was nothing foreign to him. His last two races were no exception. The official comments pulled no punches:

Penultimate race: *"Steady Decline."*

Last race of his career: *"Not a Contender."*

Ah, the cruel echo of Marlon Brando's immortal lines.

"I coulda been a contender. I coulda been *someone.*"

When JoAnn Turnbull looks for a dog to adopt for Rescue to Service, a program within her main service dog training organization, Handi-Dogs, she's understandably choosy.

She wants to see confidence. The dogs need to be comfortable going to new environments with different sights and sounds, new people, new dogs, big crowds, small groups. They can't be remotely aggressive and mustn't be skittish.

She also looks for a work ethic: Will the dogs be motivated to get up when lying down? Some dogs she has trained master tasks quickly, but if they're snoozing and their person needs them, they just look up as if to say, *Ummm, could you please do it yourself? Can't you see I'm comfortable?*

The idea of adopting dogs and making them into service dogs is a noble one. But it's not so easy to find the right dogs. About half of the dogs JoAnn and her staff adopt from shelters and rescue groups don't make it. They adopt those dogs out as pets. (The dogs get snapped up because they have excellent temperaments and they're well trained. They just may not want to be bothered to get your cane when they're sleeping.)

In the spring of 2015, JoAnn decided to look at an offering from a greyhound rescue group. His name was Wallace. He was a sable greyhound, about seventy pounds, and had recently retired from the track, where his name had been Gable Sandstorm. His foster family thought the name Wallace suited him better.

Wallace met JoAnn's standards. And he was so calm. Just the guy for someone who needed a rock of a dog. She had a special client in mind.

. . .

"What? A greyhound? A greyhound service dog?" Elizabeth said when JoAnn told her. "Aren't they known for their, um, prey drive?"

Elizabeth had come across several articles about how dogs can assist people with her conditions. She loved the idea of a dog helping her break out of the confines of her house and into the world. No drug had yet been able to do this for an extended period. Could a dog?

She decided to give the Rescue to Service program a try. It was affordable, and she liked the program's model: She would train and create her own service dog. The price was right, and she'd have something to do—something that really mattered.

After she learned she might get a greyhound, she did some research to make sure they could be good service dogs and she wouldn't go flying down the street if the dog saw a critter. The website of Greyt Hearts Service Dogs was reassuring:

> These dogs are perfectly suited for a life of Service due to the extensive training they have received since birth, their vast exposure at Greyhound racing facilities and the fact that they have a unusually long working life span as opposed to other breeds. Greyhounds are not prone to hip dysplasia, have a very low maintenance coat and do not have a "doggie" odor . . . This makes them quite user friendly and easy for a new dog handler/owner to adapt to. Greyhounds have a calm, quiet nature and bond deeply and quickly to an owner.

She laughed about the delicate "doggie odor" reference. If this dog could get her out of the house and into the world, she wouldn't care if he smelled like a skunk.

I met Elizabeth and her dog at the Tucson Mall about three years after she got him, and two years after he had passed his Canine

Good Citizen test and the public-access test and officially become a service dog through Handi-Dogs.

Elizabeth changed Wallace's briefly held name to Pippin, after one of the hobbits who accompany Frodo in *The Lord of the Rings*. Pippin helps Frodo bear the ring at the outset of his journey, and his lighthearted presence ensures a dark story doesn't get too dark.

Elizabeth has moved out of her childhood home, and she and Pippin are living with a friend and her guide dog. Elizabeth's anxiety still prevents her from driving, and she still needs her medication, but she says life is "many hundreds of percents better" than it was before Pippin.

If she's feeling depressed and can't get out of bed, Pippin gently nudges her in the face with his nose. She's taking some classes at a community college. Thanks to Pippin, she even makes it to the movies occasionally.

Before she got Pippin, she couldn't even go grocery shopping without having a panic attack. And now here she was with me at a mall. With loud teens. And children racing around. It was a weekday morning, so it was relatively quiet. But still, she never imagined she'd survive a mall before Pippin.

We walked into Forever 21 and stopped to look at some clothes. Three girls flowed toward us from behind, shrieking with laugher about a boy in their school. Pippin calmly maneuvered himself in back of Elizabeth and leaned slightly into her legs. This is meant to create a barrier as well as give Elizabeth a calming touch. The girls passed. Elizabeth remained calm in her magic invisible Pippin bubble.

She wanted to take Pippin to the Build-a-Bear store. He loves teddy bears; his favorite toy is a small beige bear with a squeaker in its tummy. At the entrance to the store, he paused to survey the fluffy toys, then quickly got to work. If a person walked to Elizabeth's left, Pippin headed to that side to provide a barrier. Any direction, and he was there. He seemed to choose the areas where more people were. He maneuvered with grace and ease.

"Off to the races!" a shopper shouted, waving from across the store. Elizabeth has heard that plenty. But she laughed because it was probably the first time the guy had said it and she wanted to be polite.

When a store is jammed with people, it can still be too much for her, even with her dog. "Exit," she'll say. She knows which stores spike her anxiety and has practiced showing Pippin the exit. At Target, for instance, if she's ready to hightail it out of there, he'll lead her to the door. She doesn't have to think. She just goes along. It helps her thwart a panic attack.

Pippin is a game changer, but he isn't a magic pill. Sometimes her illness gets the best of both of them. One day, while visiting her family, she took Pippin for a walk. Not long after they left, Pippin came running back alone, his leash trailing. A few seconds later, Elizabeth ran up crying hysterically, talking rapidly about some person she was hearing shouting at her in foreign languages. But there was no person. It was an auditory hallucination. She wouldn't calm down and had to be hospitalized. That was when she was diagnosed with bipolar disorder.

"It's heartbreaking," her mother says. "Pippin can do so much, but he can't do everything."

As we walk across the mall's shiny tile floor toward the exit, Elizabeth extends her arm and touches Pippin. He's tall and easy to reach. She says it makes her feel safe to be able to feel his warmth and his strength. Pippin now weighs a comfortable eighty pounds, and his haunches are still muscular. I tell her Pippin still looks athletic enough to race.

"Yeah, but the difference is that he doesn't have to win anymore," she said, stopping to pet him. "He's always a winner as far as I'm concerned, aren't you, Pip?"

———

Pippin is one of a growing number of dogs trained to help people with mental health issues. Psychiatric service dogs, as they're often called, are the fourth most common type of service dog in North

America, a recent University of California, Davis, study found. They rank after guide dogs for the blind, mobility assistance dogs, and dogs for the hearing impaired.

Every psychiatric service dog performs specific tasks unique to his person's conditions. Service dogs trained for people with obsessive-compulsive disorder can flag someone to repetitive behaviors with a nudge or a paw. Likewise a dog for someone who engages in self-harm, like cutting, can recognize the behavior and step in to try to put a halt to it with a paw, or a bark, or a nuzzle and request for attention.

Angus, a sweet black Lab, helps his University of Arizona student, Katharine "Kit" Heyser, with her debilitating anxiety. He has a big tool kit of ways to help keep her anxiety from getting out of control. Angus is a well-behaved boy (except for an endearing squirrel obsession), so when he's pawing at Kit or tugging at the leash or just not listening, she checks in with herself to see if trouble is brewing. It usually is. Then they work together to help her out of it.

I watched Angus guide Kit to the exit of a store on campus when she asked him to help her leave. He didn't take the most direct route, but he did an impressive job. He also practices intelligent disobedience by getting Kit's attention—sometimes by misbehaving—to distract her from rising anxiety.

"Having a dog like Angus has truly changed my life," Kit told me. "I am a different person because of him. He has helped me realize that I have a purpose to my life and need for a career to do some sort of animal-assisted therapy to help give back. It has made me more aware of the impact animals make on a person's life and how truly special that can be."

———

Skilled psychiatric service dogs like Angus and Pippin aren't the only ones who can help people with mental health. Our good old pet dogs have been doing this all along.

Anyone who has ever loved a dog treasures the incomparable

bond, the best friend who's there through hard times, the under-standing listener who doesn't judge, the fun soul who brings smiles and laughter, and, most of all, the unconditional love (a term you have come across a few times already in this book). Writer Edith Wharton put it succinctly in one of her lyrical epigrams in the *Yale Review* in 1920:

> *My little dog:*
> *A heart-beat*
> *At my feet.*

For people suffering from mental illness, that heartbeat may be the only one regularly in their lives. Science has been examining this relationship closely in recent years.

A study published in *BMC Psychiatry* in 2016 concluded that "pets should be considered a main rather than a marginal source of support in the management of long-term mental health problems . . ." When the authors asked people with serious mental illness such as schizo-phrenia and bipolar disorder who or what helped them manage their mental health, many responded that it was their pets (not just dogs but also cats, hamsters, birds, and guinea pigs).

That same study noted that pets can distract their people from "symptoms of schizophrenia such as hearing voices, from suicidal ideation or from a general sense of feeling alone," and that "pets often introduced a source of humour into difficult situations and were often the only thing that could lift participants' spirits."

A 2018 paper in the same journal reviewed seventeen studies on the role of companion animals in helping manage mental illness. The authors wrote that participants felt their pets were "a consistent source of comfort and affection. This constant presence meant that this provision was available instantaneously without request."

Thanks to their pets, many of the people in these studies had re-duced feelings of loneliness, isolation, irritability, and depression. Pets decreased worry and rumination about their illnesses, and in-creased chances for sociability.

In one of the studies in the review, people said they felt they needed less medication because of the effect their pets had on them—not that anyone is recommending taking less medication because of a pet, but it's an intriguing self-assessment that could warrant further study. And here's a hopeful explanation from the 2018 paper of how meaningful these companions can be to those with mental illness:

> Pets provided their owners with a sense of purpose and gave meaning to their lives. Often participants described how this had been diminished since diagnosis with a mental health condition but that pets helped them to overcome this and provided them with a platform for going forward with their lives. This sense of meaning and purpose included pets giving their owners a reason to live, to contributing to a sense of control and empowerment and giving individuals hope for the future.

Of course, pets aren't the answer for everyone with mental illness. The burden of caring for a pet can be too much for some. Pets can impact people financially, and the time commitment can be overwhelming. The potential or actual death of a pet was cited as being "a major source of distress" (as it is for most people without mental illness). But memories could still bring them joy.

In the studies, pets were often perceived to have a "sense" of when someone needed calming or emotional support and responded "in an intuitive way, especially in times of crisis and periods of active symptoms."

If you've had a dog, you've probably experienced this. Dogs seem to have an uncanny ability to know when something is wrong. They know us so well. They inhabit our routines, they watch our expressions and read our body language, they become accustomed to a normal tone of voice. When any—or all—of the above go out of whack, dogs can sense it.

In my book *Soldier Dogs*, I wrote about a big German shepherd named Rex. During downtime in Iraq, the military working dog always seemed to know who needed him the most, and he'd bring them his favorite toy—an empty water bottle—to crunch or toss around with him. The training manager for the Department of Defense Military Working Dog program told me he thought this kind of seemingly comforting behavior isn't so much that the dog is trying to make people feel better, but that the dog is trying to have everything become "normal" again.

That may sometimes be the case, but it doesn't really explain the dog who isn't normally affectionate but immediately snuggles into someone's side when they're feeling sick or beaten by the world. Or the dog who walks into a room of children and seems to know which child is having difficulty, and lies down at his feet, or tries to get him to play. Next thing you know, everyone's doing a little better.

Are sight and sound the only ways dogs get their signals about our state of mind? Could their sense of smell be part of it? Can dogs smell how we feel?

To help answer this, let's head to the refrigerator of Dr. Cattet at the Indianapolis headquarters of Medical Mutts. You won't find eggs, milk, or leftover pizza. This fridge is stocked with emotions.

If you riffle around, you'll find tins of anxiety, panic, fear, anger, and relaxation. Or, more accurately, tins containing cotton balls that have been swabbed on the foreheads and necks of people experiencing these states. They're among containers with the scent of diabetic hypoglycemia as well as the scent of people having seizures, which you read about earlier in the book.

The tins of emotions are in plastic bags, which are stored in sealed bins to minimize cross-contamination. These scents are normally kept in the freezer, and only thawed in the fridge when the trainers are actively working with dogs.

These literal emotional meltdowns are happening more frequently, as more people with PTSD and anxiety come to Medical Mutts for psychiatric service dogs. The organization uses scent to train all its psychiatric service dogs. The dogs are first trained with samples from a variety of other people; then in the final couple of months with scents from their future person.

Can dogs really distinguish between a "crisis" sample and a "normal" sample?

"At this point," Dr. Cattet says, "they have clearly shown that they can tell the difference between the smell of a person having an anxiety attack or even anger and the smell of the same person in a relaxed, normal state of mind."

Dr. Cattet would like to collaborate with a university group to do a study on dogs sensing mental states via olfaction. It would be groundbreaking research, although a couple of related studies from groups in Italy have already been published.

One study in *Behavioural Brain Research* with the title "The Nose 'KNOWS' Fear" found that fear body odors or "chemosignals" from humans made dogs appear more stressed than a control condition and increased their heart rates. In other words, the researchers from the University of Bari found that dogs can smell fear—something people who work with dogs in military and police settings have often assumed.*

Researchers from the University of Naples later looked at whether dogs can smell human emotion. They started with the premise that body odors can carry clues about emotional states and other information from one person to another. We're not overtly aware of this level of communication since it's "below the threshold of consciousness," notes the 2018 paper in the journal *Animal Cognition*. "Nevertheless, such transmission induces in the receiver a partial affective, behavioral, perceptual, and neural reproduction of the state of the sender."

The study concluded that dogs could distinguish happy and fearful human states purely by smell. The researchers saw a long

---

*One fascinating observation they made while doing the research: Dogs used their right nostril to sniff odors of stressed dogs. (The stress was not caused by anything horrible. The dogs were temporarily isolated from their people in an unfamiliar setting.) And the dogs used their left nostril to sniff human odors collected when the humans were feeling fearful. The researchers suggest that chemosignals communicate dog and human emotional cues "using different sensory pathways."

evolutionary story: "The fact that the oldest sensory system is tuned across these two species may suggest that the specific biochemical signature of chemosignals has remained a relatively invariable carrier of information that . . . remains a major medium of interspecies communication."

Maybe at some point dogs can help researchers find a better way of diagnosing, much as they're doing with cancer. In the meantime it's heartening to realize that dogs probably use their eyes, ears, *and* noses in their quest to figure out what's going on inside of us.

When dealing with cases of severe mental illness, it helps to use every tool at their disposal . . .

———

The voices started when Molly Wilson was six years old. At first they were quiet—a distracting breeze swirling around her head. They whispered or seemed far away, but she could usually make out what they were saying. They called her names. They said she was worthless. They didn't like her and they said no one else did either.

She tried to ignore them. She put her hands over her ears. But nothing would silence the voices. At home, in school, they were always there. She was ashamed of what they were telling her about herself, so she didn't mention them to anyone.

Over the years the voices grew louder, more invasive. She heard them as if they were coming through headphones she couldn't remove. There were usually three voices: a man, a woman, and a child. The man was the most intense and brutal. His voice was grating and full of hate. He usually yelled or screamed. The woman came and went. The child ridiculed her. Sometimes strange noises added to the cacophony.

The ugly chorus convinced her that her mother, father, sister, and brother lied to her when they told her they loved her. That her friends thought she was ridiculous. That they'd all be better off without her. They told her to hurt herself. They told her to kill herself.

At school she somehow managed to keep up her grades. She was well liked and had several close friends. At home Molly was anxious and angry. Her parents had her see a counselor for her anxiety, but she still didn't reveal anything about the voices. When she was about ten, she became panicky that someone was going to break into the house at night and kill her. She would lock her bedroom door and sleep with her light and TV on. She developed other phobias, like an extreme fear of needles—a common enough phobia, but she wasn't scared of the needles themselves; she was afraid she would be injected with something other than a vaccine or medicine. Something that would poison her.

Around sixth grade a man wearing a fedora and brown trench coat began following her. He seemed to have no face; it was always in shadow. He came back every day, sometimes joined by a roomful of others. They all seemed mentally ill and they scared her, but the man in the fedora was the one she dreaded the most. He carried a knife and threatened her. One day he stabbed her and she fell on the ground, writhing in pain and fear.

When she was fifteen, she broke down and told a friend about the voices and the man in the hat. The friend convinced her to tell her parents. On October 26, 2014, Molly wrote a two-page letter and left it on her mother's pillow. She told her about the nightmare she had been keeping secret for nearly a decade. She confessed that she had been cutting herself since she was eleven. She explained that cutting seemed to get rid of the voices, at least for a while. She had cuts on her thighs and hips, and a few on her arms, but she had stopped cutting her arms a while back because the scars were too obvious. She had worn longer sleeves even in warm weather so no one would see.

Molly's mother, Melanie, felt like she'd been punched in the gut. Not only was she heartbroken for Molly; she was also livid at herself for having no clue of her daughter's secret hell. She and her husband sought emergency help for Molly. Three days later, Molly began an eighteen-day stay at an acute-care psychiatric inpatient facility ninety minutes away, in Wilmington, North Carolina. She was diagnosed with bipolar disorder with unspecified psychosis. Her family visited her every day. They wanted to show her the voices were as wrong as could be.

On her first night back home, the man with the fedora blocked the door of her bedroom and she couldn't get out. When she finally escaped, she refused to go back into her room. She started sleeping on the couch right outside her parents' bedroom.

She didn't sleep alone. Guarding Molly was the young ninety-pound black Lab mix they'd recently adopted. They'd had three smaller dogs at the time, but Molly was smitten when she met Hank. He needed a home, so he joined the family.

Every night Molly slept on the couch, and Hank slept curled up in a tight ball at her feet. He worried and paced when she left the house and celebrated with dancing paws when she returned. She wouldn't go into her room to get clothes or supplies unless Hank was flanking her. She said she felt better with Hank there to protect her.

School wasn't going well. The man in the fedora was showing up and tapping his knife on a desk in her classrooms. It was distracting and terrifying. Her parents wished she could take Hank to school, but he was no service dog, just a pet.

Psychiatrists tinkered with her medications, but the man wouldn't leave. It got so bad that she asked to be readmitted to the hospital. This time, she stayed for fifteen days. Doctors diagnosed her with "schizoaffective disorder/severe depressive type"—a double whammy of schizophrenia and severe depression.

Her parents—desperate to help their girl—noticed that she didn't have hallucinations when she was around horses. The closest equine therapy program was three hours away from their home in Swansboro, North Carolina, so they got her a horse. Melanie had grown up with horses, and Molly had been taking riding lessons for years and had always wanted a horse. It was a financial stretch, but if a horse could help keep the bad guys away even for a while, it was worth the investment.

On May 1, 2015, Melanie left her schoolteaching job to be with

Molly and manage her care. They spent their days going to the barn and working with her horse, going to Molly's appointments, and hanging out.

On May 17, Melanie and Molly watched a couple of movies and had some laughs. Her brother needed a ride to baseball practice. Molly didn't want to go, so Melanie left her with her sister since Molly seemed in good spirits. When Melanie got home, she was fixing lunch and saw Molly walk downstairs and go into another room for a few minutes. Molly emerged, smiling, a few minutes later and walked back upstairs to her room.

Melanie finished preparing lunch and went up to Molly's room to let her know lunch was ready. Molly was resting. Melanie knew she hadn't slept the night before, so she quietly told her she could get her lunch when she woke up from her nap.

When Melanie got back downstairs, she saw she had missed three calls. They were from Molly's best friend. Then a text popped up: *"You need to check on Molly. She really needs you."*

Melanie wrote back: *"I just saw her and Molly's fine."*

The phone rang.

"Mrs. Wilson—I think Molly may have taken too much medicine."

She rushed to Molly's room. Ten minutes had passed since she took the medicine, if her friend was right.

"Molly!"

Molly's eyes were glassy.

"What did you take, Molly? Honey? What did you do?"

Molly slurred her words: "Please let me die. Please."

For the next awful few minutes the universe seemed to be answering Molly's wishes. In something that's usually reserved for nightmares, Melanie dialed 9-1-1 five times and the call wouldn't go through. She ran to her neighbor, who couldn't reach 9-1-1 either. Finally a call succeeded and the ambulance came. It had been more than a half hour, maybe forty minutes, since Molly had taken the medicine. They'd later learn that Molly had taken a large dose of Amitriptyline, which she used for her depression, and 400 mg—a half bottle—of Zyprexa, a drug for schizophrenia. Her normal dose was 10 mg.

Molly had a seizure in the ambulance, another in the emergency room. She was airlifted from the hospital to the nearest pediatric intensive care unit. She stayed for five harrowing days.

She would end up spending the next six months in a residential behavioral health center in Louisville, Tennessee. Melanie had looked all over the country for a facility that didn't feel like a hospital* or a juvenile detention center and had a doctor who specialized in schizophrenia. At Village Behavioral Health, the patients stayed in cabins and participated in healthy outdoor activities. It was the best setup for Molly, but it was eight hours from their home.

Melanie rented an apartment near Molly so she would never feel abandoned. She brought Molly's brother and Hank. The hallucinations weren't going to win.

The center allowed only short visits at first, so Melanie had plenty of time to try to come up with a plan for when Molly came home. Life had to be better for Molly—for everyone. The doctors would take care of her medications, and there would be counseling. But she was desperate for something else that could make life more manageable for her daughter.

"We will *never* give up on you," Melanie told her during a visit when Molly was feeling hopeless. "Everyone misses you, including Hank. We can't wait till you're home."

Hank! Why hadn't this occurred to her before? If he was her service dog, he could help her navigate the world when she came home.

---

*As far back as the 1800s, a "peculiar smell" has been reported to be associated with psychiatric hospitals, particularly with patients with schizophrenia. Since the 1960s there have been several attempts to find out if this scent exists and, if so, what causes it. Some researchers have found that people with types of schizophrenia have a chemical in their sweat that causes an unusual scent—a scent often undetectable by the person who has it, while others can smell it more easily. Other research points to different VOCs in the breath of people with schizophrenia. There's nothing conclusive yet, but if researchers can find biomarkers for certain types of schizophrenia, it could aid in early diagnosis.

Molly wanted to return to high school. Maybe Hank could give her the stability she needed. He'd already shown himself to be a loyal, steady friend. Melanie was sure he'd be a great service dog if she could just find someone who could help train him.

Then again, how could a dog help Molly with her hallucinations if her new medicines weren't working? How do you get a dog to stop your daughter from slashing the flesh of her arms? Would Hank be a match for the fedora man and all the people with no faces and all the hateful voices? He was just a dog. And maybe she was just a mom grasping at straws.

It was a cool spring day when Molly was finally reunited with her dog at the home of his trainer. Hank recognized Molly instantly. He ran up to her and jumped his paws onto her shoulders and wagged harder than ever. They hugged like this for a couple of minutes.

Hank had been gone for five months of intensive training with Comprehensive Pet Therapy in the Atlanta area. Melanie had shopped around for a long time with little luck. Either the organizations had no idea how to train a dog to help with Molly's level of illness, or they said they did but seemed more interested in money than outcome. Then she found out about longtime dog trainer Mark Spivak's organization. He and his small crew seemed to be able to train dogs to do almost anything. Mark had even helped teach dogs to patiently lie in an MRI for cutting-edge research at Emory University with neuroscientist Gregory Berns. Melanie thought if anyone could create a service dog to combat invisible monsters, Mark's group could.

When Molly and Hank took a break from their hugging, the woman who had been in charge of Hank's training buckled him into a service dog vest. He immediately became a different dog—serious, focused, all about being there for Molly. She and Melanie learned about the ways Hank was going to help her life. They went to a mall with the trainer to practice.

Once back home, Hank wasted no time getting to work. The family was stunned at what he could do.

Hank can tell when Molly starts to feel anxious. He'll walk up to Molly and lean into her legs. It grounds her and lets her know she's not alone.

If she starts to cut herself, Hank jumps on her legs. It's usually enough to stop her, to bring her back from wherever she is. It's like a jolt into reality, and it gives her a chance to realize she doesn't want to do this.

He can even lead her out of hallucinations. When she hallucinates, she often covers her eyes or hides her face. All Hank does is nudge her with his nose. Such a simple act, but it can be enough to rip her out of the clutches of the man in the fedora and his sinister friends.

Hank doesn't like Molly to be out of his sight. Sometimes, if her psychosis is bad, she'll shut her door on him and hide in her closet. Hank stays by her door. He won't leave. Melanie wishes she'd asked for Hank to be trained to fetch someone during the episodes, but now they just watch for him standing post and they know Molly needs help.

Then there's something unexpected. Something Molly figured out on her own. It has nothing to do with training. It's more a striking example of how dogs can become an extension of ourselves.

Hank is your typical Lab—a big, friendly, happy dog who wants to greet everyone. He has never met someone who isn't his pal. So if Molly sees or hears people and Hank doesn't acknowledge them, sometimes she realizes they probably aren't real. Their power diminishes. A young woman can stay in the world with her dog instead of the terrifying alternative.

By just hanging out calmly and being himself, Hank scares away the demons.

Hank can't stop all of Molly's troubles. Her illness is severe—too much for teams of doctors to resolve, much less a lone Labrador retriever—but he makes her life better.

Hank joined her on job interviews after she became a certified nursing assistant. There was only one problem: She never got a job offer when she brought him. But she wanted to work, so she left him home for one interview, just to see if Hank could be getting in the way of offers. She got the job.

The bosses at the rehabilitation and senior center where she works don't know about her disability. She's been doing well on clozapine, an antipsychotic used for schizophrenia. The drug usually banishes the man in the fedora. It quiets the voices, although they don't entirely go away.

She wishes she could tell her supervisors.* She's thinking about it. She wants to tell the world how much Hank has helped.

Molly hasn't cut herself since May of 2016. On her right thigh, disguising all of its scars, is a tattoo of a red-and-orange phoenix rising from the ashes.

---

*Yes, they will probably find out after this book comes out. I had my concerns about putting Molly's story out there with her real name if she wants to keep it hidden from her bosses, but Molly and her mother are OK with this, and they know the law is on Molly's side.

CHAPTER 9

AFTER THE WAR

Dogs on the Front Lines of PTSD

S teve Gagnon can never forget the faces of the dead. Or, in the worst cases, their bodies.

There was that time when IEDs blew three soldiers out of a Humvee. The bodies were flown from Iraq to Kuwait, to be processed by a Mortuary Affairs unit. Steve, a Marine staff sergeant, opened the first casket and unzipped the body bag. He reached into the bag with gloved hands and shoveled out as many ice cubes as he could. It always struck him as odd that they packed bodies in the kind of ice you put in your cocktails and sodas.

When enough ice was gone, he and a colleague lifted the body bag to a steel table. They gently coaxed the body out. The soldier had been badly burned in the explosion. In death, his hands were raised above his head, one higher than the other, palms forward. Steve realized the kid had died trying to crawl away from the inferno.

The other two soldiers came out of their body bags in similar desperate poses. The smell of burned flesh filled the small, hot room. In later years the smell of burned chicken would bring him right smack back to days like this.

Sometimes just a body part would arrive in a casket. There was the corpse that had been in the Euphrates for over a month. And then there was the time he had to count all 243 bone fragments that arrived in Ziploc bags within the body bag. Everything had to be accounted for.

While those who were killed in action had fought so tenaciously for their lives, some who came through his doors had taken their own lives—victims of undiagnosed depression, PTSD, spousal abandonment, lonely holidays.

Lives fought for and lost, lives not fought for and lost. In the end, they all came to him.

Nothing had prepared Steve for this job as logistics chief at this theater mortuary evacuation point. He had spent the majority of his career in logistics. It was pretty much a paperwork position. When he was told he'd be in logistics in Kuwait and Iraq for this deployment from fall of 2007 to spring 2008, he figured he'd be doing the usual business of tracking personnel and equipment in and out of country. Bodies were never mentioned. But Mortuary Affairs, a service within the US Army Quartermaster Corps, was understaffed at the time. They asked the Marines to pitch in, and Steve and his small logistics team got volunteered. He became logistics chief.

He thought that if he looked at his job as a logistics job, it wouldn't be so disturbing. It was another form of taking inventory—something he'd been doing for years. He looked at it as an honor to be able to get the deceased one step closer to their loved ones back home.

The dead often arrived with tourniquets, bandages, IVs, and other last-ditch medical equipment attached. The freshness of their deaths rattled him. But he tried to keep on task. He looked for ammunition, unexploded ordnance, and anything with sensitive or critical information. That meant going through pockets. Why did uniforms have to have so many pockets? He inventoried everything from personal protective equipment to personal effects: wedding rings, photographs, good-luck charms, rosaries, letters.

Of all the possessions, letters were the worst. Every time he searched a body, he prayed he wouldn't find a note. "If I don't make it . . ." they often began. He didn't want to read them. The idea that this person had felt threatened enough to write this letter, and that the letter would soon be in the hands of a devastated spouse, mother, father, or child, was too much. But reading everything was part of the security aspect of the job. He learned to scan, to look for possible unintentional security concerns while ignoring everything else—or at least trying to.

He wished he could have just scanned the faces rather than truly *looked*, but it was as if his mind took photographs of the faces. Even when he was relaxing away from the job, he'd close his eyes and see them.

He couldn't wait until he could go home and put it all behind him.

The images knew no international borders. They had worked their way deep into his memory and hitched a ride home with him after his deployment. Back in Wilmington, North Carolina, he couldn't sleep more than two or three hours a night. When he did sleep, he saw the carnage that had surrounded him for seven months. Sometimes an active shooter would storm into his dream and wake him up. It was a relief to be awake. He had no desire to go back to sleep.

A year passed. Two years. Three.

Steve was tired all the time. At home he was irritable. He fought with his wife and distanced himself from his children. His wife would tell the kids, "Be careful because you don't know Dad's mood when he wakes up." It made him feel terrible because he knew it was true, but it also made him angry.

He couldn't understand why he was always so angry. This wasn't like him. He'd tell his wife he wanted to stop feeling angry, to go back to the way it used to be. She tried to tell him it was the war that had changed him, that she thought he had post-traumatic stress disorder.

He was sure he didn't have PTSD. He hadn't gone through anything like what those poor souls on his steel tables had. He was just doing a job, far from the front lines. And besides, after his first deployment to Iraq in 2003, he was fine. His wife reminded him that he was doing regular logistics then, not performing inventory in hell.

It wasn't until 2011 that the VA diagnosed Steve with PTSD. He's among the 11 to 20 percent of Operation Enduring Freedom and Operation Iraqi Freedom veterans who have experienced PTSD. (The Vietnam War saw even more PTSD casualties—30 percent.)

Even though Steve realized he was far from alone in his diagnosis, he still didn't want to admit it. He'd been able to hide it until then—even from himself.

It took him two years to realize the diagnosis was right. He was writing a paper on PTSD for an English class, and as his fingers tapped the keyboard, it became clear that he was writing about himself. He went back to the VA and was put on some medications and started receiving counseling. It didn't work. He felt the counseling wasn't so hot, and the drugs were sucking the life out of him.

For a while he was taking eight prescriptions for his condition. "I'm being medicated to death," he'd complain. "I feel like a zombie."

One sleepless night (which could have been any night in his life at that point) he searched online for information on local organizations that provide psychiatric service dogs for veterans with PTSD. He didn't understand how a dog could help him. How could a dog know he was having nightmares or feeling anxious? It didn't make sense. But he couldn't go on like this anymore.

Three years later, Steve is having a nightmare. From the outside it doesn't look like much, just a little rustling and kicking, like someone getting more comfortable in his sleep. But somehow his dog, Siler, knows the difference. The golden retriever gets up from his dog bed and pops his front legs onto Steve's bed. The dog finds Steve's face and bumps him with his nose.

Steve doesn't wake up, so Siler bumps him a couple more times. He licks his face. Steve opens his eyes. He sees Siler's outline and realizes he is not in the mortuary room or on the road with the bombs. He is next to his wife, in his comfortable home, with his dog peering at him and wagging his tail. He rubs Siler's ears and lands back in reality. He tells him he's a good boy. When Steve seems more relaxed, Siler lies back down on his dog bed. Steve rests his hand on Siler's head and goes back to sleep.

Siler is trained to wake up if Steve is having a nightmare. The training was intensive and took months, with volunteers pretending to have nightmares—first while Siler was awake, and later while Siler had been asleep a few minutes, and finally when the dog had been asleep a couple of hours.

As Siler and Steve bonded, Siler learned that nose bumps aren't always enough to wake up Steve. Siler does not let his sleeping veteran lie. He's been known to get up on Steve's bed and lie on his side facing Steve. He'll push him hard with all four paws, shoving him until he awakens. No one trained him to do this. He just knows what he needs to do.

There are nights Steve doesn't even try to sleep in his own bed. On rough days, he knows he needs to be right next to Siler. The bed gets crowded with his wife and a seventy-pound dog, so he bunks on Siler's dog bed. With Siler next to him, he feels calmer and falls asleep more easily, despite being on a dog bed on the floor. If Steve still can't sleep, he'll go to another room to do some work or watch TV, and his canine shadow always follows.

Steve is down to two medicines. With Siler at his side, he doesn't need the others.

"This dog is my best medicine."

Siler goes to work with Steve most days. He sleeps under his desk. If he senses Steve is stressed or aggravated, he'll wake up and put his head on Steve's lap, or come out and lean against him. Something so simple, but it makes all the difference. Anger evaporates. A wounded veteran can breathe again.

There's no doubt that psychiatric service dogs for PTSD can help fix lives broken by the hell of war. Stories abound about how they

diminish the depression, anxiety, anger, negative moods, reckless behavior, sleep troubles, and disengagement that plague many veterans
with PTSD.

Until recently the success of these service dogs has been largely
anecdotal. That's usually good enough for anyone desperate enough
to seek out a service dog. But for years there's been a call for more
empirical evidence to see if specially trained dogs really do effect
measurable clinical changes in veterans—and, if so, to determine
how to best use the dogs.

Why is this data-driven evidence needed? In part because the
Department of Veterans Affairs has covered certain expenses for service dogs who help veterans with physical impairments be as independent as possible. If the VA pays for some of the mobility-assistance
dog expenses for vets with physical disabilities, the argument goes,
why not do so for veterans with mental health issues?

For that to happen, the VA wants proof—or something close to
it. This has inspired a number of studies.

A small study published in 2018 in the *Psychiatric Rehabilitation
Journal* found that PTSD service dogs reduced veterans' hypervigi-
lance, suicidal impulses, and medication use, and improved the quality and duration of sleep.

As of this writing, a large-scale National Institutes of Health
clinical trial has been going on for about one and a half of its three
years. A preliminary study by the Purdue University College of Veterinary Medicine, which is also leading the NIH-funded study,
showed promising results.

That study, published in 2018 in the *Journal of Consulting and
Clinical Psychology*, looked at 141 veterans with PTSD. Half were on
a waiting list to get a psychiatric service dog for their PTSD, and the
other half already had their service dog.

"We found that the group of veterans with service dogs had significantly lower levels of PTSD symptomology than those who did
not have a service dog," Purdue's Maggie O'Haire, PhD, who coauthored the study, said in a Purdue news release. "They also had lower

levels of depression, lower anxiety and increased social participation, meaning a willingness to leave their house and go engage with society in different activities."

The veterans with the psychiatric service dogs also had higher levels of life satisfaction and resilience, and less absenteeism from work due to health problems.

"The results of this study demonstrate not only the impact of this unbreakable bond, but that these service dogs are so much more than service dogs," wrote David Van Brunt, of Bayer Animal Health, which co-funded the research. "They are able to bring the joy of living back into veterans' lives."

One small step for dogs, one giant leap forward for the veterans they serve.

———

There are dozens of organizations around the United States that train dogs for veterans with PTSD. It's a big industry that's been growing for years. There are some top-notch organizations—large and small—that train great dogs and give their veterans the support they need. And there are some not-so-great organizations. They're often well-meaning, but the dogs and/or the veterans are sometimes not prepared when they're paired.

I learned that Steve's dog, Siler, had spent several months of his young life learning his impressive skills from inmates in prisons in West Virginia. Their crimes ranged from prescription forgery to robbery to murder. I reached out to Paws4People, the organization that brought Siler and Steve together. Danielle Cockerham, deputy executive director, told me that inmates, using positive training, taught Siler about 120 commands. They do this for all the dogs they train, regardless of what the dogs' future jobs will be.

Gus knows maybe twelve commands, and that's a record for any dog I've ever had. I wanted to meet these inmates who were training dogs with such big vocabularies. I asked Danielle if I could visit one of the prisons to see how the organization's Paws4Prisons program works. She said it would take time to secure a visit. The prisons were not as open to journalists as they had been, and there were a lot of hurdles.

Prisons have become common training grounds for training dogs since Sister Pauline Quinn, a Dominican nun, started the first inmate dog-training program in 1981.* As demand for service dogs increases, many organizations across the United States are launching their own prison programs in order to provide more dogs to more people more quickly. Everyone benefits, from the prisoners chosen for these programs to the budgets of the organizations to the people getting dogs who will change their lives.

Paws4People is based in Wilmington, North Carolina, but works with four prisons in West Virginia—a good ten-hour drive away. It's a haul, especially with dogs in tow. Why so far away? The organization launched in West Virginia years ago, when its founder was living there, and West Virginia's Department of Corrections has been supportive, so they've maintained the relationship. Cece McConnell, who oversees the Paws4Prisons program, makes the drive about every six weeks, checking on the prisoners, picking up their homework, sometimes bringing dogs back or forth and matching recipients with dogs.

A few weeks after making my request to check out the prison training program in person, I got a voicemail from Danielle.

"How would you like to go see some of the prisons with Cece? You can spend a couple of days up in West Virginia prisons and drive back with her and a bunch of dogs in a van through the Appalachians.

"It's a long drive, but it'll be an adventure."

Just my kind of business trip.

---

*There's even a Hallmark TV drama chronicling Sister Pauline's prison program. If you look for it online, don't confuse *Within These Walls*—the 2001 movie starring Laura Dern as the nun—with the 2015 horror movie by the same name. Or the 1970s TV series. Or the 1945 drama. They all have something of a prison theme, but only one has dogs and Ellen Burstyn as a tough prisoner whose own walls come down as she works with dogs. Yeah, that sounds pretty Hallmark-y, but it's not bad for a TV movie.

· · ·

The road Cece and I take from our hotel to the first prison we'll visit follows the muddy Ohio River through deep-green land studded with mobile homes past their prime. Signs encouraging the acceptance of God and Jesus—"Every Knee Shall Bow" and "Jesus is your Lord and Savior"—are nailed to trees and leaning against rusty cars that won't be going anywhere until they're hauled off or dismantled. A skinny beige dog ambles along the railroad tracks with a scruffy salt-and-pepper companion. An occasional smokestack puffs into the gray sky.

Our van weaves through this land of stark contrasts. Rich natural landscapes like this back in California would be home to multimillion-dollar houses and restaurants with one-word names. Instead, West Virginia's beauty bears witness to high rates of unemployment, poverty, and drug abuse.

The inmates we'll spend the day visiting* are often the collateral damage of this dilapidated economy: The coal miner who lost his job and got in fight after fight until one day he didn't know when to stop. The man who was protecting his twelve-year-old brother from bullies when he was nineteen and went too far. Hardscrabble childhoods leading to dead-end roads where opioids and meth and booze seem like the only way out.

Paws4Prisons is a coveted program among inmates. The only ones who won't be considered are those who have committed crimes against children, animals, or the elderly. It helps to have a decent prison record, but it doesn't have to be perfect. Cece says if someone seems like they'd be a good fit, she does what she can to make room.

Paws4Prisons is a six-month-long academic program. In addition to training the dogs using positive reinforcement, participants attend

---

*Unfortunately, we found out the night before our visit to the prisons that I wouldn't be allowed to interview any inmates, use real names, or take notes. Corrections department representatives said they wanted to protect victims of crimes from having to read about the perpetrators. We couldn't get them to budge, even with the promise to change names. I would have to leave my notebooks, recorder, and camera in the van.

classes, take tests, and write essays. It's not all about dogs either. Essays are several pages long and designed to help the inmates gain insight into their lives. Topics include "Addiction—why do you think you have it?" And "There's someone in your life you have to apologize to. Please write about this."

"The program helps the inmates to connect to the outside world. They are doing something bigger than themselves," Cece says. "Most of them have never done anything for someone else—least of all someone they don't know. The program enables them to help someone, and in return they learn to love, heal, and most of them reconnect to their families and children and show them that they aren't terrible people; they are people who made a terrible mistake or terrible decision. They learn humility, integrity, discipline, gratitude, respect, and more. They learn to love and be loved. They learn they are worthy of love."

My eyes get wet. I try not to blink until the tears evaporate. (Cece doesn't know me yet. I don't want her to think I'm not a pro.)

She tells me that despite the rigors, once the prisoners are in the program, most never want to leave. They say it's the first time they've felt a purpose in their lives. They know they've taken something from society and feel that by helping the dogs get ready to assist people with difficulties, they can help give something back. And having a dog by them nearly 24/7 is therapeutic—lessening the loneliness and isolation and providing a built-in best friend. Cece explains the bond:

"The dog doesn't judge them for what they did or who they are or where they came from or how much money they have. A dog doesn't know how to do these things. If they love a dog, feed him, take care of him, don't abuse him, a dog will give them love they may have never had."

Cece knows firsthand what it means to train a dog as an inmate: In 2007 she was sentenced to two years in federal prison in Bruceton Mills, West Virginia, for construction contract fraud. She saw the papers going through, and she signed them even though she had suspicions they weren't legitimate. In the eyes of the law, she was part of the fraud. She had to leave her two children behind.

Some inmates find God in prison; Cece found dogs. (She had already found God.) Paws4People had just rolled out its prison program. Paws4Prisons had been in Cece's prison for six months before she arrived. Three days into serving her sentence, she became part of the program. She quickly rose to the top and became a valued trainer. When she was released, the organization didn't want to let her go. She could identify with the prisoners and knew how to work with them. She became a volunteer two weeks after her prison term ended. She volunteered until 2013, when there was funding to hire her.

Our first stop this day is at Lakin Correctional Center, a women's prison that houses custody levels from minimum to maximum. Cece meets with the forty-two khaki-clad women in the program for a couple of hours and updates them on how some of their dogs are doing in the outside world.

A few women wipe away happy tears when they hear about the successes of the dogs they'd worked so hard to train. The dogs don't stay with the same prisoners the whole time, but the trainers still get attached. At the end of the meeting, Cece announces the names of the dogs who will be moving to the men's prison for their next round of training. Some of the women just nod, understanding it's part of the process to let go. A couple of others get emotional. They hug their dogs, say good-bye, and file out to lunch.

As Cece, two prison employees, and I walk out with several leashed dogs, we pass the chow hall line. One of the inmates from the program is weeping so hard that her body shudders as she watches a dog she came to love walk out of prison and out of her life forever.

The dogs won't be free for long. Ninety minutes after we leave Lakin, we arrive at St. Mary's Correctional Center, a medium-security men's prison. The dogs, seemingly unfazed by the change of venue and the fact that they're back in the slammer, wag through security, and are soon distributed among the excited trainers who have been waiting for them in the prison yard.

"Good dawg!" "You're going to like it at St. Mary's!" The head rubs and hearty greetings seem to make the dogs feel welcome as they jog off to their new quarters with their new trainers.

A half hour later, the fifty men in the St. Mary's dog program assemble in the prison's gymnasium and take their seats. Four of the inmates have dogs with them. One after the other, the men with the dogs walk up to a podium and address a Marine veteran who has flown in from North Carolina to be matched with his future psychiatric service dog, who will help him cope with PTSD. They tell their stories eloquently and compellingly. One man with thick-rimmed black glasses reminiscent of a 1960s NASA scientist bats tears back when talking about his children, and how the dogs have helped make him a better father, even from behind bars.

The Marine veteran sits riveted as he listens. When it's his turn, he tells his story of how the hell of war damaged him. On the outside he's a strapping Marine, the kind you see on recruitment posters. But just below the surface, he says, he's angry and anxious and on edge almost all the time. He's here with his mother, who hopes that adding a dog to his therapy and meds will help save him.

Now it's the dogs' turn. Working with their trainers, they show off some of their skills. A golden retriever opens a refrigerator, takes out a bottle of water, and closes the fridge. A couple of dogs show how they calm and ground someone who appears anxious. A Lab alerts to someone approaching from behind. A golden-Lab mix shows how he can summon help for someone who has passed out, and how he can help him stand back up, using his own body to aid the man's balance.

After the demos, it's time for the dogs to meet the veteran. Cece has narrowed the candidates to these four, but now it's up to the dogs. There's a kind of chemistry that she's looking for. "We've had dogs who won't go near someone I thought they'd do well with. They have this demeanor like they're giving them the middle finger almost," she says. "Then there are the dogs who walk up and almost seem to say, *This is my guy.*"

The prison version of speed dating commences. One handler at a time walks toward the veteran's chair and lets go of the leash. A chocolate Labrador retriever who moves with the lithe enthusiasm of a cartoon character becomes even more animated near the veteran. To me, it looks like love, but Cece says it's too much energy. This vet needs a calm, reassuring dog. One dog approaches him hesitantly and seems to want to leave. A Lab appears to like him well enough, sitting next to him and letting the Marine pet him. Last up is Blu, an eighteen-month-old golden retriever.

Cece had noticed that Blu "was all eyes" on the veteran during the demo. She has a good feeling about this dog. And sure enough, when it's Blu's turn to meet him, he walks right up to him, turns around, and sits between his feet—a classic "anchor" position that trained dogs take when they sense their person is anxious. The veteran strokes Blu's fur and talks to him. He looks more relaxed with Blu than he had been with the other dogs.

At the end of the session, Cece announces that Blu is the match, and that he'll be one of the dogs going back to Wilmington with us the next day. The veteran's mom breaks out in a wide smile, clasping her hands together under her chin. "I liked him best all along," she tells me quietly. Her son wouldn't be getting Blu for a while, though. In Wilmington the dog will be receiving another few months of training with a student from the University of North Carolina Wilmington Service Dog Training Program.

Before he leaves, the vet tells the inmate who's with Blu that he's grateful for everything he's done.

"Happy to pay it forward," the inmate responds. "I think you're going to really like this guy."

Blu is one of the first to jump into the van the next morning at 7:55 when we load it with twelve dogs who will be going on the journey back to North Carolina. Most of the dogs did the first leg of this round-trip van ride six to ten months earlier when they were sixteen to eighteen weeks old. They left North Carolina as preschoolers, and thanks to the prison program, they were going back with the canine equivalent of college degrees.

All but two of the dogs who aren't that keen on each other get to choose their spots on the rubber-coated van floor. The other two will ride in kennels. As we drive south, the van is remarkably quiet. Cece hopes to keep it that way. It's a ten-hour ride. She doesn't stop for the dogs to stretch their legs or go to the bathroom because it would add too much time to the already long trip, and it could be dangerous, with dogs potentially escaping as she lets others out.

She has taken dogs back and forth dozens of times ("way too many to count") and has it down to something of a science. The dogs don't get food after 5 p.m. the day before a trip. At 9 p.m. they get a little water, and are taken out to relieve themselves every two hours. By the time she picks them up in the morning, they should be fairly empty. Since they mostly just lie down and sleep for the ride, she says ten hours isn't that bad. It's rare that anyone has an accident in the back of the van.

My own bladder has not been prepped like this, and I'm hoping Cece won't mind making a stop or two along the way.

Our passengers today will soon be embarking on a variety of career trajectories, and consist of Labs of various colors, golden retrievers, and some Lab-golden mixes. As we head south, I assemble the manifest:

Blu—Matched with the veteran with PTSD
Helo—Not yet determined, but he'll be working in a health care or educational setting
Hopkins—Emotional support dog
Kennedy—Dental dog offering comfort to nervous dental patients in a rehabilitation facility
Lansing—Emotional support dog
Layton—Not yet matched
Lochlynn—Helping patients in a psychiatric facility

Noah—Emotional support dog; "he wasn't cut out for
   service dog work"
Rhode—Psychiatric/medical alert dog for a veteran
Shire—Not yet matched
Trent—Civilian psychiatric/medical alert dog
Vivian—Paws4People ambassador and demo giver

At 9:25 a.m. Lochlynn, a golden retriever, manages to get her front
half over the barrier of kennels and supply boxes Cece has set up
between our seats and the back of the van. The dog is perched on
Cece's left shoulder and is smiling as she watches the scenery through
the windshield. (Goldens almost always look like they're smiling.)

I realize how exciting it must be for this freshly sprung dog. I am
sure that in the back of the van, where I can't see, Lochlynn's tail is
wagging and whacking another dog in the face.

"Ugh, this never happens!" Cece says.

Cece tells her to go "back, back, back," but the dog won't budge.
Instead, she rests her head on Cece's shoulder. From my vantage
point, it looks like she's either giving Cece driving tips or trying to
strike a deal: *Let me stay here and I'll be the best service dog ever.*

At 9:38 a.m. Cece pulls into a Marathon gas station, gets out, and
gently pushes Lochlynn back. She adds some towels and blankets to
the top of the blockade to prevent more visits. I hop out and stretch
my legs, and when I climb back in, it smells *really* doggy. It didn't
smell like that before. Clearly I have already gone nose-blind. It
dawns on me that my luggage, in the back with the dogs and secured
in a kennel above leg-lift range, is probably sponging up the odor and
will be an olfactory souvenir of our trip.

We continue our drive down Interstate 77. Blu's head pops up over
the barrier, but Cece tells him, "HEY!" and he disappears. The rain
starts as the green hills turn to mountains. We're in the Appalachians now. Our air conditioner is going full blast to keep the dogs
cool on this muggy mid-May morning.

It gets cold fast. I pull the hood of my sweatshirt over my head to try to keep warm. As soon as I do this, a magical scarf appears around my neck. The scarf is a living, breathing dog, complete with dog breath. I look at his collar and see this is Helo. He has somehow squished his way past the barrier on my side, and his paws are draped over my shoulders. A true helicopter dog. I wonder if somehow he knows I'm cold. But he's not my miracle muffler for long. After a couple of minutes, Cece notices him and gives him a look. My scarf slinks to the back of the van.

It's quiet now except for the rain dancing on the roof of the van and the country music playing quietly on the radio. I tell Cece I don't know how she does this drive so often, alone, with so many dogs, on these winding roads perched so high up that looking down in certain spots can give you vertigo.

"I love this job and I'm driven to do it. I've got a personal reason, too."

She tells me the story of her big brother, John Champion, as we loop through the Appalachians.

First Sergeant John Champion served in the Army from 1985 to 2007. He started as a medic and worked his way into the 82nd Airborne Division, the elite infantry division specializing in parachute assault. He spent a decade with the 82nd Airborne, and eleven years as a Special Forces operator. During his career he served several combat tours, including two to Iraq and two to Afghanistan. He received a Silver Star and a Bronze Star and a long list of other honors for his courage and valor.

But for the last years of his service, it was clear to family that something was amiss. He had fought many battles overseas, but now he seemed to be fighting them in his head. There were the outbursts of anger, the screams only he heard. Usually they were the screams of children.

During his most recent deployments, boys as young as ten or eleven would come at soldiers with submachine guns or throw IEDs in their path. John didn't want to kill them. He wanted to put them on planes back to the United States and show them a good life, show them he wanted to help them, not hurt them. But sometimes there was no choice. Like the time a boy held an Uzi to his friend's head. The interpreter couldn't talk him down. The kid was about to blow his friend's life away.

Later the friend would tell Cece, "I was going to be dead any second. John did what he had to do. He saved my life."

The ghosts of the dead children stayed with John. He sought help, but there was too much red tape, and help came in the form of pills he didn't want to take. He felt that deadening the pain or sleeping wasn't the solution.

After he retired from the Army, he took a government contract job in Rwanda for two years. When the contract ended, he came back to the United States and shifted gears. He got a job as manager of a restaurant in Beaufort, North Carolina, once voted "America's Coolest Small Town." He became a member of a nearby Veterans of Foreign Wars (VFW) post and was so popular he quickly rose to post commander.

On July 6, 2009, John packed his Jeep with fishing equipment. He had everything but bait. He stopped at a local store and bought two lottery tickets, but they weren't winners. He went to Burger King.

The next morning someone at the VFW was looking for photocopy paper, which was kept in John's office. He knocked. No one answered, so he entered.

He found John there, dead from a self-inflicted gunshot wound to his head.

Cece got the news in prison. Her sentence was almost complete. She still feels remorse that she couldn't help him because she was behind bars. John had always been there for her. He was six years older and a great protector for Cece, who was born into turmoil after her father beat her mother so badly she went into early labor.

"You're the best of us, kid," John would frequently tell Cece. She can still hear him saying this. She wants to live up to his belief in her.

The road is white with rain. It's raining so hard now that we have to almost shout to hear each other. After the story of her brother, it's not the time for high-volume talking, so we fall silent for a while. I absorb the tragic story. Cece wipes away tears. The dogs don't say a word.

As we approach Raleigh, the rain lets up. As if to make up for the silence, two dogs begin barking, sharp staccato barks. Maybe they know we're nearing the end of the trip. Or maybe they just want to eat and find a nice patch of grass or a fire hydrant.

Cece stops at a gas station to fuel up for the last leg. When we hit the road again, more dogs join the bark chorus. The sleeping dogs no longer lie.

We decide to see if music might calm the dogs. We try different artists from her iPod music library. Waylon Jennings only sets the dogs to barking more. But a catchy Blake Shelton version of a song called "Ol' Red" seems to grab their attention. They fall silent. The song is about a prisoner who escapes thanks to distracting a tracking dog named Red with a female bluetick hound.

Cece tells me one of the inmates we met at St. Mary's recently trained a red dog. He'd sing this song with a big smile, even around the guards. I thought the song would pump up the dogs, but they quiet down and stay chill through the song. Maybe the tune is familiar to some of them.

The effect doesn't last, though. Once it ends, one dog barks, and then another.

"We're almost there! The home stretch! Just a few more lights!" Cece calls to them.

She selects a slow gospel song from Shekinah Glory Ministry. The dogs quiet down. The rain starts again. We pass a sign. "Welcome to the City of Wilmington, North Carolina!"

In a half hour, the dogs have been handed to their assigned student trainers, who run them out to a grassy area next to the van.

When the dogs are done with their constitutionals, one by one they trot away with their new trainers, ready to move on to the next stage of becoming someone's hero.

———

The next morning I met with Army veteran Wil Nobles and his chocolate Lab, Harnett. The dog had taken the long journey from the prisons about eighteen months earlier. Wil and I sat on rocking chairs on a covered porch in a semi-rural area of Wilmington during a rainstorm.

Every so often a puff of wind brought tiny dusty white flowers through the boards of the porch's roof. No rain came through, but the flowers descended on us like so many miniature snowflakes. Harnett ended up with an ivory pattern on his fur as he lay at Wil's feet.

Wil talked about his two deployments. His first was in 2005, when he was a fuel-supply specialist for aircraft. He worked on refueling and rearming helicopters in Camp Taji and Forward Operating Base Kalsu, both near Baghdad. The birds—Black Hawks, Apaches, Chinooks—would still be running as he and his crew swiftly performed their tasks. It was exciting, fast-paced, and relatively safe.

They took some mortar rounds. And one of the Apache crews he'd worked with got shot down. Both pilots were killed. That got to him, but he thought he processed it pretty well.

He came home and felt he was doing OK. His wife said he was more tense. He decided not to continue in active duty and joined the National Guard instead. During his second year in the National Guard, he got the news he was deploying.

"Just what I didn't want," he said.

This time he was in Mahmudiyah, south of Baghdad, working logistics. It was quieter than the first deployment. But there was this one incident where they lost three guys. The soldiers were in a convoy in a Humvee, and an IED exploded in the road. Wil was responsible for getting the response team to them, but the soldiers had burned to death, and there was nothing the team could do.*

He knew two of the soldiers. When the vehicle came back, he had to deal with it as part of his logistics job.

"The smell—the burned flesh—I'll never get it out of my head."

As he told the story, he twisted Harnett's leash in his hand. Harnett looked at him, stood up, and put his head in Wil's lap.

Wil stopped twisting the leash and stroked Harnett's head. He became visibly more relaxed as he continued his story.

When he came back from that deployment, he felt his life slipping out of control. "I kind of knew I wasn't the same," he said.

"I was tearing my family apart. I'd get angry at my wife easily. I was having multiple affairs. I didn't care about life too much. I had terrible anxiety. I didn't like crowds. I got nervous in public places. You name it."

He took some online surveys and realized he probably had PTSD. He went to the VA and ended up taking what he calls "VA candy" for years.

Wil was helping his in-laws with their business, but with all the medications, he barely felt functional. He was flat, zombied out.

"The meds made me feel like I wasn't me. I was on antidepressants, antianxiety meds, all kinds of things, five or six pills all the time," he said. "The side effects were awful, and when they realized something wasn't working, they'd give you another and see how it worked.

"There's a reason they call it *practicing* medicine. It was really sad. You're like a guinea pig."

He decided to quit, cold turkey. The withdrawals were awful. He felt like he had the flu. His stomach hurt. His body hurt. He doesn't

---

*If you read Steve Gagnon's story earlier in this chapter and noticed that these Humvee incidents bear remarkable similarities, you're not alone. I've often wondered if, by some freakish coincidence, the soldiers Wil knew were the same ones whose bodies still haunt Steve. It's not something I brought up during the interviews.

recommend others do it this way. But after it passed, he was glad he'd quit.

"I felt better just because I was *me*," he said. "The people around me didn't think I was better, though, because I was *me*."

All his anger issues came back. So did the anxiety, the night-mares, the panic attacks, the depression. But he was just relieved to be off the meds, happy to be able to feel anything.

His wife told him that if he wasn't going to take the medication, he had to do something to improve. He said the VA offered therapy only once every couple of months. And it wasn't cutting it.

Wil didn't know what to do. He looked into going for in-house therapy at a VA in Asheville, but he would have missed Thanksgiving and Christmas. One day he attended a local event for veterans and ran into a man who was there with his psychiatric service dog. The veteran saw how Wil always tapped his foot nervously when he was sitting. He could spot an anxious veteran.

"I think a service dog would probably be pretty good for you," the man told him. "It'll help you with that leg and a lot of other things that probably go with it."

Wil talked it over with his wife, and they decided to give it a try. He met someone in his church who had a service dog through Paws4People and applied for the program. His application moved along quickly, and a few months later, he was introduced to Harnett at St. Mary's. Wil liked Harnett from the start, but it was a matter of how much Harnett liked him.

Harnett acted like he'd known Wil a long time. They just fit.

They'd been together about a year when we met. He said that between Harnett and regular counseling he's getting now (a stipulation of the program is that veterans have to be getting some kind of counseling), his life has become infinitely better. So has his family's.

"Having Harnett is the biggest thing every day. I can't even de-scribe it," he said. Harnett keeps Wil calm in public; if Wil senses his anxiety levels rising, Harnett is just a command away from being able to help him. Often Harnett does it on his own. He'll "anchor" while standing in line or "visit" while Wil is sitting, as he did when he put his head in Wil's lap.

But of all the commands Wil uses with Harnett, "cuddle" is his favorite. "It's the best. Sometimes that's all I need, to feel his weight and his warmth right next to me.

"My wife loves him, but I think she feels like he's a second spouse," he said and laughed. "I'm more affectionate now in general, more in tune with my emotions, so she really appreciates that. I've hardly had any angry outbursts since Harnett. He's brought out the real me. Medicine only hid it."

Wil has a tattoo on the inside of his left arm. It's a long arrow with the word "warrior."

I asked him about it.

For years he didn't feel like a warrior, he said. "Really, I felt like the opposite of a warrior, whatever that is. Powerless and helpless."

Then along came a dog who'd done time in prison.

———

It's easy to think about PTSD only in relation to veterans who have seen combat. But that's just part of the story.

More than twice as many women as men are affected by PTSD. The US Department of Veterans Affairs, which keeps track of the latest studies on PTSD, reports that about 10 percent of women and 4 percent of men will develop PTSD during their lifetime. The VA PTSD website states that one-third of women will experience sexual assault or childhood sexual abuse, making these the most common traumas for women—traumas that can lead to PTSD.*

One balmy spring day, I was in Southern California to see how Little Angels Service Dogs trained seizure-alert dogs. As I was

---

*The VA reports a particularly disturbing statistic for women in the armed forces: Twenty-three percent of women who use VA services have been sexually assaulted while in the military. Many women veterans who get a dog for PTSD do so at least in part because of sexual assault. And women aren't the only ones being sexually assaulted. Recent statistics compiled by the Defense Department show that for every four women who report sexual assault, one man does.

watching Dexter gleefully perform his tasks, I noticed a young English cream retriever lying on the sidelines. She seemed to be hanging out with Judy, one of the trainers. (You met Judy and Dexter in Chapter 2.) In between Dexter's romps with the life-alert button and the medicine pouch, I asked Judy about this other pup.

"This is Oprah," she said. "I love telling people I hang out with Oprah all day. They always do a double take."

But this wasn't the time or place to go into who Oprah was and why she was with Judy. Their story would unfold over the coming months.

The abuse started when Judy was five years old. She somehow found herself alone with her abuser. After that, it happened every few summers. She dreaded going on vacation, but she couldn't tell her parents. Her abuser—and, eventually, abusers—said that terrible things would happen to her and to anyone she told.

So she stuffed her anger and fear and disgust and guilt and pain away as best as she could. After several years, summer vacations changed, and she thought it was behind her.

She had a pretty good run of it for a few years, but then, in college at the University of San Diego, something else happened. Different person, same results. She was old enough now that she felt she should have more control, so the guilt overwhelmed her. And the depression took over. She got some counseling, but she wouldn't part with her secrets. She was diagnosed with attention deficit disorder.

Comedy was the only therapy that worked. She took to the stage as a stand-up comic at school and was a hit. She became known as the Catholic Comedian and performed her faith-based routines to packed audiences. On the stage, the rest of her world went out of focus, and the burden of her past disappeared.

After college she toured full-time, bringing laughter to military bases, conferences, churches, top comedy clubs, and TV. Her unique brand of humor landed her a spot on *The Dennis Miller Show*. She opened for comic legends Paula Poundstone, Margaret Cho, and Mark Curry. Life should have been good.

But behind the scenes, she was barely functional. She couldn't shake the mysterious depression. And there were the flashbacks. She wanted some way to get rid of the part of her that she hated. Death seemed like the only way to shed it all.

She couldn't deliberately kill herself, though; suicide was off the table because she's devoutly Catholic. But she realized there were other escape doors—ones that might not feel so overtly suicidal. She was hardly sleeping, and she wasn't really eating. Maybe one Power-Bar all day. And she was running several miles daily. She knew she was running from something and, at the same time, hoped she was running toward the final finish line.

"I really thought I'd run to death," she says.

If she wasn't running, she was most likely in bed. She went through periods where she didn't want to wake up, or go out, or see anyone. She managed to rally herself for her shows and usually pulled herself together for church. Otherwise she was running or hiding.

In 2012, she didn't have the strength to hold back the secret of her years of sexual abuse any longer. She finally told her story to a therapist. The therapist diagnosed her with PTSD. A psychiatrist later confirmed the diagnosis. Judy didn't understand.

"I thought it was something guys from the Vietnam War got, not women in Southern California," she says. "How could I have PTSD?"

While she was coming to terms with her diagnosis, she ran across an article on psychiatric service dogs for veterans with PTSD. She thought if they could help men and women coming back from war, they might be able to help her. Something inside her told her she had to pursue this—that it might be her last chance.

But finding an organization that provided PTSD service dogs to people who'd never gone to war wasn't easy. Every call she made ended with a little less hope. Everything was riding on this. She couldn't give up.

"In my mind, it was either a dog or death," she says.

A winding path led to a small organization only about an hour east of her home. The owner of Little Angels Service Dogs took Judy's need for a dog seriously. After all, Judy had the same symptoms as war veterans—flashbacks, nightmares, anxiety, depression—and unlike soldiers on battlefields, she had to face her enemy alone. "We've got to do something for you," she told Judy.

Daisy is a yellow Lab with light brown eyes Judy describes as "looking right past all the BS other people see and getting straight to the heart." When she was Judy's service dog, she was part therapist, part best friend, and you could even say part pharmaceutical. She did what nothing and no one else has been able to during Judy's long fight with PTSD.

Daisy gently brought Judy out of flashbacks and nightmares and calmed her, often by applying the canine version of deep-pressure therapy: She'd lie on Judy with all or most of her weight. If Judy was sitting, she'd get on her lap and snuggle tight, or stand with her back paws on the ground and her front half curled around her in something like a hug.

When Daisy sensed Judy's anxiety rising, she'd bump her with her nose. (Originally Daisy's signal for anxiety was alerting with her paw. But she was too enthusiastic. "I looked like a mixed martial artist who sucked at being a mixed martial artist," Judy says. So they switched the alert to the nose nudge.)

If possible, Judy would sit, and Daisy would work her magic. Judy hugged her and put her head down on her. Her tension dissipated. The deep pressure helped Judy remain in the present and reminded her she was not alone.

"It was like Valium," she says. "Actually, better than Valium."

Daisy also had her back while she stood in lines, offering a buffer between Judy and others. And on rougher days, she helped her get out of bed. Some of this was Daisy simply being driven by her stomach. When she was hungry for breakfast, she nuzzled Judy until she woke up. Then she covered her face with kisses. If that didn't work, she'd stand over her and bark until she moved.

"I love her more than anything or anyone, and being able to focus on her needs and off of mine helped me get up and get going to tackle the day with her," Judy says.

Daisy also had another job: She was Judy's mobility-assistance dog. She helped stabilize and brace Judy when she was feeling beat up from her bum back: Judy had spinal fusion of a few vertebrae, and while she maintained an active lifestyle, sometimes she needed a little extra help.

"God knew he didn't have to send me a person, a therapist, or a drug. He knew what I could handle and sent me a dog," she says.

When Judy first brought Daisy home after their initial training weeks, she could sense life beginning to shift in her favor. "I hadn't felt this normal and safe for a long, long, long, long, long time," she says.

Psychiatric service dogs need frequent feedback from their people to let them know if they're helping and how they're doing. It's not like they have a single concrete scent to work with, as medical alert dogs do. Continually working with Daisy to be in tune with her mental state helped Judy to check in with herself—something she had never done before.

"I had this seventy-five-pound psychologist checking in with me all the time, so I had to be aware of things I used to try to bury," she says. "She enabled me to talk about this horrible stuff that a few years ago I'd rather have taken a bullet than admit it.

"Daisy saved my life."

But even the most dedicated heroes have their limits.

It was the kind of perfect mid-September San Diego day that calls surfers to the Pacific. The water temperature was comfortable, and the waves were a few feet and glassy, just right for an easy ride.

Judy was driving her Ford Escape to pick up a longboard at her parents' house and meet some friends at the beach. She had undergone the back surgery a year earlier, and thanks to regular physical therapy, and mobility help from Daisy, she was doing well and happy to be able to surf again.

Daisy loves the beach as much as any other red-blooded Labrador retriever. She was hooked into her harness in the back seat and enjoying the breeze that made her ears flap like small velvet wings. It was going to be a fun day for both of them.

Judy came to a stop behind a truck at a traffic signal. When the light turned green, she slowly accelerated, and there was the oddest sensation. Her SUV sped off out of control at an angle to the right. She realized it was nothing she was doing. *Oh my God, I think we're in a car accident.* A small truck going thirty to forty miles per hour had smashed into them.

Even though Daisy was buckled in a harness, she flew into the front seat. They were about to crash down a steep embankment when Judy pulled to the left.

Everything stopped.

Judy managed to call 9-1-1. Soon a fire engine, ambulance, and sheriff arrived. Judy felt a sharp pain in her back and neck. EMTs wanted to transfer her to the ambulance.

"I'm not going unless my service dog can ride with me," she told them.

"Of course she can, that's not a problem."

They carefully moved Judy onto a gurney. As soon as she was loaded into the ambulance, a firefighter brought Daisy over. Judy and Daisy rode together to the emergency room. Daisy seemed shaken and pressed close to Judy. Once at the hospital's ambulance entrance, Daisy flanked the gurney as they wheeled Judy in. Staff warmly greeted Daisy first, then Judy.

Physically, Judy and Daisy were lucky. Nothing was broken, and no damage had been done to the hardware in Judy's back from her spinal fusion. But soft-tissue damage led to new nerve pain in her neck and back. She had to start physical therapy from scratch.

Daisy would never be the same dog. Even though she hadn't been seriously hurt physically, something inside her—something that can't be detected by X-rays or MRIs—had broken.

On walks, noises she had never reacted to before would make her jump. Daisy could no longer join Judy on the stage during her comedy acts. Before, she had slept during Judy's stand-up routine (this always provided Judy with self-deprecating material). After the accident, Daisy would shake uncontrollably. Judy gave up on bringing her to the stage.

At home Daisy sought refuge in the bathtub. Judy could tell when Daisy was in the tub when she saw the shower curtain trembling.

She took Daisy to veterinarians and behaviorists. They diagnosed her with PTSD and did what they could. But nothing—not any combination of medicines, not prescribed rest, not any of the suggestions offered by behaviorists—made much difference.

For a while, the beach seemed to be the only place where Daisy's anxiety decreased. But then she started barking at seaweed and surfers.

"She went from being my energetic rock to being a bowl of Jell-O," says Judy. "My poor service dog needs her own service dog."

Instead of alerting to Judy's anxiety, Daisy seemed to be alerting to her own anxiety. Roles reversed. Judy found herself helping Daisy as Daisy had once helped her. She woke Daisy from nightmares, calmed her with deep pressure, and tried to be her rock. She didn't want to give up on her.

But every time she brought Daisy out as her service dog, she felt like she was bringing a shadow to Little Angels, where she had started working as a trainer after going through an extensive program there.

"She was a broken wheelchair," she says.

One day she looked at her shaking dog wearing a service dog vest, and she knew what she had to do. She needed to get another service dog and retire Daisy. The idea of finding a new service dog, training her, and seeing if it was a good match was overwhelming. The idea of leaving Daisy at home or with her parents while she went out in the world with the new dog was worse.

"I'd take a bullet for Daisy," she says. "I felt like I was abandoning her. How would she handle it? How would I handle it?"

She didn't have to worry. Daisy now spends her days relaxing with Judy's retired parents in their Southern California home. She enjoys occasional dips in their pool and adores Judy's parents, especially her mother. She follows her around the house and gets rewarded with plenty of treats just for being Daisy.

Judy visits nearly every day, and often joins her in the pool. Sometimes they go to the beach. Daisy seems more like her old self, but sometimes there's a sharp noise and she's back to trembling. When Judy's parents use their fireplace, something about the little crackles and pops gets to her, and she seeks refuge in or next to their bathtub.

But for the most part Daisy's retirement is going much better than Judy thought it would. At least it is for Daisy. Judy misses her terribly, but she's relieved that she's happy.

Daisy has found a new calling. She's teaching Oprah, Judy's service dog in training. She keeps her in line when she gets too hyper and mentors Oprah during beach time. Daisy swims and gives Oprah the confidence to swim. She has taught Oprah how to deal with waves and carry a ball at the same time. While Daisy is helping her protégée, she seems transformed. She lives in the moment, and the moment is joyous.

CHAPTER 10

STAND BY ME

Dogs in Times of Crisis and Disaster

The victims of former USA Gymnastics and Michigan State University doctor Larry Nassar came forward for seven days. One at a time, 156 women steeled their courage and shared their stories of how the once-revered doctor sexually assaulted them during treatments for sports injuries.

They made their raw, searing, impassioned statements as part of Nassar's sentencing in a Michigan court. They were not just talking to the judge. They addressed Nassar himself, who sat only feet away as he listened to one young woman after another tell of the damage he did.

Kyle Stephens, who said she was repeatedly abused by Nassar starting when she was six years old, was the first to give her impact statement.

"Perhaps you have figured it out by now," she said at the end of her statement, "but little girls don't stay little forever. They grow into strong women that return to destroy your world."

Parents also approached the podium. One was the mother of a girl who committed suicide as a result of his abuse. Like so many others, she was there hoping to have an influence on Nassar's sentencing.

For many, it was the first time going public with the anguishing secrets they had kept locked away for years. Some had tried to get authorities to listen, but the doctor was too vaunted and their accusations were not taken seriously. Coming forward and facing their abuser was both empowering and emotionally exhausting.

Circuit Court Judge Rosemarie Aquilina, who called his former patients survivors, not victims, offered empathy, comfort, and sometimes advice for each of the young women who spoke.

"The monster who took advantage of you is going to wither, much like the scene in *The Wizard of Oz* where the water gets poured on the witch and the witch withers away," Judge Aquilina told one of them. "That's what's going to happen to him, because as you get stronger, as you overcome—because you will—he gets weaker and he will wither away."

She told another victim, "I wish my robe came with a magic wand so I can wave it over you and heal you."

Judge Aquilina's supportive, personalized comments bolstered the women and their families in the courtroom.

And when they left the courtroom, someone else was waiting for them if they needed a little extra comfort or a break from the grueling process.

He was not a judge. Quite the opposite, actually. He was there to offer nonjudgmental support. He's listed (last) on the staff page of Small Talk Children's Assessment Center. During his time outside the courtroom, he wore a blue bandanna and a blue necktie dappled with little white bones.

Preston, a black Labrador retriever, was sworn in as an official canine advocate in 2016 and has been helping young victims of crime for Small Talk since. His bandanna or tie—or, in the case of the Nassar sentencing, both—help him know he's on the clock. Preston saves his more energetic Lab qualities for when his outfit comes off.

A detective who had worked with Preston in other abuse cases had recommended him for the Nassar sentencing. Preston proved to be a popular pup. He was frequently surrounded by people wanting some of what he offered. Many of the young women and families coming out of the courtroom stopped to visit with him, pet him, or hug him. They found refuge in his friendly, kind, soothing demeanor.

"Having Preston here has just been a joy," former Central Michigan University gymnast Samantha Ursch told ABC News. "He really seeks out wanting to comfort people."

Attorneys sought him out as well. Even news reporters befriended him—and wrote stories about him.

"People were looking for him and so happy when they found him," says Ashley Vance, his handler, who is also a crisis counselor for Small Talk. "We definitely saw plenty of tears flowing.

"Preston seems to know when someone is in pain. He just somehow picks up on it and knows what he needs to do. Sometimes he nuzzles, sometimes he gets playful, it just depends. He was in his element at the sentencing and helped a lot of people just by being Preston."

The Nassar case was a one-off for Preston. He usually spends his forty-hour workweek helping young victims of abuse. The majority of children he works with have been sexually abused. He hunkers close to them on the witness stand in courtrooms and stays by their side at the Small Talk office in Lansing.

The children he helps are as young as three years old.

Children's advocacy centers like Small Talk strive to make the child-abuse investigation and court process as easy for children as possible by providing a sensitive and child-friendly atmosphere. They try to conduct only one forensic interview with one interviewer to avoid revictimizing children with repeated sessions. Individual counseling and group therapy are available for free.

From the time children walk into Small Talk until they're done with the court process, Preston is there for them. He's a constant and steady presence at the center. If they're interested—and they usually are—he'll hang out with them. In group therapy, if the children want him to be part of the group, he's happy to stay with them in the room, getting pats and hugs or just being a calming or funny presence.

Children love giving him snacks in exchange for him doing something they ask, like "shake" or "lie down." These snacks aren't just any dog treats, but healthy dried-green-bean treats. He's mad about them. The staff tried raw carrots at first, but that was too messy, with drooly carrot bits ending up all over the floor. The kids think it's hilarious that he loves green beans, and they enjoy getting him to do tricks for them.

It can be just enough of a reset for them to forget their troubles long enough to catch their breath.

Preston is considered a facility dog or a facility therapy dog. Facility dogs are highly trained dogs who partner with people working in certain settings. Educational and mental health professionals, social workers and advocates, different types of therapists, first responders, and clergy are among the people who might qualify to have a facility dog.

These dogs are owned by the facility, but taken care of by an employee who works with the people the agency serves—much as happens in the world of police dogs. That person becomes the dog's handler and best friend. Many of these handlers tend to stay on the job longer than they might otherwise because they don't want to give up their dog. Preston and other facility dogs can be a boon for employee retention.

Since one of Preston's primary duties is to be there to help crime victims before they have to testify and then in courtrooms, he's also known as a canine advocate or courtroom dog. These canine courtroom comforters are growing in popularity as child advocates and prosecutors see their benefits. The Courthouse Dogs Foundation, with 216 dog team members in thirty-eight states and Canada, has seen its membership double in the last three years.

An article on the website of the American Bar Association from back in 2009 helped get the word out about this relatively new role for dogs with observations like these:

Prosecutors and judges are finding that the presence of a well-trained dog aids witness testimony by providing the victim with emotional support and comfort both in the witness room and in the courtroom. Success stories are beginning to emerge demonstrating that the use of canines in the courtroom not only provides the victim with a more positive outcome but also offers the victim a positive, life-changing experience.

It's hard to imagine appearing in court against the person who committed atrocious crimes against you as a positive and life-changing experience. But if anyone can help make this happen, it's not surprising that dogs can.

"If you do everything properly beforehand, those kids are so empowered they go in and kick butt," says Dan Cojanu, founder of the Canine Advocacy Program (CAP), the nonprofit agency that provided Preston to Small Talk.

"Many children who would not have otherwise taken the witness stand have been able to summon their courage because of a dog. The dog made them feel strong and safe. They can be proud of what they were able to do, and sometimes they can call on this strength in the future."

Celeste Walsen, DVM, executive director of the Courthouse Dogs Foundation (CAP and CDF are not affiliated), says children learn to trust both the dogs and those who work with the dogs. They see how kindly the dogs are treated by the handlers, and they realize the dogs are good and the handlers are kind and caring.

CDF dogs are highly trained. They know dozens of commands and often play fun games with the children, like holding puzzle pieces for them as they put together a puzzle, or even rolling dice. "The children can end up leaving a center talking about the amazing dog, and not being so focused on what happened to them," Dr. Walsen says. "That's huge."

The dogs help children feel more comfortable during forensic interviews, she says. The interviewer has to stay neutral and can't do much beyond handing a child a Kleenex. Anything more could be seen as leading the child, she says.

"But having a dog on a couch with a child is a legally neutral way a child can feel so much more comfortable. Dogs can raise oxytocin levels, and make the child feel more relaxed. They can prevent the child from shutting down when they're talking about the horrible crime committed against them."

And the more details a child can provide about a crime, the more evidence for detectives, and the better and more thorough the investigation. Sometimes a child talks to the dog instead of the interviewer. That's OK. Children could talk to the wallpaper. As long as they talk about what happened.

"A lot of perpetrators think that a four-year-old won't tell. That they're hiding and won't say anything," says Dr. Walsen. "A dog can change that completely."

She says sometimes a dog can even help a case not go to trial, sparing the child the trauma of facing the accused perpetrator in court.

"If a defense attorney sees that a child can talk and that a dog can go with them to court, they'll think twice about taking it to trial," she says.

As helpful as dogs are in this environment, they can't always work miracles. Sometimes a child will freeze at the last minute and be unable to testify, even with the help of their trusty friend.

Dan remembers hearing from one of his canine advocates about a little boy who fell apart and couldn't take the stand. Not even the boy's canine advocate, a Labrador named Dodger, could give him the strength to go in front of a judge, jury, and the accused.

"I'm sorry," the boy said. "Do you think Dodger is still proud of me?"

"Of course he is," Dodger's handler told him. "He thinks you are the best."

. . .

The children Preston and other canine advocates accompany to court
have to recount the worst moments of their lives. And not in prepared statements, like the victims of Larry Nassar, but in their own
words, prompted by questions from attorneys. Sharing their stories
is hard enough, but being questioned by the attorney representing
the accused can be especially difficult.

Besides counseling and weeks of support to help prepare them for
their day in court, Preston's young friends also receive a fourteen-
page activity book. It's called *Preston's Guide to Court*. It portrays him
on the cover as a calm, confident cartoon canine walking to a courtroom. (A wooden sign points in the direction of the courtroom, so
we know where he's going.)

It's clear from his expression that Preston's got this.

Activity books are usually the stuff of childhood fun: connecting
dots, coloring, drawing, winding through mazes. Contentment and
crayons. Innocence and idle time.

Preston's book is cute and cheery, which may be the reason it's
also utterly heartbreaking. It exists only because dark and terrible
crimes were committed against the children who hold the book in
their hands.

On the first page, happy Preston asks children to write their
name. That's pretty standard. But then he asks for the names of their
advocate, their prosecutor, and their detective. Not the stuff of regular activity books. He ends the page on a light note, asking, "What
is your favorite treat?" ("Mine is green beans," he tells them.)

Some pages of the book are just like those of a regular activity
book. They feature simple activities with Preston, like coloring his
picture, drawing his outline in a connect-the-dots, helping him get
to the judge's gavel in a maze, and finding the Preston who doesn't
match. Others are unflinchingly court-centered. On one page Preston smilingly talks about important rules to follow in court (telling
the truth, letting someone know if you have to use the restroom,

etc.). On another he tells them, "I felt nervous the first time I went to court. Circle the feelings you have."

A word search later in the book contains words like "safe," "courage," "brave," "prosecutor," "judge," and, of course, "Preston." Children can even color a courtroom that shows them where everyone from the jury to the court recorder sits.

In real life, when a child's day in court comes, Preston will already be that child's friend. The child will walk into the courtroom—like the one he or she colored—and onto the witness stand with Preston.

Preston's main job is to lie down near the child in the witness box. That's all. Sometimes a child reaches down and pets Preston. Little ones occasionally rest their feet on him.

"He is amazing in the courtroom. Nothing ruffles him. I think he really knows how important his job is to the children he's helping," says Ashley.

Dan says the twenty-seven dogs his agency has produced for child advocacy centers and prosecutors have all been like Preston in temperament. But a couple of these mellow dogs have let it be known that they don't think much of a defense attorney.

"The dogs can be very protective of the kids, in their own quiet way," he says. "They have a sense of what's going on, I'm sure."

They signal their disapproval silently. It's by no means aggressive. There's no growling or bared teeth. It's nonconfrontational body language. Although the CAP dogs are trained to lie down near the child and never so much as raise their heads on the witness stand, a dog Dan worked with for years—a chocolate Lab named Amos—apparently had enough of a defense attorney one afternoon.

"The defense attorney was raising her voice to a child, and Amos was lying down quietly as usual. But this wasn't OK with him," Dan says. "He got up. Just sat up and stared at her silently. He gave her such a look. Like, *Really? REALLY?!* She lowered the volume and eased up, and Amos went back to lying down again."

Defense attorneys sometimes used Amos to meet a child on his or her own terms. "They don't want to hurt the child. By talking a little about Amos and being warmer, they may be able to ask questions without a kid rolling into a ball and crying," Dan says.

Amos served hundreds of children during his career. He was CAP's first canine advocate. Like all the other dogs trained by his agency, Amos had initially been slated to be a guide dog with Leader Dogs for the Blind. He was a great dog. But he was a big puller and scared of stairs—potentially disastrous traits in that profession. He had to change careers.

He came to CAP well trained by Leader Dogs. Dan worked with a trainer and taught him not to pull and got him used to stairs. It took a couple of months to make him walk calmly enough that a child could hold his leash, but Dan had plenty of time to devote to getting Amos ready for his career; his own career as a counselor and then supervisor of victim services at the Oakland County Prosecutor's Office in Pontiac, Michigan, had come to an end when they offered financial incentives to retire. So he combined his love of being an advocate for victims and his love of dogs to create his organization.

Dan says he hasn't made a dime in the eight years he's been running CAP. Some income would help, but when he thinks about moving on and finding someone to take over, his wife reminds him, "When you come home from being with the dogs and the kids, you're on fire."

He and Amos used to do crisis work at a juvenile detention center to relax the youth before therapy. Even the first time Amos joined a group, it looked like he knew who needed the most help.

"He went right up to two of the kids in the group and licked their faces immediately," Dan says. "It turned out that both of them had lost a parent that week. How could he know? But he seemed to be that tuned in. His intuitiveness knocked my socks off."

One of Amos's earliest court advocacy experiences was with a girl who was petrified of dogs. The girl, about ten years old, had been mauled by a dog three years earlier and had scars on her neck and behind an ear. At first she and her mother turned down the offer of a dog who might be able to help her in the courtroom. But then they saw Amos. Dan assured her he was a really good dog who would never hurt her. The girl's apprehension decreased, and she said it was OK for him to come close.

Amos didn't just sit and wait for her to pat him. He pulled out all the stops. He flipped onto his back and wiggled around. "The girl started laughing hysterically. He looked like such a boob, but she started petting his belly and a few minutes later she was so comfortable with him.

"Later that day I hear a scream. 'AMOS!' It was the girl. She'd just spotted him and was thrilled." Dogs weren't allowed in that judge's courtroom at the time, so Amos got her right up to the point of testifying, and she faced the defendant with a confidence she didn't have before.

Something as simple as a child holding the dog's leash can make all the difference.

"It gives children control and power in a powerless situation," Dan says. "We tell them that this is their dog for as long as they're here today. This gives them enormous power. All they've been doing is listening to people telling them what they have to do. Now they get to be in charge of a dog."

Older children were bolstered by Amos, too. A sixteen-year-old girl was about to face a man Dan says had been "pimping her out for years." Dan had told her she needed to get to the witness box and not look at the guy until she was told she had to do so to identify him.

She and Amos walked up together and took their places. When she finally had to look at the man, she was overcome. She dropped the leash and was inconsolable. She cried so hard her false eyelashes fell off.

But then a funny thing happened.

She reached down to touch Amos and stared at the man. Slowly she grew stronger. Every time she answered a question, she seemed more self-assured. Whenever she was struggling, she felt Amos. She

stared the man down. By the end, Dan said, she seemed embold-
ened, almost a different person than the frightened girl who had first
laid eyes on the man.

Judge Kelley Kostin, a 52nd District Court judge in Oakland
County, Michigan, witnessed this sort of transformation as soon as
she opened her courtroom's doors to Amos and other advocate dogs.

"I've seen it over and over again where a child is scared to death.
It's intimidating to come into a courtroom. But there's something
about having a dog there. I recommend this 100 percent to other
judges," says Judge Kostin, who has also worked with these dogs in
her veterans treatment court.

Judge Kostin often suggests to children reluctant to speak that
they talk directly to the dog. "The prosecutor or DA would ask questions and I'd say, 'You can tell Amos. He'll listen to you.'" He always did.

Amos worked with hundreds of children during his eight-year
career. He was going strong at age ten. He loved to go to work and
adored meeting new children. His home life was happy and cozy.

On June 16, 2018, it all came crashing to an end. On June 17, this
led a CAP Facebook post:

> It is with deep sorrow and profound sadness that we share
> with you our beloved Amos has crossed the rainbow
> bridge.
>   Yesterday, Amos suffered a severe neurological event
> that left him in pain, paralyzed and unable to control his
> bodily functions. After wonderful medical care and con-
> sultation, we made the swift, but mindful decision to let
> him go. It is our belief that a hero such as Amos should
> have his dignity at the end.

Dan wrote these words of remembrance:

> His legacy will continue to live on through the other ca-
> nine advocates as they continue to pave the way for change

in the criminal justice process for our young and most vulnerable victims.

————

The use of trained therapy-style dogs for trauma or a crisis hasn't received much attention from researchers. But that may be changing. In 2018 a study in *Frontiers in Psychology* mentioned it was probably the first study to investigate how and if therapy dogs can help in the aftermath of a traumatic event.

The researchers used an eleven-minute compilation of extremely disturbing scenes from the film *Irreversible*, which critic Roger Ebert described "a movie so violent and cruel that most people will find it unwatchable." The authors of the study wrote that the film has been shown in their laboratory and others "to reliably induce physiological and subjective stress responses as well as intrusive memories." They found that the group of participants who interacted with a therapy dog for fifteen minutes after the film reported lower anxiety, less negative affect, and more positive affect (basically fewer negative emotions and more positive emotions) than groups that did not.

It was an intriguing study. But those who volunteer their highly trained dogs to help in the wake of disasters and mass traumatic events could have predicted the outcomes. With all the natural disasters of late, these dogs and handlers have been getting plenty of experience. But it's not just trained dogs who can make a difference. Even our humble pet dogs can sometimes be what it takes to keep us going after we've lost everything.

On October 9, 2017, the Tubbs fire in Northern California robbed an old friend of almost everything in her life. Joan Hoerner escaped with her little dog, her purse, and her car. It was the day before her eighty-fourth birthday, and also the day before she was going to finalize the sale of her house in a tree-filled neighborhood in Santa Rosa.

Whipped forward by furious winds, the flames blazed their way

to her address on the first night of what would become the most
destructive wildfire in the history of California—at least until the
following year. At around 2 a.m., she and Tiger woke up to neighbors
pounding on the door and telling her she needed to evacuate. A fire
that had started just a few hours earlier in the wine-country town of
Calistoga was now threatening their neighborhood.

It had made its terrifying twelve-mile run in less than four hours.

She hurried to change and followed the neighbors' car in her 1998
Chrysler Sebring convertible—a car she'd hung on to because it was
cool and reliable. Tiger rode, as usual, on his plaid blanket on the
back seat. She figured they'd return in a few hours, but was glad to
see that Tiger, an old dog not used to late-night outings, had dozed
off straightaway.

They all drove to a friend's house high on a hill a couple of miles
away. For the rest of the night they watched the fire snake and pour
its way through the night—orange against black, like some nightmare from Halloween. They couldn't see their neighborhood, but
they couldn't imagine how it would be spared when the fire was so
swift and greedy.

Joan called me at 5 a.m. and said the fire was getting too close and
they would be evacuating once again later that morning. They
planned to drive north to the town of Windsor, where her neighbors'
family lived. We made a plan to meet there and bring her back to San
Francisco.

The drive would normally take about ninety minutes. But Highway 101 was closed as I approached Santa Rosa, so I had to try to
make my way north on suburban streets instead of the highway. In
some places the curtain of smoke was so gray and thick that it hurt
to breathe. Every few minutes I'd have to take another route because
the fire was scorching areas all around. Sirens sounded in stereo as
crews scrambled to close roads and detour traffic.

When I finally arrived, Joan was holding Tiger, her fifteen-year-
old Maltese-poodle-mystery mix. She had been stoic all night and

morning, but broke down in my arms. When she could talk, she told me, "You smell fresh, like nice shampoo."

I was dreading the ride back on the unpredictable and dangerous streets, but just as we approached Santa Rosa, the highway reopened and we were able to stay on 101.

At first this seemed like good news.

But within a couple of minutes, I noticed something disconcerting. The guardrails were on fire. The posts were made of wood, and as they burned, the steel railings drooped, either from lack of support or because they had softened. You wouldn't want to have to pull over here.

For a few miles it was like a highway through hell. I felt like we were driving in a Bruegel painting of the underworld. Structures were still on fire or smoldering, and endless smoke—black plumes, gray plumes—pushed into a butterscotch-pudding sky.

Even in San Francisco—although we were a good fifty-five miles away, and two blocks from the Pacific Ocean—the air choked with smoke, and ashes sprinkled cars for days.

Joan didn't feel like eating. Gus, who weighs ten times as much as Tiger, kept approaching them with toys. It looked like he wanted to make them feel better. But his size and enthusiasm were too much for Joan in her exhausted state, so I had him settle.

The next day, as we were about to leave for her birthday dinner at Original Joe's, which she hadn't been to in years, I got a Facebook message. Her neighbor had written with news that Joan's home was gone. A friend had sneaked into the area and said pretty much all the homes had burned, and nothing was left.

I decided not to say anything until we had photos to confirm. Why give Joan bad news on her birthday when her spirits were up if we didn't know for sure? She ate heartily and had a glass of wine. She said she wasn't going to let some fire ruin her celebration.

The neighbor messaged the photos the next morning. All that

remained of Joan's house were bricks from the patio and fireplace, and twisted metal remnants of a porch swing and loungers in the backyard. One house after the other looked like this. The fire had swept through and obliterated several blocks. It didn't seem possible that this had once been a cozy, tree-filled neighborhood with pretty yards.

Everything she owned was smoke and ashes—eighty-four years of life, so much of it irreplaceable. Photos, an old leather-bound family Bible with her family's history tucked inside, and favorite recipes were the first items she thought of, but it was the everyday items she missed the most. Her clothes, her jewelry, her books.

She rarely cried in the days that followed, breaking down only when someone she didn't know learned what had happened and showed her empathy. That always got her, and it embarrassed her to show her emotions like this. She had warriored her way through two serious cancers and her husband's death and had barely shed a tear.

As she came to grips with her losses, I realized how lucky she was to have escaped alive. If not for her neighbors, she might have ended up trapped and unable to get out before it was too late.

Twenty-two people were killed as a result of the Tubbs fire. Carmen Berriz, seventy-five, died in a backyard pool in the arms of her husband, who survived. They had met in Havana, Cuba, when she was twelve and he was thirteen. Arthur Grant, ninety-five, and Suiko Grant, seventy-five, perished in their wine cellar. The fire also stole the life of Christina Hanson, twenty-seven, who was confined to a wheelchair because of spina bifida. Valerie Evans, seventy-five, died trying to save her dogs.

The fire destroyed 5,636 structures and 36,807 acres. Other California wildfires had destroyed far more acreage, but at that point no fires had come close to decimating this many structures.

Santa Rosa housing had been scarce before the fire. Now it was proving impossible for many trying to find rentals in the area. Joan was picky about what she wanted. It had to be something on the first floor, with an enclosed yard. It was all about Tiger.

Tiger was constantly at her side after the fire, far more than he used to be. She toted him around, plopping him on her lap while watching TV. They had chats about this and that, and she promised him she'd have a yard for him just like in their old house. She told everyone, from my kind neighbors who had taken her into their large in-law unit to the people she met while trying to replenish her wardrobe, that she was determined to keep going and not give up. Not for herself, but for Tiger. He was like her child, and he had become the focus of her desire to continue trying. The reason to live.

"He needs me and I have to stay alive and be strong for him," she said.

I'm pretty sure that Tiger, all eight pounds of him, did more to keep her going than all of her friends and family combined.

Shortly before the fire, I had been looking into flying to Texas to watch some dogs who help people recover from disasters and other crises. Hurricane Harvey, with its catastrophic flooding, had destroyed or damaged three hundred thousand structures in the state. Hundreds of thousands of Texans had been without electricity for too long. More than a hundred people statewide had died as a result of the storm.

I knew that dogs were working there because during my visit to Japan, I'd spent a few days exploring the Kyoto area. On a walk through the Arashiyama Bamboo Forest early one morning when it was uncharacteristically low on visitors, I asked a rare passerby if he could take my photo with the stunning giant bamboo backdrop— something I couldn't do without a selfie stick or very long arms. It turned out he was an American and was there in part recuperating from the loss of his beloved dog.

We talked dogs for a while, and when he found out why I was in Japan, he shared that he was a physician in Houston, and that he was intrigued by the healing power of animals, especially dogs.

"Besides their companionship, they have real skills," Jim Kelaher, MD, told me as we strolled through the towering green bamboos. "I have this interest in whether dogs change their behavior when their humans get sick, and maybe even before they're diagnosed, how dogs grieve, and everything else that makes them special."

It turns out he had been a volunteer with an organization that uses dogs to help survivors of disasters, and he told me about some of the work he had done when he was still active with the group.

That in the middle of a bamboo forest in Japan I should meet an American doctor who is fascinated by dogs and volunteered to help disaster survivors with a crisis-dog organization is one of those enchanting coincidences of travel. I knew about dogs who do this work and had been planning on including them in this book, but this fell right into my lap—or at least into my notebook, where I wrote down the info he gave me.

Once back home, I reached out to Hope Animal-Assisted Crisis Response to learn more about the group Dr. Kelaher had told me about. It's one of a few organizations in the United States that has rigorous standards for screening and training dogs and their people to help in the aftermath of disasters.

The hurricane and flood recovery was under way after Harvey, and Hope's dog teams were traveling from across the country to assist. As I was looking at dates for a possible trip to Texas to watch some of these teams in action, the Tubbs fire broke out. A dozen other fires were ravaging Northern California at the same time. They were collectively known as the Northern California firestorm.

I wouldn't have to travel to Texas to see crisis-response dogs at work. The firestorm would bring them close to my backyard. In fact, about ten days after Joan lost her home, I needed to bring her up to the Local Assistance Center, a partnership of local, state, and federal agencies set up as a disaster-assistance one-stop shop.

I learned from Pam Bertz, a regional director of Hope, that they'd have some crisis-assistance dogs there. So along with Joan's insurance info and the few papers she had in her purse, I brought my notebook and camera. This would be a multipurpose trip.

As we got close to downtown Santa Rosa, Tiger sat up on his

plaid blanket on the back seat of my yellow Honda Fit and looked out the window. I wondered if his olfactory memory made him real-ize he was in his old town, or if the smell took him back to the strange day when he went for many rides in the car while the air was heavy with smoke, and maybe even with the smell of fear.

We couldn't get into Joan's neighborhood. It was still closed, waiting for authorities to inspect it to see if it was safe for residents to visit. Joan wanted to check if anything was salvagable. Maybe some jewelry or sentimental collectable porcelain dolls.* With that part of our visit scratched, we headed for the disaster center.

It was set up on the first floor of the *Santa Rosa Press Democrat* building. Dozens of government agencies and support services, in-cluding FEMA, the American Red Cross, housing-assistance groups, and building permitting agencies, were represented at tables in several expansive rooms.

As we spoke with people at a number of agencies, we realized that Joan was far from an outlier: Nearly everyone milling about and go-ing from table to table had lost their homes. There were hundreds of people, from young children to men and women far older than Joan. Many seemed in remarkably good spirits. But others were worn-out, walking around dazed under the fluorescent lighting in clothing someone had given them because they had nothing.

Joan was working with a FEMA counselor and would be busy for a while. They didn't need my help, so I set out to look for some Hope dogs. Several pet dogs were wandering the rooms with their people, but the dogs I was looking for would be wearing green vests. I learned that two of them were off at a first-responder staging area, giving comfort to those who had been risking their lives to get the fire un-der control. After a while I spotted an Australian shepherd walking beside a woman wearing official-looking credentials on a lanyard

---

*Eventually all that could be recovered on her property were some concrete garden figures: a turtle, a couple of gnomes, and a memorial plaque someone had given her after one of her sons died of esophageal cancer on Thanksgiving several years earlier.

around her neck. The dog's fur was so thick that I couldn't see a vest, but when I got closer, I saw that it stood out from his fluffy coat.

This was Cody. It said so in bold yellow letters on top of his vest. His handler and other half, Kathy Felix, told me she and Cody normally volunteer with other organizations for more typical therapy dog gigs. They go to libraries to help children learn to read, and to schools for disabled children. They visit medical clinics, and they spend time at college campuses to help reduce stress during finals.

The two had recently gone through Hope's intensive screening and multiday training in Southern California. They were tested in a mock disaster situation typical of what they might see on a "callout," where there were frantic people, traumatized children, and chaotic scenes at every turn.

"I came home a little awed by the responsibility of being with persons hurting so badly," Kathy told me.

This was only their second time at a disaster site. She was moved by how people were coping with their profound losses. She told me about something that had happened earlier that day.

A man approached her and asked if he could pet her dog. As he snuggled with Cody on the floor, Kathy asked if he had a dog.

Yes, he answered, he had a dog. But he had lost his dog in the fire. And he had lost his wife as well.

"He experienced such tragedy, and he only wanted to hug Cody," she said. "It's so heartbreaking. I hope Cody made him feel a little better for a few minutes."

As we were talking, a burly man in his thirties approached Kathy and asked if he could pet Cody. As he did, he told Kathy his story. He had been between jobs and could no longer afford renter's insurance. He and his wife had let the insurance go, reasoning it was more important to pay for rent and food. "It wasn't the priority," he told her. "Hindsight is everything, I guess."

By now he was kneeling down with Cody, who was sitting and looking at him with the most empathetic dog eyes I'd ever seen.

Kathy listened in a natural, caring, nonintrusive way, never prodding, just being there.

The home he and his family had been renting on a vineyard had burned to the ground. They'd seen the fire approaching in the dark—an orange glow rapidly growing brighter. He called 9-1-1 several times and finally got through. The dispatcher told him they couldn't help, that the whole area was a tinderbox, and to get to safety immediately.

He and his wife and twelve-year-old son gathered some clothes, a few cherished items, essential papers like birth and marriage certificates, and loaded the car with their kelpie–black Lab mix and one of their two cats. The other cat had run off toward the blaze. He promised his son the cat would survive, that he'd come back and the cat would be there waiting for him.

Flames engulfed the vineyard's larger house. He realized theirs would be gone soon. They could feel the heat as they ran to the car. The fire was encroaching from all around now.

"It all happened so fast. If we didn't get out right then, we'd be trapped," he said. "We got out of there just in time, I think."

As he spoke, he seemed to be unconsciously grabbing onto the loose skin of Cody's neck every couple of seconds and releasing it. Cody didn't mind. He looked like he was enjoying a massage.

The man began talking to Cody.

"We were really lucky. Material things can be replaced. We have a new place to stay for a while. But it doesn't allow dogs, isn't that a bad rule?

"So our dog is staying with friends. We'll hopefully have him back soon when we get a new place. We're all safe, and it's going to be OK. Right, Cody?"

Cody's expression remained the same.

The man went back to talking to Kathy.

"Yeah, I promised that the cat would be OK, and when I went back, there he was. He flicked his tail at me and gave me one of those *It's about time!* looks."

The man beckoned his son, who had been standing nearby.

Kathy introduced herself and Cody and asked the boy about his dog and cats. He told her their names, and said he missed his dog. She invited him to pet Cody. At the invitation, he sat down on the carpet, and Cody went from sitting to lying down. He faced the boy and, in a move that seemed like he was a caring therapist ready to listen to a patient, crossed his soft white paws.

Kathy joined them on the floor, occasionally petting Cody as they talked. I backed off and let them have their conversation.

As I watched, the boy edged closer to Cody, and almost imperceptibly, Cody inched his head closer to the boy. The boy talked to Kathy, who had the demeanor of a gentle and kind grandmother. Then he fell silent. He reached out and touched Cody's paw. Cody gazed at him. The boy stroked his paws with great tenderness while looking into Cody's eyes. He didn't say anything to Cody. He didn't need to. They were in the same moment.

"Crisis-response dogs are the PhDs of therapy dogs," Pam says. "They have been through so much training and know how to be calm and comforting in all types of disaster or crisis situations. They can work longer hours than regular therapy dogs.

"Therapy dogs are very special. Crisis-response dogs are off the charts."

Pam says Hope is the largest crisis-response dog organization in the country, with about 250 dog teams from coast to coast. Its founder was inspired to start the organization after a 1998 Oregon high school shooting that left two dead and twenty-five wounded. She and some other therapy dog handlers had visited to comfort the students. Afterward she realized that she and her dog, and some of the other handlers and their dogs, had soaked up too much emotion.

"It was clear that for crisis work, they needed better-trained dogs and handlers, especially when dealing with issues that can affect mental health," Pam says. They gradually came up with the type of training that would help volunteers and their dogs weather the storm, or earthquake, or whatever they'd be facing.

Each dog-and-handler team has an "SOS card" they give the

team leader when they arrive at a disaster site. It lists the unique signs of stress for the dog and the handler. The team leader and the handlers continually assess the dogs while they're on the callout. If they see any signs of stress, the dog is pulled and given a rest. The team leader will also pull handlers who appear stressed.

To get dogs ready for some of the sights and sounds they'll come across, and to keep stress levels down during callouts, they're exposed to situations they'll face after real-life disasters. Besides mock disaster-center scenarios like the ones Kathy and Cody went through, there's also special training for helping first responders. Since the dogs are often requested to visit firefighters and others at base camps, part of their schooling involves going to fire stations and being around equipment, with engines running and an occasional siren blaring.

A firefighter in full gear, including a mask respirator, will approach a dog with treats in gloved hands. Dogs can be apprehensive at first, but firefighters work to show the dogs that they're just regular people. Sometimes they kneel at dog level to give the treats, or take off the mask. They're happy to help acclimate the dogs.

"In a deployment, you've got these big strong firefighters at base camp on a shift change, and some will come right off a vehicle and fall to their knees when they see our dogs," Pam says. "They just melt. The dogs help bring a piece of home to these men and women who are often hundreds of miles from their own homes."

As long as the canine comfort teams are available and they're invited by an organization like FEMA, the American Red Cross, or a state office of emergency services, they'll go to any disaster or crisis where they can help as people are starting to recover. Most of the financial burden is on the volunteers, who pay for their own airfare, rental cars, and a portion of their lodging.

"It takes a very special person to do this kind of volunteer work," Pam says. "Those who can do it are game changers."*

---

*Unfortunately, Kathy and Cody and the other Hope volunteers are staying busy with natural disasters. As I was wrapping up this chapter a little more than a year after the fire, we had to keep the windows of the house shut because of thick smoke

There are the little children who won't say much to anyone after a disaster, and then a volunteer introduces a dog. "You can tell him anything," the handler may say. "He won't tell anyone else, I promise." After petting the dog for a while, the child lifts up the dog's ear (if it's a floppy-eared dog) and quietly gives him the lowdown.

Dogs have had a similar effect when they visit after a school shooting. Students cry into a dog's neck, hug the dog, and may start talking. Maybe not to the dog, but to counselors, or the handler, or one another.

Then there are the people who are so upset and distraught that they're unable to function at a disaster-recovery center—not the easiest places to navigate even in the best of times. "Would you like a little puppy love?" a handler may ask. A little petting—or, better yet, a head in the lap—can be all it takes to defuse the person's anxiety.

Pam, like so many who work with dogs, marvels at the way some dogs seem to know who needs help.

"Sometimes you walk into a room with all these people and your dog is already headed toward someone. Maybe they're giving off smells of stress and the dog knows this is a person who needs them. They'll pull you to these people."

She tells the story of a handler who arrived with a dog at an emergency disaster shelter in San Bernardino County after a devastating fire in 2003. The woman's Cavalier King Charles spaniel, Duke, immediately began pulling. She couldn't get him to stop. This wasn't like him. He was usually the model of obedience.

Duke pulled the handler to a boy lying on a cot. The boy reached out and stroked Duke. He invited Duke up to his cot. Duke hopped up and lay down next to the boy. Duke's handler found out the boy was by himself in the shelter. His mother had passed away a month before. His father had brought him there, but something happened

---

overwhelming San Francisco from another wildfire. This one, in Butte County, about three hours from San Francisco, is known as the Camp fire. It now holds the awful record of being the most deadly and destructive wildfire in California's history.

and he had to be taken to a hospital by ambulance. The boy's cat had died in the fire.

The boy was running a fever. A Red Cross volunteer had come to his cot to see him, but she thought he needed to be assessed by a nurse, who couldn't leave her station except for an emergency. The boy didn't want to go to the first aid station. He had been refusing to get up, silently shaking his head.

After hugging Duke for a while, he had an idea. "I'll go," he said, "if Duke can go with me. Could he?"

"Of course! He'd love to go with you," Duke's handler said. Duke helped escort the boy to the first aid station. Duke checked in on him throughout the afternoon.

The boy's father came back later that day, and they had a teary reunion. He thanked Duke and his handler for how they had helped his son.

Duke received a Red Cross Bravo for Bravery Award for his work with the boy.

"When it comes to helping people in crisis, well-trained dogs can make a huge difference in someone's demeanor and their ability to handle stress," Pam says.

Or even not-so-well-trained dogs.

As I write this, it's been nearly a year since Joan lost everything in the fire. She decided not to rebuild. She used some of her insurance money to buy a small place about twenty-five minutes south of Santa Rosa.

Tiger got his yard.

Tiger hasn't had formal crisis-response training. I'm not sure he even knows how to sit on command. But he definitely knows how to give an eighty-four-year-old woman a reason to get up each morning.

All he has to do is be a dog.

BEDSIDE MANNER REDEFINED

I magine you're enjoying a pleasant stroll through the park when you hear someone say, "My owner needs your attention! Please follow me!" You look around and see no one; then you look down and see a dog staring up at you. You think someone's pulling a fast one. But then the dog reaches around and his mouth tugs something on the yellow vest he's wearing, and you hear it again.

"My owner needs your attention! Please follow me!" the dog seems to say again, looking at you plaintively and now beckoning with body language for you to follow him. You do, and he leads you to someone who's having a severe allergic reaction, a seizure, or some other medical emergency.

Welcome to the new world of dog-human communication, where technology is allowing dogs to "speak" in ways we can easily understand when it really counts. If that same dog had run up to you Lassie-style and tried to get your attention without the voice, you might not have followed him. You might have reached down to pet him or thrown a pinecone for him while his person suffered alone nearby.

The vest is one of several emerging technologies a few universities are developing that could forever change the way working dogs (and probably pet dogs, down the road) can communicate with people—and the way people can communicate with dogs.

I wanted to see how these devices work, so I flew to Atlanta to visit the Georgia Institute of Technology (Georgia Tech), the epicenter of this field in the United States. One of the first researchers I met was Sky, a supersmart border collie who happens to be the dog of Melody Jackson, PhD, director of the school's Animal-Computer Interaction Lab and also director of the FIDO project.* FIDO focuses on creating wearable technologies as well as other ways to open the lines of communication between dogs and humans. Sky is the star tester and demonstrator of the devices produced by Dr. Jackson and her team.

When Dr. Jackson and Sky greeted me in the lobby of the university's genius-filled Technology Square Research Building, Sky inspected me with his intelligent border collie eyes and gave me a few sniffs. If he could talk (beyond the talking vest, that is), he might have said something like this:

Barely remembers long division. Why is she here? Does not compute! Don't let her upstairs!

But he couldn't. So we went up to Dr. Jackson's office. Sky was wearing a bright yellow Georgia Tech vest and a matching Georgia Tech collar. He had the school spirit, but this was not the vest I'd come to see. When we got to Dr. Jackson's office, she rustled up a couple of prototypes of the talking vest.

"Working dogs are smart, and they have important information they need to tell their handlers or someone else. But they're limited in what they can do," she said, handing me a small yellow vest with the words "FIDO research team" on the side. "This is just the beginning of helping them communicate."

She explained that when the vest is ready for use in the real world, the electronics will all be covered and disguised. But for now, as it gets tweaked and improved, the guts are exposed. The talking vest, in this bare-bones prototype, would get a dog stopped at any security

---

*The acronym is more user-friendly and memorable than the actual name, Facilitating Interactions for Dogs with Occupations, which may have been conceived after a few beers among colleagues. The idea of talking dogs did happen over beers, actually.

checkpoint. On the top of the vest is a plastic-and-metal controller box about the size of a deck of cards. Out of this stream red and black wires and a couple of white conductor ribbon cables. Some of the wires end in a hard plastic tube that protrudes from the side of the vest.

Dr. Jackson asked me to touch the blue surface of the tube. If I were a dog, I'd just tap it with my nose. I expected to hear the slightly robotic female voice I'd heard on a video of Sky using one of the vests.

"My owner needs your attention!" a man's voice announced with a slight Southern twinge. "Please follow me!"

"A man? A Southern man?" I asked, laughing in surprise. Dr. Jackson explained that during testing, users said they wanted their dog's voice to match their dog's gender. So they got one of the department's male researchers to be the voice of Sky's technology. I envisioned the day the vests would come with customized accents and local parlance. Gus could have the California version, ending with "Dude, follow me!"

More important than the voice is the message. Dr. Jackson told me that in real life, the dog would be trained to "say" the emergency message twice.

"In our tests, usually the first time people hear it they jump back or just don't believe what they've heard," she said.

At this point the talking vest is a one-trick pony. But future vests will likely incorporate a few tabs and pulleys for dogs to "say" whatever information is most important for his or her job.

A seizure-alert dog could tell her person to find a safe place before a seizure by pulling on one tab. She could summon help if necessary by nosing another. This would be especially handy in busy public settings when the dog's normal alert signal might not be as obvious to the handler and where there's no life-alert button as there might be at home.

The messages could be customized depending on the disability. Diabetic-alert dogs who detect both low and high blood sugar might have an easier job of communicating if they can "say" their person is going high or low.

The technology could even apply to military working dogs and police dogs. After alerting to an explosive, Dr. Jackson said, the dog could communicate if it's a particularly unstable type, like triacetone triperoxide (TATP), or something more stable, like C-4.

At the time of my visit there were no real-world applications of the technology in place, but that was about to change. The team was working on a vest for a service dog organization that wanted to try it for children with autism. A dog would be trained to use it to supplement a few tasks in his normal repertoire. If the dog sensed an impending meltdown, he could nuzzle into the child and use his usual body language to try to calm him or her. But with the talking vest, he could also gently ask the child directly, "Could you please pet me now?" or some such phrase. The vest will be a full-size service dog vest with the best sensors the team has developed.

The FIDO team has spent a few years creating the kinds of sensors that would stand up to dog mouths and a variety of environments, including water. Another prototype on Dr. Jackson's desk is more friendly looking, with a simple tug toy attached to it. A paper describing the research on the tug-toy sensor in the *Journal on Technology & Persons with Disabilities* delves into the technical details of the model, then describes the tug-toy sensor as being equipped with a gloriously nontechnical-sounding Kong Wubba—a goofy name for a product sold by the Kong pet toy company. On the next page the paper gets technical again, with a description of voltage-divider schematics.

Other sensors developed by FIDO include one a dog has to gently bite to set off a voice, and another a dog just has to pass his nose next to, as we do with our hands under touchless faucets.

"We've come a long way, but we still have a way to go," Dr. Jackson said as she recounted some of the frustrating and amusing issues they've faced.

There have been crunched sensors and drowned sensors. The

proximity sensor was sometimes triggered by random objects the dogs would pass in their environment, or if they scratched an itch. These last two resulted in many false alerts, with dogs inadvertently calling for help as, say, they groomed themselves—the ultimate twenty-first-century version of crying wolf.

Georgia Tech scientists are no strangers to the challenges of creating reliable wearable technology. In fact, who should be sitting in the lounge area outside Dr. Jackson's office but Thad Starner, PhD, founder and director of the school's Contextual Computing Group. The wearable computing pioneer and technical lead for the infamous Google Glass was dressed in his trademark plain black T-shirt and black pants, eating a Subway sandwich and working on his computer, his smartphone, and a one-handed keyboard called the Twiddler—all at the same time, it appeared. He was also wearing Google Glass, the "smart glasses" he had helped develop.

Dr. Jackson and I sat down to talk with him briefly on our way to see Sky do a demo of some other communications prototypes. Dr. Starner has been instrumental in developing several of the FIDO devices. He has three advanced degrees from MIT. Dr. Jackson has two advanced degrees from Georgia Tech. It was heartening that these are the kinds of brains that want to help dogs better communicate important information to humans.

At the end of our conversation, Dr. Starner took my contact info. Or, rather, he found it somehow by looking into his Google Glass. Maybe an email had been cc'd to him? Then he asked me to look at him so he could take a photo with his Google Glass to go with my contact info. It was like magic—and slightly disconcerting—to have someone take a photo of me just by looking in my direction.

But that's not what ended up happening. Google Glass didn't take the photo. Something went wrong. Dr. Starner took off his glasses and tried to figure out the problem.

"Wearable computing is mind-blowing," he said as he tinkered. "Especially when it works."

I have little doubt this team will succeed in helping working dogs "talk" in a potentially lifesaving manner. But what about pet dogs? What if they could really talk instead of communicating with us the way they currently do with their eyes and body language and their own canine utterances? What if our pet dogs were able to "say" things they couldn't before?

Isn't part of the bliss of dogs that they listen to us as if they truly understand? We can tell them anything, and they don't offer advice or try to fix things or blabber it to someone else. They're just there, with their unconditional love and understanding.

Several years ago when I was news editor at Dogster.com, a Japanese company came out with a gadget that was purported to interpret barks. It was more of a gimmick than anything, but it started a conversation about whether we would really want our dogs to be able to talk.

Would Gus beg at the dinner table with more than his eyes? (*Want! Please!*) Would he suggest I stop using deodorant and toothpaste so I would smell better? (*No, don't do that! Stop!*) Or would he, given the chance, just keep listening, only chiming in for important communications?

Taking this a step further, maybe in the future there will be vests for people who want their dogs to help them reach goals. I'd get the "writer on deadline" vest. Gus could be trained to sense by my body language or my scent that I was getting distracted and about to head to the fridge or checking my social media accounts. He would then pull the Kong Wubba on his vest. "Don't even *think* of procrastinating! This book isn't going to write itself," it would say. Or an encouraging "You've got this!" And there's always the popular "Sit! Stay!"

There wouldn't be many phrases because the real estate on a talking vest is limited. There are only so many sensors that can be placed on a vest before it gets uncomfortable or unwieldy. So the FIDO team is working on other ways to expand what dogs can tell us.

The team designed motion-detecting collars, and they've trained dogs to "gesture" by moving their heads or bodies in certain ways. Mini electronics in the collar would interpret the gestures and put into words what the dog is trying to get across. It's like the talking vest, only without a dog having to do anything with her mouth. It just requires a little choreography on the part of the dog.

And then there's touchscreen technology. At this point the touchscreen the FIDO folks are using is the size of a medium flat-screen TV. The screen in a real-life scenario could be significantly smaller. Depending on its use, it might be only the size of a large tablet if portability is important.

Dr. Jackson and Sky showed me how it works. "Help!" Dr. Jackson said, undramatically, while looking at Sky. He immediately reached back to pull a sensor on his vest, but this wasn't the right vest. Realizing he was outfitted in his nontalking vest, he performed his other "help" function without missing a beat.

He ran over to the screen, where the numbers "9-1-1" appeared in white, against three circles colored bright blue, yellow, and green. Sky touched them in sequence, but nothing happened. Dr. Jackson explained that his nose hadn't hit them just right. He tried again, and this time the screen switched to a notification that an alert had been sent.

I asked if it would be easier to just have a large "HELP" button dogs could bump with their noses in an emergency. Dr. Jackson said it would be too easy, with dogs calling 9-1-1 or other emergency contacts if they accidentally touched it with their nose.

As service dogs like Terri Krake's Brody can tell you, there are already devices dogs can use to summon help in an emergency. Brody, as you may recall, runs over and presses a big life-alert button with his paw if Terri is in trouble from a seizure. A notification goes to a chain of family and friends, or 9-1-1, or both.

The 9-1-1 feature of the Georgia Tech touchscreen is partly a trial to see if dogs can work with touchscreens and how touchscreens react to dogs. Slobber was a confounding factor for a while, but they've worked out some fixes.

FIDO researchers are investigating ways working dogs might be able to communicate using this technology. They've been exploring how dogs react to the colors, shapes, size, and placement of icons. The goal is to see if dogs can be trained to use a touchscreen to communicate information specific to their job.

Dr. Jackson says icons could be linked to a text or voice message for easy conveyance of what a dog is trying to communicate. She envisions touchscreen applications being a useful tool for dogs who help the hearing impared. They could alert their deaf handlers to different sounds by pressing icons that would send them text messages like "doorbell is ringing" or "tornado siren."

Dogs have already proven to be rapid and enthusiastic learners of touchscreen technology. Researchers in Budapest and Vienna have trained more than two hundred pet dogs to nose-touch certain images on a screen. The results are promising, with researchers concluding: "The power of the touchscreen as a training tool is in its flexibility, reliability and controllability, and in its ability to provide novel motivational experiences. The number of cognitive training possibilities are limitless . . ."

Other researchers have used touchscreens to determine if dogs can discriminate between emotional expressions in human faces. With continuing research into dogs interacting with screens, it may not be long before your dog is asking (via her pleading eyes or a talking vest) for an iPad of her own.

Depending on what researchers learn in their ongoing quest to find the scent of cancers, dogs might be able to use icons or even an onscreen slider—like those we use for volume, only easier to manipulate—to communicate the strength of the scent. This might tell researchers something about the stage of the cancer. Or dogs could even identify the type of cancer if it turns out cancers do have distinct odors.

Applications go well beyond the health and service dog field. Bomb dogs might be able to give more specific information about what they're smelling. They could tap their nose on an icon they've learned to associate with a specific explosive scent, and let their handler or the explosive ordnance disposal technician know what they've detected. Same with narcotics dogs.

It's easy to see how touchscreen technology might evolve to become popular with people and their pets. Just the other evening, Gus bolted down to the front door and barked as if Godzilla himself (or herself? The debate rages on) were trying to get into the house. I was annoyed because I was delving into some complex research for the book and didn't want to break my concentration. But he wouldn't stop, so I headed downstairs to check what was going on. The stripe of fur along Gus's spine had bristled to make him look vaguely larger, and he was barking and growling at something invisible to my eyes.

"*What* are you barking at?" I asked. In response he barked some more until I got him to stop and shooed him upstairs. This is where a Georgia Tech touchscreen of colorful icons could have come in handy.

I'd hand Gus his slobber-proof screen, where he could choose from the following options, symbolized by icons he'd been trained to recognize.

Cat!
Someone raiding our recycling bin!
Bad guy!
Raccoon!
Evil mail carrier!
Skunk!
Evil UPS worker!
Godzilla!
I have no idea!

In England, computer scientists are having a different conversation with dogs. It's a conversation led by dogs, so instead of words, the dogs are conveying their side of the story with their noses.

The biodetection canines at Medical Detection Dogs seem to do an excellent job at detecting the scent of cancer, but founder Claire Guest felt there was a breakdown in the flow of communication that—if fixed—could make them even more accurate.

Claire met Clara Mancini, PhD, at an MDD open house several years ago. Dr. Mancini is the founder and head of the Animal-Computer Interaction (ACI) Lab and the Pervasive Interaction Lab at the Open University (UK). Her research focuses on animal-centered approaches to design and research. She wants working animals to be able to do their tasks in a manner that's more natural to them. It's better for the animals and could lead to improved results.

Claire told Clara that she and the other trainers felt they were missing opportunities for the biodetection dogs to be able to convey more information than just a simple yes or no. She thought if researchers could provide dogs with a new way of answering the question of whether cancer is present in a sample, the dogs might be able to tell them more.

They discussed the possibility of dogs being able to show not only whether a sample was positive or negative, but also how sure they were of their assessment. Some samples might be in between, and that's important information to be able to convey.

Researchers think that in some cases an unsure response could mean a dog is picking up on very early cancer. If the trainers don't know a sample has the VOCs of the beginnings of cancer, the dog won't get rewarded and might be confused about what to do. MDD's trainers were troubled by the times they could tell a dog had accidentally passed a positive cancer sample and seemed to want a do-over. A dog would flick her head in its direction or alert at the next position, which wouldn't get her any reward. There are no do-overs, so data may not always reflect what a dog knows.

The ACI team tried to figure out the best way for dogs to communicate the nuances they might be detecting. They bounced around the idea of a keyboard system, where dogs could use their paws to tap a small number of large buttons to show whether a sample was positive, negative, or in between. They'd seen this kind of setup work for dogs to ask for food, water, or going out.

But this solution didn't seem natural for the dogs. Dogs usually interact with objects using their mouths and noses, not their paws. The researchers wanted the dogs to stay focused to do their best job, and not come off a scent to perform an activity that could be distracting.

Eventually the researchers realized that the dogs were interacting with samples spontaneously, often pressing their noses more strongly into the ones that were positive and lingering longer. So they designed and developed an interface with pressure sensors connected to the metal plates that hold the samples. They recorded the degree of pressure the dogs were exerting with each sample and graphed the results. The beauty of it was that they gained more information without any additional training.

Instead of cancer samples, ACI scientists have recently been using amyl acetate, a compound that smells like bananas and is sometimes used as a flavoring agent. It's better for initial research because it's consistent, and easy to control the concentrations.

The results so far have been encouraging. It's easy to see the positives, the negatives, and the ones where the dogs were unsure. Do-overs aren't necessary with a system like this. Researchers can refer to the graphs to see how a dog reacted.

"I'm very happy with how it's going," Dr. Mancini says. "By engaging with animals on their own terms, our research can provide the opportunity to better understand animals, their capacities and perspective. . . . It is wonderful what you can learn from dogs if you just know how to listen."

Dogs have been listening all along. It's part of what makes their bedside manner so appealing.

People who work at the intersection of dogs and science believe that doctor dogs will soon be ready to take their place at a kind of global bedside; that dogs have what it takes to help keep the world safer from natural scourges—stopping the spread of deadly disease outbreaks before they become epidemics or, worse, pandemics. They may even be able to protect us from bioterrorism. It's a matter of being able to train dogs, test them, and deploy them where they're needed.

"Dogs are portable rapid detectors. There's real potential for expanding their detection of biological targets," says Dr. Angle, of Auburn University. "But there are real challenges, too."

In a paper in *Frontiers in Veterinary Science*, Dr. Angle and his coauthors urged researchers to realize "there are intricacies in training dogs on biological targets that are complex and unlike any skill set utilized in other aspects of dog training. A detection dog is a highly complex sensory technology, and not understanding its full capabilities and its influences could skew study results to not reflect the true potential of a dog."

It's up to us to get it right. Fortunately, dogs, being dogs, will help us along the way.

What would it look like to have dogs on the front lines of containing a disease?

No one can say for sure, but it might be something as simple as dogs working at a checkpoint for malaria and sniffing everyone who passes through. Think airport dogs, only in a variety of settings, and sniffing for disease, not explosives. If an explosives-detection dog at an airport alerts on someone, that person will be thoroughly checked out before being permitted to proceed. Similarly, if a malaria dog alerts on someone, the person would probably need to be tested before being allowed to enter an area that has eradicated or greatly reduced malaria.

It gets more complicated for some other diseases. Take the Ebola virus. Instead of checkpoints where dogs would smell people passing through, Dr. Angle thinks dogs could expedite testing of people behind the scenes.*

If dogs could be trained to detect Ebola from cheek swabs placed inside individual containers, for instance, they could sniff large quantities quickly. As with malaria, if a dog alerts, the donor would need further testing.

"They can't run blood tests on a thousand people moving through an area," Dr. Angle says, "but they can do a quick swab, and dogs could act as an initial screen. It could greatly help containment."

It's going to take time and a deep commitment and investment in research to get to the point where dogs could one day help save lives on a massive scale. Fortunately, the work has already begun.

The pathogen hunt has started in hospitals, but walls won't contain these doctor dogs for much longer. If all goes well with the malaria study, we could be seeing dogs helping beat down this disease in Africa within a few years.

As dogs succeed, there will likely be no shortage of ideas for how they can help detect other diseases. And not just ones that cause illness in humans. Dr. Angle thinks dogs could be invaluable in detecting pathogens in livestock, crops, and soil.

Meanwhile cancer-detection dogs will be hard at work in their quest to find the odor of cancer in exchange for their favorite toy or treat. Researchers will keep looking for ways to improve screening. More researchers from a variety of disciplines are joining the quest all the time.

I recently received an email from the Royal Dutch Guide Dog Foundation, which provides guide dogs and other service dogs and trains cancer-detection dogs. I had visited the Amsterdam-area

---

*The CDC reports that dogs can be infected with Ebola, but that there is no evidence they have symptoms or that they can spread it to people or other animals. (Sadly, in 2014, authorities in Spain—against overwhelming public outcry from around the world—overreacted and euthanized the dog of a nurse infected with Ebola.)

organization and watched its dogs sniff for colorectal cancer as part of a pilot study. The group has now been asked by the Leiden University Medical Center to see if biodetection dogs can find cancer in blood samples of women under age forty who have a common breast cancer gene. Patrick Hilverink, the head of medical detection dogs for the foundation, wrote me that mammography is "far from effective for this group, with only 40 percent sensitivity."

Their goal is to find breast cancer early and reliably. "It would of course be fantastic if these dogs could make a valuable contribution here and save lives," he wrote.

If all goes well, those of us at higher risk for cancers that are hard to detect early will be able to have our blood, urine, or saliva analyzed by a reliable dog scan that will give us peace of mind for six months or a year or more. (This is assuming that researchers can get past the significant challenges of screening discussed in Chapter 3.) If something like this were around for ovarian cancer, I'd be less likely to consider going under the knife prophylactically.

Dr. Angle understands this line of reasoning: "If someone is on the fence 50-50 about having an organ or gland removed because of their cancer risk, and there were solid data showing dogs are 85 to 90 percent capable of detecting it at an early stage during screenings, they might opt to keep getting checked by cancer-detection dogs.

"In your case," he told me, "you might end up being able to kick the can down the road if dogs give you the clear."

We're not there yet, though. Right now, because of the lack of good testing for this cancer, I'm kicking the can in the dark. I could end up over a cliff if I'm not careful. I'm not alone. There are people with much higher cancer risks than mine who would benefit even more than I could from having dogs detect cancer early.

In the war on cancer, dogs could be there to keep as many people as possible from danger—just as they do on the battlefields. It's a comforting and hopeful thought.

But with the way e-nose technologies are advancing, cancer-sniffing devices may be here before the dogs deploy as a significant force against cancer. The olfaction technologies dogs are helping develop could have far-reaching impacts—even beyond cancer.

MIT's Dr. Mershin thinks the e-nose his team is working on for cancer could easily be adapted for other uses.

"There's no limit. Remember that if it smells, we can find it. Whatever dogs' or other noses have ever been used for before, nano-noses can be used, only they will be faster, better, and eventually cheaper—although they are currently prohibitively expensive, same as early cameras and computers."

He's in good company with his ideas about expanding e-nose technology beyond cancer. A certain queen of the United Kingdom recently brought this up to him.

On the day Medical Detection Dogs gave its demonstrations at Buckingham Palace's Royal Mews, Dr. Mershin was among the lucky attendees who got to meet Queen Elizabeth.

"I was blown away," he says of their meeting. It wasn't necessarily her refinement and grace that won his admiration. It was the way the nonagenarian monarch seemed truly and intelligently interested in the miniaturized version of MIT's e-nose.

"She held the nose in her hand. Her elegant, gloved hand. And she asked me really good questions. She was genuinely curious. She wanted to know how the dogs are working to help what we're doing.

"She even asked if we could put a device like this in airports for malaria," he says. "I've met a lot of celebrities at MIT. They're great, but you don't expect to get ideas from them. But here was the ninety-two-year-old queen with this brilliant thought."

His answer was yes, absolutely. This delighted the queen.

It seems we all love a good dog story. But if the happy ending involves small, lifesaving devices that dogs helped humans invent, that's OK, too.

One day we may look back at this era with nostalgia. We will tell our children or grandchildren, who may tell their children and grandchildren, that there was once a time when people were getting sick and dying from many diseases, but that our best friends were at our side, helping us figure out what was wrong. The dogs did what they loved to do—they used their incredible noses—and we rewarded them with love and toys and treats.

We communicated as best as two species could, and eventually the dogs led us to the scents of danger. They helped us develop advanced machines that became widely available and easy for almost anyone to use.

Thanks to the dogs, and the researchers who believed in them, the world became a healthier place.

———

As I sit at my desk seven months after the publication of the hardcover edition of this book, some details of everyday life remain the same. The model of the dog's nose Gus once coveted is still tucked out of his reach on a shelf. Gus lies sleeping in the sun in his favorite spot just outside the open cottage door.

But now, to my left lie three plastic storage bins. They're crammed with beans, rice, pasta, soup, oatmeal, flour, nuts, and other foods with a long shelf life. An envelope of surgical masks sits atop a giant package of paper towels. It looks more like a dry goods store than my peaceful writing cottage.

The word "coronavirus" has made its way into our lexicon, and the disease has profoundly changed the way people live. There have been more than five million cases, with almost 300,000 deaths. The virus's fallout will soon be much higher.

The news is filled with grim statistics and frightening stories. We long to get back to a normal life, or something resembling it. As we wait for a vaccine, no matter how busy and upbeat we try to keep, it's easy to feel down, worried, at times even hopeless.

And that's where dogs come in. That's where dogs always seem to come in—when we need them most.

For the past few weeks, some of the best medical detection dog institutions in the world have been training dogs on the scent of

SARS-CoV-2, the virus that causes COVID-19, in laboratory samples. As reported in Chapter 6, dogs at the Canine Performance Sciences program at Auburn University have already been able to detect viruses, and even to tell the difference between viruses. Those dogs were sniffing out bovine viruses, but it's promising.

If the proof-of-concept trials succeed, the next step will be to see if dogs can sniff out actual people with COVID-19. At this point no one knows if they'd be smelling the virus, the body's response to the virus, or both. This phase will be trickier, because there are so many unknowns, such as whether asymptomatic people have the same scent as those with symptoms. Even extraneous factors, like what someone ate that day, or if they have another illness, might be distractors that affect the results.

But if dogs can do this with a decent degree of accuracy, it could be a game changer. If enough dogs become COVID detectors, they could be responsible for a great reduction in community spread of the virus. They may be stationed as screeners at places like airports, sporting events, and other venues where there are large numbers of people. If it goes well, who knows—COVID dogs may even be coming to a mall near you, helping to ensure shoppers are virus-free.

The London School of Hygiene & Tropical Medicine's Dr. Logan thinks dogs have the potential to be a "new diagnostic tool" that "could revolutionize our response to COVID-19." The school is once again working with Claire Guest and the crew at Medical Detection Dogs, after their successful trials with dogs detecting malaria on clothing. Scientists and trainers in Australia, Iran, Spain, France, Finland, and the Netherlands are immersed in their own COVID detection dog studies.

Even though at this point only three dogs in the world are thought to have contracted the virus, the safety of COVID detection dogs is a source of much concern. Researchers at Canine Performance Sciences have developed methods to capture viral target odors and sterilize them to a safe level for the dogs. Other venues are doing what they can.

Penn Vet Working Dog Center's Dr. Otto is leading a team that's determining if eight Labrador retrievers will be able to detect the virus. When the school announced the study earlier this month, Dr. Otto fielded dozens of media interviews from around the globe, with resulting stories appearing in nearly four hundred news outlets— evidence of how hungry we are for something to make the world safer, to revive tanking economies, to bring us a little closer to the lives we once knew but maybe didn't always appreciate.

If all goes as hoped, the term "good dog" will take on extra meaning for the world as our intrepid best friends help curb the spread of COVID-19, saving untold numbers of lives, and having a ball (or favorite treat) doing it.

SOURCES

All interviews for this book took place between January 2017 and January 2019, mostly in person but also by phone, FaceTime, Skype, email, texts, Facebook, WhatsApp, Line, and (true story) snail mail.

What follows is a list of my main sources by chapter. You may notice there are no dog books. This is because I relied on primary sources when possible, and because other dog books have not dealt with most of the contents of this book. But my knowledge of dogs has been enriched over the years by dozens of books, and I'd like to share a few of the more relevant ones in case you'd like further reading.

For more on a dog's sense of smell, check out *Being a Dog*, by Alexandra Horowitz, and if you want to become a super dog-nose nerd, I'd recommend the more technical but fascinating *Canine Olfaction Science and Law*, edited by Tadeusz Jezierski, John Ensminger, and L. E. Papet. Favorite books that have helped me learn about the way dogs think and the way they sense the world include *The Genius of Dogs*, by Brian Hare and Vanessa Woods; *How Dogs Love Us*, by Gregory Berns; *How Dogs Think*, by Stanley Coren; *Dog Sense*, by John Bradshaw; *Dog Behaviour, Evolution, and Cognition*, by Ádám Miklósi; *Inside of a Dog*, by Alexandra Horowitz; and *The Other End of the Leash*, by Patricia McConnell.

You may also notice that within each chapter's list of people I interviewed, there are no dogs. It seems my publisher doesn't include dogs in the "people" category. Gus apologizes to all of the dogs in this book, from Ajax to Zen.

INTRODUCTION: THE DOCTOR'S NOSE

Agence France-Presse in Paris. "Bomb Detector Works Better with Fake Dog Nose on the End." *The Guardian*, 1 December 2016. www.theguardian.com/science/2016/dec/02/bomb-sniffer-works-better-with-fake-dog-nose-on-the-end.

Alberge, Dalya. "Dogs Trained to Sniff Out Ancient Treasures Looted from Syria." *The Guardian*, 11 March 2018. www.theguardian.com/artanddesign/2018/mar/11/dogs-trained-to-sniff-out-ancient-treasures-looted-from-syria.

Amann, Anton, et al. "The Human Volatilome: Volatile Organic Compounds (VOCs) in Exhaled Breath, Skin Emanations, Urine, Feces and Saliva." *Journal of Breath Research* 8, no. 3 (September 2014): 034001, doi:10.1088/1752-7155/8/3/034001.

American College of Obstetricians and Gynecologists (ACOG). "ACOG Statement on FDA Safety Communication on Ovarian Cancer Screening Tests." News release, 8 September 2016. www.acog.org/About-ACOG/News-Room/Statements/2016

/ACOG-Statement-on-FDA-Safety-Communication-on-Ovarian-Cancer
-Screening-Tests.

Angle, Craig, et al. "Canine Detection of the Volatilome: A Review of Implications for
Pathogen and Disease Detection." *Frontiers in Veterinary Science* 3 (24 June 2016),
doi:10.3389/fvets.2016.00047.

"Canines for Conservation." *Steve Austin: Canine Training and Behaviour.* Accessed 2 February 2018. www.steveaustindogtrainer.com/services/canines-for-conservation/.

"Conservation Canines." Center for Conservation Biology, University of Washington. Accessed 1 August 2018. conservationbiology.uw.edu/conservation-canines/.

Costello, B. de Lacy, et al. "A Review of the Volatiles from the Healthy Human Body." *Journal of Breath Research* 8, no. 1 (March 2014): 014001, doi:10.1088/1752-7155/8/1/014001.

Craven, Brent A., et al. "The Fluid Dynamics of Canine Olfaction: Unique Nasal Airflow
Patterns as an Explanation of Macrosmia." *Journal of the Royal Society Interface* 7,
no. 47 (9 December 2009): 933–943, doi:10.1098/rsif.2009.0490.

"Cremains Recovery after California Wildfire." Institute for Canine Forensics. Accessed
1 November 2018. https://www.icfk9.org/cremains-recovery.

Cuthbert, Lori. "How Sniffer Dogs Find Cremated Human Remains after Wildfires."
National Geographic, 30 October 2018. www.nationalgeographic.com/animals
/2018/10/sniffer-dogs-human-remains-california-wildfires-cremation-news/.

Daley, Jason. "Sniffer Dogs Represent the Latest Weapon in the Fight Against the Illegal
Ivory Trade." *Smithsonian*, 28 August 2018. www.smithsonianmag.com/smart
-news/sniffer-dogs-and-new-technology-team-save-elephants-180970143/.

Donahue, Michelle Z. "Meet the Dogs Sniffing Out Whale Poop for Science." *Smithsonian*,
8 February 2016. www.smithsonianmag.com/science-nature/meet-dogs-sniffing
-out-whale-poop-science-180958050/.

Fiegl, Amanda. "Meet Migaloo, World's First 'Archaeology Dog.'" *National Geographic*,
11 December 2012. news.nationalgeographic.com/news/2012/12/121210-archae
ology-dogs-australia-conservation-canines/.

Geggel, Laura. "Elephants Can Outsniff Rats and Dogs." *LiveScience*, 22 July 2014. www
.livescience.com/46940-elephant-genes-sense-of-smell.html.

Gray, Richard. "The Many Reasons Why Dogs Might Roll in Smelly Poo." *Earth*, BBC
News, 8 June 2017. www.bbc.com/earth/story/20170608-the-many-reasons-why
-dogs-might-roll-in-smelly-poo.

"Hero Rats." YouTube video, 1:19, published by iloveratrats, 4 July 2011. https://youtu.be
/WS1gh3QtB44.

Interviews with Matthew Staymates, PhD, fluid dynamicist and mechanical engineer,
National Institute of Standards and Technology; Craig Angle, PhD, codirector,
Canine Performance Sciences, College of Veterinary Medicine, Auburn Univer-
sity; Cindy Otto, DVM, PhD, founder and executive director, Penn Vet Working
Dog Center, University of Pennsylvania; Naoto Anzue, Guide Dog & Service Dog
& Hearing Dog Association of Japan; Marie-José Enders, PhD, Royal Dutch
Guide Dog Foundation; Dina Zaphiris, In Situ Foundation; Leone, Renato, and
Zeljka Brašnić; Takayuki Uozumi, PhD, and Kazuko Matsubara, PhD, Hirotsu
Bio Science; Robyn Stark, program manager, Steve Austin Conservation Canines;
and Clive Wynne, PhD, Canine Science Collaboratory, Arizona State University.

Japan Assistance Dog Welfare Association. Accessed October 2017. http://www.kaijoken
.or.jp/about/index.html.

Jenkins, Eileen K., et al. "When the Nose Doesn't Know: Canine Olfactory Function
Associated with Health, Management, and Potential Links to Microbiota." *Frontiers in Veterinary Science* 5 (29 March 2018), doi:10.3389/fvets.2018.00056.

"Key Statistics for Ovarian Cancer." American Cancer Society. Accessed November 2018.
www.cancer.org/cancer/ovarian-cancer/about/key-statistics.html.

Kimball, Bruce A., et al. "Avian Influenza Infection Alters Fecal Odor in Mallards." *PLoS One* 8, no. 10 (16 October 2013), doi:10.1371/journal.pone.0075411.

Levenson, Richard M., et al. "Pigeons (*Columba livia*) as Trainable Observers of Pathology and Radiology Breast Cancer Images." *PLoS One* 10, no. 11 (18 November 2015), doi:10.1371/journal.pone.0141357.

Mangaly, Jennifer. "About a Wolf's Sense of Smell." *Sciencing*, last modified 24 April 2017. sciencing.com/wolfs-sense-smell-4565769.html.

Niimura, Yoshihito, et al. "Extreme Expansion of the Olfactory Receptor Gene Repertoire in African Elephants and Evolutionary Dynamics of Orthologous Gene Groups in 13 Placental Mammals." *Genome Research* 24, no. 9 (September 2014): 1485–1496, doi:10.1101/gr.169532.113.

Perlman, Howard. "A Million Gallons of Water—How Much Is It?" USGS Water Science School, last modified 6 September 2018. water.usgs.gov/edu/mgd.html.

Seidel, Jamie. "Could Cats Replace Search-and-Rescue Dogs? If We Can Motivate Them." News.com.au, 11 October 2017. www.news.com.au/technology/science /animals/could-cats-replace-searchandrescue-dogs-if-we-can-motivate-them/news -story/57b549f5a2f77399485412c696fdb84b.

Shirasu, Mika, and Kazushige Touhara. "The Scent of Disease: Volatile Organic Compounds of the Human Body Related to Disease and Disorder." *Journal of Biochemistry* 150, no. 3 (September 2011): 257–266, doi:10.1093/jb/mvr090.

Shreve, Kristyn R. Vitale, and Monique A. R. Udell. "Stress, Security, and Scent: The Influence of Chemical Signals on the Social Lives of Domestic Cats and Implications for Applied Settings." *Applied Animal Behaviour Science* 187 (February 2017): 69–76, doi:10.1016/j.applanim.2016.11.011.

Staymates, Matthew E., et al. "Biomimetic Sniffing Improves the Detection Performance of a 3D Printed Nose of a Dog and a Commercial Trace Vapor Detector." *Scientific Reports* 6, no. 1 (December 2016), doi:10.1038/srep36876.

Stingl, Jim. "Dog Sniffs Out Her Owner's Ovarian Cancer Three Times, and She Is Right on the Nose." *Milwaukee Journal Sentinel*, 30 November 2018. www.jsonline.com /story/news/columnists/jim-stingl/2018/11/30/womans-dog-detects-her-ovarian -cancer-three-times/2154700002/.

Strauch, Martin, et al. "More than Apples and Oranges—Detecting Cancer with a Fruit Fly's Antenna." *Scientific Reports* 4, no. 1 (6 January 2014), doi:10.1038/srep03576.

"13 Fun Facts about Bicycles in Amsterdam." *Awesome Amsterdam*. Accessed 9 October 2018. awesomeamsterdam.com/facts-about-bicycles-in-amsterdam/.

Tyson, Peter. "Dogs' Dazzling Sense of Smell." *NOVA*, PBS, 4 October 2012. www.pbs .org/wgbh/nova/article/dogs-sense-of-smell/.

University of Konstanz. "The Scent of Cancer: Detecting Cancer with Fruit Fly's Antenna." *ScienceDaily*, 24 January 2014. www.sciencedaily.com/releases/2014/01 /140124082702.htm.

Viegas, Jen. "Here's Why Cats Might Make Skilled Search and Rescue Animals." *Seeker*, 22 February 2017. www.seeker.com/why-cats-could-make-skilled-search-and -rescue-animals-2277969871.html.

Wasser, Samuel K, et al. "Scat Detection Dogs in Wildlife Research and Management: Application to Grizzly and Black Bears in the Yellowhead Ecosystem, Alberta, Canada." *Canadian Journal of Zoology* 82, no. 3 (March 2004): 475–492, doi:10.1139 /z04-020.

Williams, Caroline. "Crittervision: What a Dog's Nose Knows." *New Scientist*, 17 August 2011. www.newscientist.com/article/mg21128262-000-crittervision-what-a-dogs -nose-knows/.

World Health Organization. *Global Tuberculosis Report: 2018.* Accessed 2 January 2019. apps.who.int/iris/bitstream/handle/10665/274453/9789241565646-eng.pdf.

CHAPTER 1: STOP THE ROLLER COASTER, I WANT TO GET OFF

Alkeminder, Elisabeth. "Your Urine and Diabetes: What You Should Know." Diabetes Council, last modified 15 September 2018. www.thediabetescouncil.com/urine-and-diabetes/.

Blake, Donna. "The Evolution of Insulin Pumps." *Voice of the Diabetic* 15, no. 3 (Summer 2000). nfb.org/Images/nfb/Publications/vod/vsum0001.htm.

Brulliard, Karin. "Company Sold $25,000 'Service Dogs' That Were Really Just Untrained Puppies, Virginia Says." *Washington Post*, 8 May 2018. www.washingtonpost.com/news/animalia/wp/2018/05/08/company-sold-25000-service-dogs-that-were-really-just-untrained-puppies-virginia-says/.

"Cat Saves Man's Life." YouTube video, 1:26, published by Adam Knapik, 22 November 2011. https://youtu.be/v9_eGg7rD8Y.

Centers for Disease Control and Prevention. "New CDC Report: More Than 100 Million Americans Have Diabetes or Prediabetes." News release, 18 July 2017. www.cdc.gov/media/releases/2017/p0718-diabetes-report.html.

Centers for Disease Control and Prevention. "National Diabetes Statistics Report, 2017." www.cdc.gov/diabetes/pdfs/data/statistics/national-diabetes-statistics-report.pdf.

Chen, Mimi, et al. "Non-Invasive Detection of Hypoglycaemia Using a Novel, Fully Biocompatible and Patient Friendly Alarm System." *BMJ* 321, no. 7276 (23 December 2000): 1565–1566, doi:10.1136/bmj.321.7276.1565.

Dehlinger, Ky, et al. "Can Trained Dogs Detect a Hypoglycemic Scent in Patients with Type 1 Diabetes?" *Diabetes Care* 36, no. 7 (July 2013), doi:10.2337/dc12-2342.

"Diabetic Ketoacidosis." My VMC, last modified 31 May 2018. www.myvmc.com/diseases/diabetic-ketoacidosis/.

Eknoyan, Garabed, and Judit Nagy. "A History of Diabetes Mellitus or How a Disease of the Kidneys Evolved into a Kidney Disease." *Advances in Chronic Kidney Disease* 12, no. 2 (April 2005): 223–229, doi:10.1053/j.ackd.2005.01.002.

Fernando, Richard. "'There Are Ants in My Urine!'" *Philippine Daily Inquirer*, 1 August 2015. business.inquirer.net/196299/there-are-ants-in-my-urine.

Gonder-Frederick, Linda, et al. "Diabetic Alert Dogs: A Preliminary Survey of Current Users." *Diabetes Care* 36, no. 4 (April 2013), doi:10.2337/dc12-1998.

Gonder-Frederick, Linda A., et al. "Variability of Diabetes Alert Dog Accuracy in a Real-World Setting." *Journal of Diabetes Science and Technology* 11, no. 4 (July 2017): 714–719, doi:10.1177/1932296816685580.

Hardin, Dana S., et al. "Dogs Can Be Successfully Trained to Alert to Hypoglycemia Samples from Patients with Type 1 Diabetes." *Diabetes Therapy* 6, no. 4 (December 2015): 509–517, doi:10.1007/s13300-015-0135-x.

"Insulin Pumps." Diabetes.co.uk. Accessed 5 July 2018. www.diabetes.co.uk/insulin/Insulin-pumps.html.

Interviews with Clay, Karin, and Ken Ronk; Mark Ruefenacht, Ralph Hendrix, Mona Elder, and Carrie Treggett, Dogs4Diabetics; Kim Denton; Ben O'Neill and Dwight Cawthon, Ukiah High School; Jennifer Cattet, PhD, Medical Mutts; Luke and Dorrie Nuttall; Crystal Cockroft, Canine Hope for Diabetics; Steven Wolf, MD; Paolo Incontri (a.k.a. Bhante Upali) and Valentina Braconcini, L'Associazione Italiana Cani d'Allerta; and Lidia Calabro.

Kaplish, Lalita. "Diagnosing Diabetes: A Wee Taste of Honey." Wellcome Library, 14 November 2013. blog.wellcomelibrary.org/2013/11/diagnosing-diabetes-a-wee-taste-of-honey/.

Karamanou, Marianna, et al. "Milestones in the History of Diabetes Mellitus: The Main Contributors." *World Journal of Diabetes* 7, no. 1 (10 January 2016): 1–7, doi:10.4239/wjd.v7.i1.1.

Kearney, T., and C. Dang. "Diabetic and Endocrine Emergencies." *Postgraduate Medical Journal* 83, no. 976 (February 2007): 79–86, doi:10.1136/pgmj.2006.049445.

Los, Evan, et al. "Reliability of Trained Dogs to Alert to Hypoglycemia in Patients with Type 1 Diabetes." *Journal of Diabetes Science and Technology* (28 August 2016), doi: 10.1177/1932296816666537.

Luke & Jedi (website for *Luke & Jedi* documentary film). Accessed 7 September 2018. www.lukeandjedi.com/.

Maranda, Louise, et al. "A Novel Behavioral Intervention in Adolescents with Type 1 Diabetes Mellitus Improves Glycemic Control." *Diabetes Educator* 41, no. 2 (April 2015): 224–230, doi:10.1177/0145721714567235.

Maranda, Louise, and Olga T. Gupta. "Association between Responsible Pet Ownership and Glycemic Control in Youths with Type 1 Diabetes." *PLoS One* 11, no. 4 (22 April 2016), doi:10.1371/journal.pone.0152332.

Neupane, Sankalpa, et al. "Exhaled Breath Isoprene Rises During Hypoglycemia in Type 1 Diabetes." *Diabetes Care* 39, no. 7 (July 2016), doi:10.2337/dc16-0461.

O'Connor, M. B., et al. "A Dog's Detection of Low Blood Sugar: A Case Report." *Irish Journal of Medical Science* 177, no. 2 (June 2008): 155–157, doi:10.1007/s11845-008-0128-0.

Petry, N. M., et al. "Perceptions about Professionally and Non-Professionally Trained Hypoglycemia Detection Dogs." *Diabetes Research and Clinical Practice* 109, no. 2 (August 2015): 389–396, doi:10.1016/j.diabres.2015.05.023.

Realsen, Jaime, et al. "Morbidity and Mortality of Diabetic Ketoacidosis with and without Insulin Pump Care." *Diabetes Technology & Therapeutics* 14, no. 12 (2012), doi:10.1089/dia.2012.0161.

Rooney, Nicola J., et al. "Investigation into the Value of Trained Glycaemia Alert Dogs to Clients with Type I Diabetes." *PLoS One* 8, no. 8 (7 August 2013), doi:10.1371/journal.pone.0069921.

Seewoodhary, Jason, et al. "The Role of Diabetic Alert Dogs in the Management of Impaired Hypoglycaemia Awareness." *Practical Diabetes* 31, no. 8 (October 2014): 323–325, doi:10.1002/pdi.1895.

Tucker, Miriam E. "Can Diabetes Alert Dogs Help Sniff Out Low Blood Sugar?" NPR, 29 July 2016. www.npr.org/sections/health-shots/2016/07/29/487772706/can-dogs-help-sniff-out-low-blood-sugar-in-diabetes.

Twilley, Nicola. "Urine Flavour Wheels." *Edible Geography*, 19 October 2012. www.ediblegeography.com/urine-flavour-wheels/.

"Type 1 Diabetes." American Diabetes Association. Accessed 7 July 2018. www.diabetes.org/diabetes-basics/type-1/.

Weber, K. S., et al. "Do Dogs Sense Hypoglycaemia?" *Diabetic Medicine* 33, no. 7 (July 2016): 934–938, doi:10.1111/dme.12975.

Wells, Deborah L., et al. "Canine Responses to Hypoglycemia in Patients with Type 1 Diabetes." *Journal of Alternative and Complementary Medicine* 14, no. 10 (December 2008): 1235–1241, doi:10.1089/acm.2008.0288.

Wells, Deborah L., et al. "Feline Responses to Hypoglycemia in People with Type 1 Diabetes." *Journal of Alternative and Complementary Medicine* 17, no. 2 (February 2011): 99–100, doi:10.1089/acm.2010.0704.

CHAPTER 2: IT'S ABOUT TO HIT THE FAN

Barriaux, Marianne. "Dogs Trained to Warn of an Imminent Epileptic Fit." *The Guardian*, 16 October 2006. www.theguardian.com/business/2006/oct/16/lifeandhealth.medicineandhealth.

"Cancer Statistics." National Cancer Institute, last modified 27 April 2018. www.cancer.gov/about-cancer/understanding/statistics.

Catala, Amélie, et al. "Dog Alerting and/or Responding to Epileptic Seizures: A Scoping Review." *PLoS One* 13, no. 12 (4 December 2018), doi:10.1371/journal.pone.0208280.

Catala, Amélie, et al. "Dogs Demonstrate the Existence of an Epileptic Seizure Odour in Humans." *Scientific Reports*, 28 March 2019. www.nature.com/articles/541598 -019-40721-4?fbclid=lwAR1Uy_kfxu8qFrZoJSV40SNf75ev4bpDjwgplrJlx6lrZRep WBI34.

Charous, Steven J., et al. "The Effect of Vagal Nerve Stimulation on Voice." *The Laryngoscope* 111, no. 1 (November 2001): 2028–2031, doi:10.1097/00005537-200111000-00030.

Chitale, Radha. "Trauma, Depression Can Cause Seizures." ABC News, 1 May 2009. abcnews.go.com/Health/MindMoodNews/story?id=7473832.

"Croatian Rock Band Psihomodo Pop Touring USA & Canada." *Croatia Week*, 16 August 2018. www.croatiaweek.com/croatian-rock-band-psihomodo-pop-touring-usa -canada/.

Dalziel, Deborah J., et al. "Seizure-Alert Dogs: A Review and Preliminary Study." *Seizure* 12, no. 2 (March 2003): 115–120, doi:10.1016/s105913110200225x.

Davis, Jeanie Lerche. "Dogs Anticipate Epileptic Seizures." WebMD, 21 June 2004. www .webmd.com/epilepsy/news/20040621/dogs-anticipate-epileptic-seizures.

Doherty, Michael J., and Alan M. Haltiner. "Wag the Dog: Skepticism on Seizure Alert Canines." *Neurology* 68, no. 4 (23 January 2007): 309, doi:10.1212/01.wnl.0000252369 .82956.a3.

Dreier, Natalie. "Woman Mauled, Killed by Dog While She Had Seizure." KIRO, 24 August 2018. www.kiro7.com/news/trending-now/woman-mauled-killed-by-dog -while-she-had-seizure/819857372.

"Egyptian Man Goes into Seizure, Attacked and Killed by His Dogs." Al Arabiya English, 5 December 2016. english.alarabiya.net/en/variety/2016/12/05/Egyptian-man -goes-into-seizure-attacked-and-killed-by-his-dogs-.html.

"Epidogs International Inventory of Seizure Alert Dogs." ClinicalTrials.gov, NIH US National Library of Medicine, 31 August 2018. clinicaltrials.gov/ct2/show/NCT03655366.

"Epilepsy Foundation's Position on Seizure 'Predicting' Dogs." Epilepsy Foundation. Accessed 15 September 2018. www.epilepsy.com/learn/seizure-first-aid-and-safety /staying-safe/seizure-dogs/seizure-predicting-dogs.

"FAQs." Canine Assistants. Accessed July 2018. www.canineassistants.org/faqs/.

Interviews with Davor, Sanja, Matea, and Zdravko Kobešćak; Lea Devčić and Damir Vučić, Croatian Guide Dog and Mobility Association; Leslie and Brandon Fong; Judy McDonald, Little Angels Service Dogs; Natalie and Lisa Tapio; Tonya Guy, Canine Partners for Life; Terri Krake and Lora Kennedy; Mona Elder; Alan Peters, Can Do Canines; and Nathaniel Hall, PhD, director, Canine Olfaction Research and Education Laboratory, Texas Tech University.

Kirton, Adam. "Pseudoseizure Dogs." *Neurology* 68, no. 23 (5 June 2007): 2045–2046, doi:10.1212/01.wnl.0000268590.95483.74.

Kirton, Adam, et al. "Seizure-Alerting and -Response Behaviors in Dogs Living with Epileptic Children." *Neurology* 62, no. 12 (22 June 2004): 2303–2305, doi:10.1212 /wnl.62.12.2303.

Kirton, Adam, et al. "Seizure Response Dogs: Evaluation of a Formal Training Program." *Epilepsy & Behavior* 13, no. 3 (October 2008): 499–504, doi:10.1016/j.yebeh.2008 .05.011.

Krauss, Gregory L., et al. "Pseudoseizure Dogs." *Neurology* 68, no. 4 (23 January 2007): 308–309, doi:10.1212/01.wnl.0000250345.23677.6b.

Lou, Nicole. "Can Dogs Predict Seizures?" *NOVA*, PBS, 20 July 2017. www.pbs.org/wgbh /nova/article/seizure-alert-dogs/.

Magness, Josh. "'When Is Mommy Coming?' Woman Mauled to Death by Her Dog as

4-Year-Old Calls for Help." *Miami Herald*, 24 August 2018. www.miamiherald
.com/news/nation-world/national/article217265390.html.

Moawad, Heidi. "An Overview of Lennox-Gastaut Syndrome." *Verywell Health*, last modified 12 February 2019. www.verywellhealth.com/lennox-gastaut-syndrome
-overview-4172378.

Ortiz, Rafael, and Joyce Liporace. "'Seizure-Alert Dogs': Observations from an Inpatient
Video/EEG Unit." *Epilepsy & Behavior* 6, no. 4 (June 2005): 620–622, doi:10.1016/j
.yebeh.2005.02.012.

Piña-Garza, Jesus Eric, et al. "Challenges in Identifying Lennox–Gastaut Syndrome in
Adults: A Case Series Illustrating Its Changing Nature." *Epilepsy & Behavior Case
Reports* 5 (11 February 2016): 38–43, doi:10.1016/j.ebcr.2016.01.004.

Ramos, Stephanie. "Pet Dogs Detect Seizures Before They Happen." ABC News. Accessed 14 September 2018. abcnews.go.com/Health/Technology/story?id=118221.

"Seizure Alert Dogs." Canine Partners for Life. Accessed 4 June 2018. k94life.org/seizure
-alert/.

"Seizure-Alert Dogs—Just the Facts, Hold the Media Hype." Epilepsy Foundation,
1 November 2007. www.epilepsy.com/article/2014/3/seizure-alert-dogs-just-facts
-hold-media-hype.

"Seizure Alert Dogs." Little Angels Service Dogs. Accessed 4 May 2018. www.littlean
gelsservicedogs.org/seizure-alert-dogs/.

Shafer, Patricia O. "New Terms for Seizure Classification." Epilepsy Foundation, last
modified 23 December 2016. www.epilepsy.com/learn/types-seizures/new-terms
-seizure-classification.

Shafer, Patricia O., and Patricia M. Dean. "Vagus Nerve Stimulation (VNS)." Epilepsy
Foundation, last modified 12 March 2018. www.epilepsy.com/learn/treating
-seizures-and-epilepsy/devices/vagus-nerve-stimulation-vns.

Singer, Emily. "Dogs Can Predict Epileptic Seizures." *New Scientist*, 21 June 2004. www
.newscientist.com/article/dn6047-dogs-can-predict-epileptic-seizures/.

Strong, Val, et al. "Effect of Trained Seizure Alert Dogs® on Frequency of Tonic-Clonic
Seizures." *Seizure* 11, no. 6 (September 2002): 402–405, doi:10.1053/seiz.2001.0656.

Strong, Val, et al. "Seizure-Alert Dogs—Fact or Fiction?" *Seizure* 8, no. 1 (February 1999):
62–65, doi:10.1053/seiz.1998.0250.

Strong, Val, and Stephen W. Brown. "Should People with Epilepsy Have Untrained Dogs
as Pets?" *Seizure* 9, no. 6 (September 2000): 427–430, doi:10.1053/seiz.2000.0429.

Warner, Jennifer. "Dogs Respond to Non-Epileptic Seizures." WebMD, 22 January 2007.
www.webmd.com/epilepsy/news/20070122/dogs-respond-non-epileptic-seizures.

"Worldwide Cancer Data." World Cancer Research Fund, 12 September 2018. www.wcrf
.org/dietandcancer/cancer-trends/worldwide-cancer-data.

CHAPTER 3: A DOCTOR DOG IN THIS FIGHT

Alexander, Jack. "Pet Dog Sniffs Out Gal's Cancer." *Weekly World News*, 2 May 1989. books
.google.com/books?id=g-wDAAAAMBAJ&pg=PA17&lpg=PA17&dq=%22bonita
+whitfield%22+england&source=bl&ots=0woD2Fzr4H&sig=P8JOj-nX2fmbs1FJTa
pTTUN1F_Y&hl=en&sa=X&ved=2ahUKEwiE4v-ilr7dAhUGbawKHfX1AqYQ6
AEwBHoECAAQAQ#v=onepage&q=%22bonita%20whitfield%22%20england&f
=false.

Amundsen, Tore, et al. "Can Dogs Smell Lung Cancer? First Study Using Exhaled Breath
and Urine Screening in Unselected Patients with Suspected Lung Cancer." *Acta
Oncologica* 53, no. 3 (2014): 307–315, doi:10.3109/0284186x.2013.819996.

Associated Press. "Hirohito Dies, Ending 62 Years as Japan's Ruler." *Los Angeles Times*,
8 January 1989. articles.latimes.com/1989-01-08/news/mn-196_1_emperor-hirohito.

Associated Press. "Police Dog Trained to Sniff Out Cancer." *Los Angeles Times*, 21 January 1996. articles.latimes.com/1996-01-21/news/mn-27027_1_skin-cancer.

"Bacteria That Can Lead to Cancer." American Cancer Society, last modified 11 July 2016. www.cancer.org/cancer/cancer-causes/infectious-agents/infections-that-can-lead -to-cancer/bacteria.html.

Bedford, Tom. "The iPhone 11 or Apple Watch 5 Could Monitor Your Body Smells." *TechRadar*, 5 April 2019. www.techradar.com/news/the-iphone-11-or-apple-watch -5-could-monitor-your-body-smells.

Bird, Isabella L. *Unbeaten Tracks in Japan* (Mineola, NY: Dover Publications, 2005).

Butts, David. "Japanese Doctors Lie about Cancer." UPI, 18 December 1988. www.upi .com/Archives/1988/12/18/Japanese-doctors-lie-about-cancer/6461598424400/.

Campbell, Leon Frederick, et al. "Canine Olfactory Detection of Malignant Melanoma." *BMJ Case Reports* 2013 (14 October 2013), doi:10.1136/bcr-2013-008566.

"Cancer Cell Lines." *Sigma-Aldrich*. Accessed 10 September 2018. www.sigmaaldrich .com/life-science/cell-culture/cancer-cell-lines.html.

Chen, Angus. "We Unravel the Science Mysteries of Asparagus Pee." NPR, 14 December 2016. www.npr.org/sections/thesalt/2016/12/14/505420193/we-unravel-the -science-mysteries-of-asparagus-pee.

Church, John, and Hywel Williams. "Another Sniffer Dog for the Clinic?" *The Lancet* 358, no. 9285 (15 September 2001): 930, doi:10.1016/s0140-6736(01)06065-2.

Cornu, Jean-Nicolas, et al. "Olfactory Detection of Prostate Cancer by Dogs Sniffing Urine: A Step Forward in Early Diagnosis." *European Urology* 59, no. 2 (February 2011): 197–201, doi:10.1016/j.eururo.2010.10.006.

D'Amico, Arnaldo, et al. "An Investigation on Electronic Nose Diagnosis of Lung Cancer." *Lung Cancer* 68, no. 2 (May 2010): 170–176, doi:10.1016/j.lungcan.2009.11.003.

"Diagnosis of Cancer Through Dogs." Accessed 22 February 2019. http://www.dogprog nose.co.il/.

"Doctors Intrigued by Dog That Found a Tumor." Associated Press, 3 April 1989. www .apnews.com/09c7ccd2d83a30179239721751d3c6fd.

Eldridge, Lynne. "What It Means If You Have Precancerous Cells." *Verywell Health*, last modified 18 December 2018. www.verywellhealth.com/what-are-precancerous -cells-2248796.

Elliker, Kevin R, et al. "Key Considerations for the Experimental Training and Evaluation of Cancer Odour Detection Dogs: Lessons Learnt from a Double-Blind, Controlled Trial of Prostate Cancer Detection." *BMC Urology* 14, no. 1 (27 February 2014), doi:10.1186/1471-2490-14-22.

Finamore, P., et al. "Analysis of Volatile Organic Compounds: An Innovative Approach to Heart Failure Characterization in Older Patients." *Journal of Breath Research* 12, no. 2 (April 2018): p. 026007, doi:10.1088/1752-7163/aa8cd4.

Fischer-Tenhagen, Carola, et al. "A Proof of Concept: Are Detection Dogs a Useful Tool to Verify Potential Biomarkers for Lung Cancer?" *Frontiers in Veterinary Science* 5 (14 March 2018), doi:10.3389/fvets.2018.00052.

Gasparri, Roberto, et al. "Volatile Signature for the Early Diagnosis of Lung Cancer." *Journal of Breath Research* 10, no. 1 (9 February 2016): 016007, doi:10.1088/1752 -7155/10/1/016007.

Gordon, A. C., and R. D. Spicer. "Impregnated Via a Bullet?" *The Lancet* 333, no. 8640 (1 April 1989): 737, doi:10.1016/s0140-6736(89)92264-2.

Gordon, Robert T., et al. "The Use of Canines in the Detection of Human Cancers." *Journal of Alternative and Complementary Medicine* 14, no. 1 (30 January 2008): 61–67, doi:10.1089/acm.2006.6408.

Hackner, Klaus, et al. "Canine Scent Detection for the Diagnosis of Lung Cancer in a

Screening-like Situation." *Journal of Breath Research* 10, no. 4 (27 September 2016): 046003, doi:10.1088/1752-7155/10/4/046003.

Hackner, Klaus, and Joachim Pleil. "Canine Olfaction as an Alternative to Analytical Instruments for Disease Diagnosis: Understanding 'Dog Personality' to Achieve Reproducible Results." *Journal of Breath Research* 11, no. 1 (9 January 2017): 012001, doi:10.1088/1752-7163/aa5524.

Horvath, György, et al. "Characteristic Odour in the Blood Reveals Ovarian Carcinoma." *BMC Cancer* 10, no. 1 (24 November 2010): doi:10.1186/1471-2407-10-643.

Horvath, György, et al. "Cancer Odor in the Blood of Ovarian Cancer Patients: A Retrospective Study of Detection by Dogs during Treatment, 3 and 6 Months Afterward." *BMC Cancer* 13, no. 1 (26 August 2013), doi:10.1186/1471-2407-13-396.

Horváth, I., et al. "Exhaled Biomarkers in Lung Cancer." *European Respiratory Journal* 34, no. 1 (July 2009): 261–275, doi:10.1183/09031936.00142508.

Interviews with Bonita and Jane Whitfield; Hywel Williams, MD, DSc, professor of dermato-epidemiology, Centre of Evidence Based Dermatology, University of Nottingham; Claire Guest, Rob Harris, and Jenny Corish, Medical Detection Dogs; Patrick Hilverink and Danielle de Jonge, Royal Dutch Guide Dog Foundation; Craig Angle, PhD, codirector, Canine Performance Sciences, College of Veterinary Medicine, Auburn University; Cindy Otto, DVM, PhD, founder and executive director, Penn Vet Working Dog Center, University of Pennsylvania; Jennifer Essler, PhD, and Pat Kaynaroglu, Penn Vet Working Dog Center; Klaus Hackner, MD, Krems University Hospital, Austria; Glenn Ferguson, CancerDogs; Akiei Shibata, Kaneyama town clinic official; Masao Miyashita, MD, PhD, Nippon Medical School Chiba Hokusoh Hospital; Yuji Sato, St. Sugar Japan; Wataru and Sayoko Inoue; Hiroshi Suzuki, Kaneyama mayor; Eiko Tan; Tsuruko Chigahara; Keimi Miura; Kyoichi Seo, MD; Seitero and Sanae Miura; Andreas Mershin, PhD, research scientist and director, Label Free Research Group, Massachusetts Institute of Technology; and George Preti, PhD, analytical organic chemist, Monell Chemical Senses Center, Philadelphia.

"Japanese Say Cancer Victims Shouldn't Be Told." UPI, 3 April 1989. www.upi.com /Archives/1989/04/03/Japanese-say-cancer-victims-shouldnt-be-told/1020607579 200/.

Jezierski, Tadeusz, et al. "Study of the Art: Canine Olfaction Used for Cancer Detection on the Basis of Breath Odour. Perspectives and Limitations." *Journal of Breath Research* 9, no. 2 (June 2015): 027001, doi:10.1088/1752-7155/9/2/027001.

"KDOG Cancer Detect Group." Institut Curie. Accessed 11 July 2018. kdog.institut-curie .org/.

"Key Statistics for Ovarian Cancer." American Cancer Society, last modified 8 January 2019. www.cancer.org/cancer/ovarian-cancer/about/key-statistics.html.

Kitiyakara, Taya, et al. "The Detection of Hepatocellular Carcinoma (HCC) from Patients' Breath Using Canine Scent Detection: A Proof-of-Concept Study." *Journal of Breath Research* 11, no. 4 (13 September 2017): 046002, doi:10.1088/1752-7163/aa7b8e.

Kwak, Jae, et al. "Volatile Biomarkers from Human Melanoma Cells." *Journal of Chromatography B* 931 (15 July 2013): 90–96, doi:10.1016/j.jchromb.2013.05.007.

Lassya, Samhita, and Hans J. Gross. "The 'Clever Hans Phenomenon' Revisited." *Communicative & Integrative Biology* 6, no. 6 (November 2013), doi:10.4161/cib.27122.

McCulloch, Michael, et al. "Diagnostic Accuracy of Canine Scent Detection in Early- and Late-Stage Lung and Breast Cancers." *Integrative Cancer Therapies* 5, no. 1 (1 March 2006): 30–39, doi:10.1177/1534735405285096.

"Medical Detection Dogs Receive Green Light for First Canine Prostate Cancer Trial in UK." Medical Detection Dogs. Accessed 28 September 2018. www.medicaldetection

dogs.org.uk/medical-detection-dogs-receive-green-light-for-first-canine-prostate-cancer-trial-in-uk/.

Mikkelson, David. "Woman Became Pregnant from a Civil War Bullet?" Snopes, last modified 22 June 2014. www.snopes.com/fact-check/son-of-a-gun/.

Mukherjee, Siddhartha. *The Emperor of All Maladies: A Biography of Cancer* (New York: Scribner, 2010).

Onion, Amanda. "Dogs Being Trained to Detect Cancer." ABC News, 11 June 2002. abcnews.go.com/Technology/story?id=97979.

"Oregon Woman Says Cat Detected Her Breast Cancer." KXAN, 5 November 2018. www.kxan.com/news/national-news/oregon-woman-says-cat-detected-her-breast-cancer/1573751209.

Palmer, Richard. "Prince Charles and Camilla Meet Medical Experts with a Nose for Trouble." *Express*, 11 March 2014. www.express.co.uk/news/royal/464270/Prince-Charles-and-Camilla-meet-Medical-Detection-Dogs.

Pickel, Duane, et al. "Evidence for Canine Olfactory Detection of Melanoma." *Applied Animal Behaviour Science* 89, nos. 1–2 (November 2004): 107–116, doi:10.1016/j.applanim.2004.04.008.

Pirrone, Federica, and Mariangela Albertini. "Olfactory Detection of Cancer by Trained Sniffer Dogs: A Systematic Review of the Literature." *Journal of Veterinary Behavior* 19 (May–June 2017): 105–117, doi:10.1016/j.jveb.2017.03.004.

Pomerantz, Alan, et al. "The Possibility of Inventing New Technologies in the Detection of Cancer by Applying Elements of the Canine Olfactory Apparatus." *Medical Hypotheses* 85, no. 2 (August 2015): 160–172, doi:10.1016/j.mehy.2015.04.024.

"Regional Disparities of Cancer Incidence." *Chuokoron* (Japan) 6 (2016).

"Skin Fun Facts." Forefront Dermatology, 24 October 2017. forefrontdermatology.com/skin-fun-facts/.

Sonoda, Hideto, et al. "Colorectal Cancer Screening with Odour Material by Canine Scent Detection." *Gut* 60, no. 6 (31 January 2011): 814–819, doi:10.1136/gut.2010.218305.

Spector, Paul. "Canines and Cancer Detection: The New PET Scan?" *HuffPost*. 12 May 2015. www.huffpost.com/entry/dog-cancer-detection_n_7254746.

"The Strange Powers of Animals—Mysterious Universe 1994." YouTube video, 24:03, published by Sromba, 8 September 2015. https://youtu.be/_BC0vH0jrXY.

Taverna, Gianluigi, et al. "PD19-01 Prostate Cancer Urine Detection through Highly-Trained Dogs' Olfactory System: A Real Clinical Opportunity." *Journal of Urology* 191, no. 4s (April 2014), doi:10.1016/j.juro.2014.02.1520.

Taverna, Gianluigi, et al. "Sniffing Out Prostate Cancer: A New Clinical Opportunity." *Central European Journal of Urology* 68, no. 3 (15 October 2015), doi:10.5173/ceju.2015.593.

Walczak, Marta, et al. "Impact of Individual Training Parameters and Manner of Taking Breath Odor Samples on the Reliability of Canines as Cancer Screeners." *Journal of Veterinary Behavior* 7, no. 5 (September–October 2012): 283–294, doi:10.1016/j.jveb.2012.01.001.

Williams, Hywel, and Andres Pembroke. "Sniffer Dogs in the Melanoma Clinic?" *The Lancet* 333, no. 8640 (1 April 1989): 734, doi:10.1016/s0140-6736(89)92257-5.

Willis, Carolyn M., et al. "Olfactory Detection of Human Bladder Cancer by Dogs: Proof of Principle Study." *BMJ* 329 (23 September 2004), doi:10.1136/bmj.329.7468.712.

"You've Heard of the CAT Scan? Now, Here's the Dog Scan: Canine Helps with Cancer Detection." Imaginis, last modified 15 January 2001. www.imaginis.com/breast-health-news/you-146-ve-heard-of-the-cat-scan-now-here-146-s-the-dog-scan-canine-helps-with-cancer-detection-date-1.

CHAPTER 4: DOG, MD

Biagini, D., et al. "Determination of Volatile Organic Compounds in Exhaled Breath of Heart Failure Patients by Needle Trap Micro-Extraction Coupled with Gas Chromatography-Tandem Mass Spectrometry." *Journal of Breath Research* 11, no. 4 (30 November 2017): 047110, doi:10.1088/1752-7163/aa94e7.

Cikach, Frank S., and Raed A. Dweik. "Cardiovascular Biomarkers in Exhaled Breath." *Progress in Cardiovascular Diseases* 55, no. 1 (July–August 2012): 34–43, doi:10.1016/j.pcad.2012.05.005.

Coren, Stanley. "Beware the Howling Dog." *Modern Dog*. Accessed 29 October 2018. moderndogmagazine.com/articles/beware-howling-dog/42779.

Erlinger, Catherine. "The Health Benefits of Having a Dog." Heart Foundation, 9 March 2018. theheartfoundation.org/2018/03/09/the-health-benefits-of-having-a-dog/.

Faulkner, Lisa A. "Cardiac Alert Dog Saves Handler from Stroke." *Anything Pawsable*, 26 June 2013. www.anythingpawsable.com/cardiac-alert-dog-saves-handler-from-stroke/.

Finamore, P, et al. "Analysis of Volatile Organic Compounds: An Innovative Approach to Heart Failure Characterization in Older Patients." *Journal of Breath Research* 12, no. 2 (6 February 2018): 026007, doi:10.1088/1752-7163/aa8cd4.

Goodavage, Maria. *Soldier Dogs: The Untold Story of America's Canine Heroes* (New York: Dutton, 2012).

Hinton, William, et al. "Insulin Therapy in Type 3c Diabetes—More Common in Chronic Rather than Acute Pancreatitis." *Diabetes* 67, suppl. 1. July 2018. doi.org/10.2337/db18-1047-P.

Interviews with Deanne (DeeDee) Kramer; Nick and Tammy Blackford, North Coast K9; Tina Brassel; Alan Stryker; Mary McNeight, Service Dog Academy; "Kevin Turner," who asked me to use an alias, as explained in the book; and Paul and Vivian Willis.

Klein, Karin. "What Is Type 3c Diabetes?" A Sweet Life. 7 November 2017. asweetlife.org/what-is-type-3c-diabetes/.

Lee, Donovan. "Multi-Purpose Canine Program Proves Invaluable." DVIDS, 15 May 2015. www.dvidshub.net/news/167653/multi-purpose-canine-program-proves-invaluable.

Levine, Glenn N., et al. "Pet Ownership and Cardiovascular Risk." *Circulation* 127, no. 23 (9 May 2013): 2353–2363, doi:10.1161/cir.0b013e31829201e1.

Marcus, Dawn A., and Amrita Bhowmick. "Survey of Migraine Sufferers with Dogs to Evaluate for Canine Migraine-Alerting Behaviors." *Journal of Alternative and Complementary Medicine* 19, no. 6 (June 2013): 501–508, doi:10.1089/acm.2012.0234.

Miles, Otesa. "Migraine Statistics." Migraine.com, last modified November 2010. migraine.com/migraine-statistics/.

"The Strange Powers of Animals—Mysterious Universe 1994." YouTube video, 24:03, published by Sromba, 8 September 2015. https://youtu.be/_BC0vH0jrXY.

"The Top 10 Causes of Death." World Health Organization, 24 May 2018. www.who.int/news-room/fact-sheets/detail/the-top-10-causes-of-death.

"What Are the Ehlers-Danlos Syndromes?" Ehlers-Danlos Society. Accessed 19 May 2018. www.ehlers-danlos.com/what-is-eds/.

CHAPTER 5: FAINTING IN FRONT OF THE QUEEN

Centers for Disease Control and Prevention. "Sleep and Sleep Disorders." 5 June 2017, www.cdc.gov/sleep/about_us.html.

Dauvilliers, Y., and R. Lopez. "Narcolepsy with Cataplexy: Type 1 Narcolepsy." *La Revue du Praticien* 66, no. 6 (June 2016): 671–676. www.ncbi.nlm.nih.gov/pubmed/27538328.

Eckstein, Sandy. "Dogs and Cats Sleeping in Your Bed—Is It Healthy?" WebMD. Accessed September 2018. pets.webmd.com/features/pets-in-your-bed#1.

Engelhaupt, Erika. "You Can Smell When Someone's Sick—Here's How." *National Geographic*, 18 January 2018. news.nationalgeographic.com/2018/01/smell-sickness -parkinsons-disease-health-science/.

"From Nose to Diagnostics: Development of an Accessible Screening Platform for Early Diagnosis of Parkinson's Disease" (research grant, 2017). Michael J. Fox Foundation for Parkinson's Research. Accessed 5 November 2018. www.michaeljfox.org/found ation/grant-detail.php?grant_id=1672.

Hartley-Parkinson, Richard. "The Queen Met Some Life-Saving Dogs Today and She Loved It." *Metro* (UK), 6 June 2018. metro.co.uk/2018/06/06/queen-looks-super -excited-watches-life-saving-medical-detection-dogs-7609996/.

Interviews with Jodie and Jane Griffin; Lisa Holt, PADs for Parkinson's; Jack Bell, PhD, analytical chemist and professor, University of Washington; Jenny Corish, Medical Detection Dogs; Jamie Eberling, PhD, director of research programs, Michael J. Fox Foundation for Parkinson's Research; Danielle Brooks; Tonya Guy, Canine Partners for Life; and Mary Rose, PsyD, clinical associate professor, Baylor College of Medicine, and staff psychologist, TIRR Memorial Hermann.

Knapton, Sarah. "Dogs Could Sniff Out Parkinson's Disease Years before Symptoms Appear." *The Telegraph*, 9 July 2017. www.telegraph.co.uk/science/2017/07/09/dogs -could-sniff-parkinsons-disease-years-symptoms-appear/.

Mayo Clinic. "Are You Barking Up the Wrong Tree by Sleeping with Your Dog?" ScienceDaily. 7 September 2017. www.sciencedaily.com/releases/2017/09/170907144553 .htm.

McFadden, Joan. "Meet the Woman Who Can Smell Parkinson's Disease." *The Telegraph*, 19 December 2017. www.telegraph.co.uk/health-fitness/body/meet-woman-can -smell-parkinsons-disease/.

Miller, Jen A. "Out of the Doghouse, Into the Bed." *New York Times*, 13 March, 2018. www.nytimes.com/2018/03/13/well/family/dog-cat-pets-sleep-bed-insomnia .html.

"Narcolepsy." National Sleep Foundation. Accessed 24 July 2018. www.sleepfoundation .org/sleep-disorders-problems/narcolepsy-and-sleep.

"Narcolepsy Type 1." *Orphanet:* The Portal for Rare Diseases and Orphan Drugs, last modified October 2009. www.orpha.net/consor/cgi-bin/OC_Exp.php?Lng=EN&Expert=2073.

Patel, Salma I., et al. "The Effect of Dogs on Human Sleep in the Home Sleep Environment." *Mayo Clinic Proceedings* 92, no. 9 (September 2017), 1368–1372, doi:10.1016/j .mayocp.2017.06.014.

"Postural Orthostatic Tachycardia Syndrome." Dysautonomia International. Accessed 16 July 2018. www.dysautonomiainternational.org/page.php?ID=30.

"The Queen and the Duchess of Cornwall Meet Our Life-Saving Dogs." *The Sniff* 15 (November 2018): 8–9. www.medicaldetectiondogs.org.uk/sniff-magazine/.

Quigley, Elizabeth. "Scientists Sniff Out Parkinson's Disease Smell." BBC News, 18 December 2017. www.bbc.com/news/uk-scotland-42252411.

Rose, Mary, et al. "Dogs and Their Promising Roles in Sleep Disorders Therapy." *Sleep Review*, 22 June 2015. www.sleepreviewmag.com/2015/06/dogs-promising-roles -sleep-disorders-therapy/.

Sexton-Radek, Kathy. "A Look at Worldwide Sleep Disturbance." *Journal of Sleep Disorders & Therapy* 2, no. 3 (20 April 2013), doi:10.4172/2167-0277.1000115.

Slowik, Jennifer, and Allison Yow. *Narcolepsy* (Treasure Island, FL: StatPearls Publishing, 2018). www.ncbi.nlm.nih.gov/books/NBK459236/.

Williams, Glenn. "What's the Relationship Between Sleep and Headache?" *Neurology*

Reviews 18, no. 4 (April 2010): 7. www.mdedge.com/neurology/article/72601/sleep -medicine/whats-relationship-between-sleep-and-headache.

CHAPTER 6: HIDDEN ENEMIES

Ali, Naheed Shoukat. "Aldehydes." Fragrantica. Accessed 4 August 2018. www .fragrantica.com/notes/Aldehydes-165.html.

Angle, T. Craig, et al. "Real-Time Detection of a Virus Using Detection Dogs." *Frontiers in Veterinary Science* 2 (8 January 2016), doi:10.3389/fvets.2015.00079.

"The Basics of CF." Cystic Fibrosis Center at Stanford. Accessed 27 September 2018. med .stanford.edu/cfcenter/education/english/BasicsOfCF.html.

Bomers, M. K., et al. "Using a Dog's Superior Olfactory Sensitivity to Identify *Clostridium Difficile* in Stools and Patients: Proof of Principle Study." *BMJ* 345 (13 December 2012), doi:10.1136/bmj.e7396.

Branswell, Helen. "The Dogs Were Supposed to Be Experts at Sniffing Out C. Diff. Then They Smelled Breakfast." *STAT News*, 22 August 2018. www.yahoo.com/news /dogs-were-supposed-experts-sniffing-084025353.html.

Bryce, E., et al. "Identifying Environmental Reservoirs of *Clostridium Difficile* with a Scent Detection Dog: Preliminary Evaluation." *Journal of Hospital Infection* 97, no. 2 (October 2017): 140–145, doi:10.1016/j.jhin.2017.05.023.

Cafasso, Jacquelyn. "Pseudomonas Infections." *Healthline*, last modified 28 June 2016. www.healthline.com/health/pseudomonas-infections.

"*C. Difficile* Infection." Mayo Clinic, 18 June 2016. www.mayoclinic.org/diseases-conditions /c-difficile/symptoms-causes/syc-20351691.

"CDiff Smell?" Allnurses, 4 January 2007. allnurses.com/cdiff-smell-t145849/.

Centers for Disease Control and Prevention. "Malaria's Impact Worldwide." Last modi- fied 4 January 2019. www.cdc.gov/malaria/malaria_worldwide/impact.html.

Centers for Disease Control and Prevention. "Nearly Half a Million Americans Suffered from *Clostridium difficile* Infections in a Single Year." News release, 25 February 2015. www.cdc.gov/media/releases/2015/p0225-clostridium-difficile.html.

Cornwall, Warren. "Malaria Infection Creates a 'Human Perfume' That Makes Us More Attractive to Mosquitoes." *Science*, 16 April 2018. www.sciencemag.org/news/2018/04 /malaria-infection-creates-human-perfume-makes-us-more-attractive-mosquitoes.

"Cystic Fibrosis." Mayo Clinic, 13 October 2016. www.mayoclinic.org/diseases-conditions /cystic-fibrosis/symptoms-causes/syc-20353700.

Davies, J. C., et al. "P048 'Dr Dog' Will See You Now? First Steps in Assessing the Util- ity of Trained Sniffer Dogs to Detect *Pseudomonas Aeruginosa* (*Pa*) Airway Infec- tion in Non-Expectorating CF Patients." *Journal of Cystic Fibrosis* 17, supplement 3 (June 2018): S72–S73, doi:10.1016/s1569-1993(18)30345-x.

"Detecting and Treating Infection in Cystic Fibrosis." YouTube video, 17:51, published by Imperial College London, 28 July 2017. https://youtu.be/RHhH5_ZMzfI.

"Etymologia: *Clostridium difficile*." *Emerging Infectious Diseases* 16, no. 4 (April 2010): 674. https://wwwnc.cdc.gov/eid/article/16/4/e1-1604_article.

Gander, Kashmira. "Malaria Changes Humans' Scent, Making Them More Attractive to Mosquitoes." *Newsweek*, 17 April 2018. www.newsweek.com/malaria-attracts -mosquitos-human-perfume-888750.

Greenwood, Veronique. "Which Bacteria Smell Like Tortillas, Flowers, or Delicious Browned Butter?" *Discover*, 5 July 2012. blogs.discovermagazine.com/discoblog /2012/07/05/which-bacteria-smell-like-tortillas-flowers-or-delicious-browned -butter/#.XFR5Pc9Kg3F.

Interviews with Claire Guest, Jenny Corish, and a few biodetection dog trainers, Medical Detection Dogs; Craig Angle, PhD, codirector, Canine Performance Sciences,

College of Veterinary Medicine, Auburn University; Teresa Zurberg, Vancouver General Hospital; Diane Roscoe, MD, and Elizabeth Ann Bryce, MD, Division of Medical Microbiology and Infection Control, Vancouver General Hospital; James Logan, PhD, head, Department of Disease Control, London School of Hygiene & Tropical Medicine; and Steve Lindsay, PhD, public health entomologist, Durham University.

Jabbar, Umair, et al. "Effectiveness of Alcohol-Based Hand Rubs for Removal of Clostridium Difficile Spores from Hands." *Infection Control & Hospital Epidemiology* 31, no. 6 (June 2010): 565–570, doi:10.1086/652772.

Koivusalo, M., et al. "Canine Scent Detection as a Tool to Distinguish Meticillin-Resistant *Staphylococcus aureus*." *Journal of Hospital Infection* 96, no. 1 (9 March 2017): 93–95, doi:10.1016/j.jhin.2017.03.005.

Kumm, Jaklyn. "Classification of *Clostridium difficile*." Clostridium Difficile: A "Difficult" Human Pathogenic Bacterium (student website, University of Wisconsin–LaCrosse), last modified April 2009. bioweb.uwlax.edu/bio203/s2009/kumm_jakl/classification.htm.

Maurer, Maureen, et al. "Detection of Bacteriuria by Canine Olfaction." *Open Forum Infectious Diseases* 3, no. 2 (9 March 2016), doi:10.1093/ofid/ofw051.

Mwesigwa, Julia, et al. "On-Going Malaria Transmission in the Gambia Despite High Coverage of Control Interventions: A Nationwide Cross-Sectional Survey." *Malaria Journal* 14 (14 August 2015), doi:10.1186/s12936-015-0829-6.

O'Hare, Ryan. "Biosensors Detect Harmful Bugs in the Lungs of Cystic Fibrosis Patients." Imperial College London, 6 October 2017. www.imperial.ac.uk/news/182271/biosensors-detect-harmful-bugs-lungs-cystic/.

"Pseudomonas Aeruginosa." Science Direct. Accessed 17 August 2018. www.sciencedirect.com/topics/medicine-and-dentistry/pseudomonas-aeruginosa.

"'Remarkable Drop' in C. Difficile Infections at Canadian Hospitals." *Canadian Press*, 25 June 2018. www.cbc.ca/news/health/c-difficile-hospitals-cmaj-1.4720485.

Robinson, Ailie, et al. "*Plasmodium*-Associated Changes in Human Odor Attract Mosquitoes." *Proceedings of the National Academy of Sciences* 115, no. 18 (16 April 2018): E4209–E4218, doi:10.1073/pnas.1721610115.

Sawe, Benjamin Elisha. "The 50 US States Ranked by Population." *World Atlas*, last modified 14 September 2018. www.worldatlas.com/articles/us-states-by-population.html.

Smallegange, Renate C., et al. "Malaria Infected Mosquitoes Express Enhanced Attraction to Human Odor." *PLoS One* 8, no. 5 (15 May 2013), doi:10.1371/journal.pone.0063602.

"Strategic Research Centre: Personalised Approach to *Pseudomonas aeruginosa* (PAPA)." Cystic Fibrosis Trust. Accessed 12 October 2018. www.cysticfibrosis.org.uk/the-work-we-do/research/research-we-are-funding/strategic-research-centres/src-14-davies.

Taylor, Maureen T., et al. "Using Dog Scent Detection as a Point-of-Care Tool to Identify Toxigenic *Clostridium difficile* in Stool." *Open Forum Infectious Diseases* 5, no. 8 (August 2018), doi:10.1093/ofid/ofy179.

Yong, Ed. *I Contain Multitudes: The Microbes within Us and a Grander View of Life* (New York: Ecco, 2016).

CHAPTER 7: THE DOG WHISPERERS

Becker, Joanna L., et al. "Animal-Assisted Social Skills Training for Children with Autism Spectrum Disorders." *Anthrozoös* 30, no. 2 (16 May 2017): 307–326, doi:10.1080/08927936.2017.1311055.

Bergstrom, Ryan, et al. "Behavioral Intervention for Domestic Pet Mistreatment in a

Young Child with Autism." *Research in Autism Spectrum Disorders* 5, no. 1 (March 2011): 218–221, doi:10.1016/j.rasd.2010.04.002.

Berry, Alessandra, et al. "Use of Assistance and Therapy Dogs for Children with Autism Spectrum Disorders: A Critical Review of the Current Evidence." *Journal of Alternative and Complementary Medicine* 19, no. 2 (February 2013): 73–80, doi:10.1089 /acm.2011.0835.

Burrows, Kristen E., et al. "Factors Affecting Behavior and Welfare of Service Dogs for Children with Autism Spectrum Disorder." *Journal of Applied Animal Welfare Science* 11, no. 1 (2008): 42–62, doi:10.1080/10888700701555550.

Burrows, Kristen E., et al. "Sentinels of Safety: Service Dogs Ensure Safety and Enhance Freedom and Well-Being for Families with Autistic Children." *Qualitative Health Research* 18, no. 12 (27 October 2008): 1642–1649, doi:10.1177/1049732308327088.

Byström, Kristina M., and Cristina A. Lundqvist Persson. "The Meaning of Companion Animals for Children and Adolescents with Autism: The Parents' Perspective." *Anthrozoös* 28, no. 2 (9 December 2016): 263–275, doi:10.1080/08927936.2015.11435401.

Centers for Disease Control and Prevention. "Data & Statistics on Autism Spectrum Disorder." Last modified 15 November 2018. www.cdc.gov/ncbddd/autism/data .html.

Cole, Janet, et al. "Service Dog or Therapy Dog: Which Is Best for a Child with Autism?" *Autism Speaks*, 5 July 2016. www.autismspeaks.org/expert-opinion/service-dog-or -therapy-dog-which-best-child-autism.

Coren, Stanley. "How Therapy Dogs Almost Never Came to Exist." *Psychology Today*, 11 February 2013. www.psychologytoday.com/us/blog/canine-corner/201302/how -therapy-dogs-almost-never-came-exist.

Dufresne, Todd. *Killing Freud: Twentieth-Century Culture and the Death of Psychoanalysis* (New York: Continuum, 2006).

Grandgeorge, Marine, et al. "Does Pet Arrival Trigger Prosocial Behaviors in Individuals with Autism?" *PLoS One* 7, no. 8 (1 August 2012), doi:10.1371/journal.pone.0041739.

Harrison, Kelley, and Thomas Zane. "Is There Science Behind That? Autism Service Dogs." Association for Science in Autism Treatment. Accessed 19 December 2018. asatonline.org/for-parents/becoming-a-savvy-consumer/autism-service-dogs/.

Interviews with Christine LaMott; Alan Peters and Leslie Flowers, Can Do Canines; Angela Tseng, PhD, University of Minnesota; Damir Vučić and Lea Devčić, Croatian Guide Dog and Mobility Association; and Ira, Kosjenka, and Renato Petek.

Martin, François, and Jennifer Farnum. "Animal-Assisted Therapy for Children with Pervasive Developmental Disorders." *Western Journal of Nursing Research* 24, no. 6 (October 2002): 657–670, doi:10.1177/019394502320555403.

"Meeting Boris Levinson: Ellen's Passion for 'Pet Therapy.'" FriendshipWorks, 24 April 2014. www.fw4elders.org/ellens-introduction-to-pet-therapy/.

Silva, Karine, et al. "Can Dogs Prime Autistic Children for Therapy? Evidence from a Single Case Study." *Journal of Alternative and Complementary Medicine* 17, no. 7 (July 2011): 655–659, doi:10.1089/acm.2010.0436.

Snider, Kellie. "Tethering." Service Dog Central. Accessed 5 March 2018. www.servicedog central.org/content/node/80.

Viau, Robert, et al. "Effect of Service Dogs on Salivary Cortisol Secretion in Autistic Children." *Psychoneuroendocrinology* 35, no. 8 (September 2010): 1187–1193, doi:10.1016/j .psyneuen.2010.02.004.

CHAPTER 8: A HEARTBEAT AT MY FEET

Brewer, Warrick J., et al. "Olfactory Sensitivity through the Course of Psychosis: Relationships to Olfactory Identification, Symptomatology and the Schizophrenia

Odour." *Psychiatry Research* 149, nos. 1–3 (5 December 2006): 97–104, doi:10.1016/j
.psychres.2006.03.005.

Brooks, Helen, et al. "Ontological Security and Connectivity Provided by Pets: A Study
in the Self-Management of the Everyday Lives of People Diagnosed with a Long-
Term Mental Health Condition." *BMC Psychiatry* 16, no. 1 (9 December 2016),
doi:10.1186/s12888-016-1111-3.

Brooks, Helen Louise, et al. "The Power of Support from Companion Animals for People
Living with Mental Health Problems: A Systematic Review and Narrative Synthesis of the Evidence." *BMC Psychiatry* 18, no. 1 (5 February 2018), doi:10.1186
/s12888-018-1613-2.

D'Aniello, Biagio, et al. "Interspecies Transmission of Emotional Information via Chemosignals: From Humans to Dogs (*Canis lupus familiaris*)." *Animal Cognition* 21,
no. 1 (January 2018): 67–78, doi:10.1007/s10071-017-1139-x.

"GABLE SANDSTORM." Trackinfo. Accessed 9 July 2018. trackinfo.com/dog
.jsp?runnername=GABLE SANDSTORM.

Gilbert, Josiah Hotchkiss. *Dictionary of Burning Words of Brilliant Writers: A Cyclopedia of
Quotations* (New York: Treat, 1906): 567.

Greyt Hearts Service Dogs Inc. Accessed 6 July 2018. www.greythearts.org/.

Hrustic, Alisa. "Why Your Sweat Smells So Bad When You're Stressed." *Men's Health*,
4 April 2017. www.menshealth.com/health/a19544884/why-stress-sweat-smells-so
-bad/.

Interviews with Elizabeth and Sharon Horner; "Henry," Greyhound racing expert who
requested not to use his real name; JoAnn Turnbull, Handi-Dogs; Katharine "Kit"
and Amanda Heyser; Jennifer Cattet, PhD, Medical Mutts; Melanie and Molly
Wilson; and Mark Spivak, Comprehensive Pet Therapy.

Nikos-Rose, Karen. "Service Dogs Increasingly Used for Mental Health." UC Davis, 1
May 2017. www.ucdavis.edu/news/service-dogs-increasingly-used-mental-health/.

Nutt, Amy Ellis. "Why Kids and Teens May Face Far More Anxiety These Days." *Washington Post*, 10 May 2018. www.washingtonpost.com/news/to-your-health/wp/2018
/05/10/why-kids-and-teens-may-face-far-more-anxiety-these-days/.

"Pippin Took: The Lord of the Rings." *CharacTour: Everyone's a Character.* Accessed 10 July
2018. www.charactour.com/hub/characters/view/Pippin-Took.The-Lord-of-the
-Rings-The-Fellowship-of-the-Ring.

Shirasu, Mika, and Kazushige Touhara. "The Scent of Disease: Volatile Organic Compounds of the Human Body Related to Disease and Disorder." *Journal of Biochemistry* 150, no. 3 (1 September 2011): 257–266, doi:10.1093/jb/mvr090.

Siniscalchi, Marcello, et al. "The Dog Nose 'KNOWS' Fear: Asymmetric Nostril Use
during Sniffing at Canine and Human Emotional Stimuli." *Behavioural Brain Research* 304 (1 May 2016): 34–41, doi:10.1016/j.bbr.2016.02.011.

Temple, Emily. "Some Things You May Not Have Known about Edith Wharton's Dog
Obsession." *Literary Hub*, 14 January 2017, lithub.com/some-things-you-may-not
-have-known-about-edith-whartons-dog-obsession/.

Walther, Sandra, et al. "Assistance Dogs: Historic Patterns and Roles of Dogs Placed by
ADI or IGDF Accredited Facilities and by Non-Accredited U.S. Facilities." *Frontiers in Veterinary Science* 4 (19 January 2017), doi:10.3389/fvets.2017.00001.

Wisdom, Jennifer P., et al. "Another Breed of 'Service' Animals: STARS Study Findings
about Pet Ownership and Recovery from Serious Mental Illness." *American Journal
of Orthopsychiatry* 79, no. 3 (July 2009): 430–436, doi:10.1037/a0016812.

Wolfson, Jeanie. "Chemical in Sweat and Inability to Smell It May Be Schizophrenia
Marker." *Schizophrenia Daily News Blog*, 7 March 2017. www.schizophrenia.com
/sznews/archives/004743.html.

CHAPTER 9: AFTER THE WAR

Ash, Allison. "Veteran with PTSD Says Her Service Dog Didn't Help Her Anxiety, He Made It Worse." 10 News, 22 May 2017. www.10news.com/news/team-10/veteran -with-ptsd-says-her-service-dog-didnt-help-her-anxiety-he-made-it-worse.

Brulliard, Karin. "For Military Veterans Suffering from PTSD, Are Service Dogs Good Therapy?" *Washington Post*, 27 March 2018. www.washingtonpost.com/national /health-science/for-military-veterans-suffering-from-ptsd-are-service-dogs-good -therapy/2018/03/27/23616190-2ec1-11e8-b0b0-f706877db618_story.html.

Catholic Comedian: Judy McDonald. Accessed 6 July 2018. www.judymcdonald.net/index .html.

"Daisy 1." YouTube video, 2:31, published by Judy McDonald, 28 January 2013. https://youtu .be/0DLlzi1iXe8.

Doerr, Kevin, and Megan Huckaby. "NIH Funds PVM Study of Service Dogs' Effects on Veterans with PTSD." Purdue University College of Veterinary Medicine, 9 June 2017. vet.purdue.edu/newsroom/2017/170609-pvm-ptsd-research.php.

Ferdinando, Lisa. "DoD Releases Annual Report on Sexual Assault in Military." US Department of Defense, 1 May 2018. dod.defense.gov/News/Article/Article/1508127 /dod-releases-annual-report-on-sexual-assault-in-military/.

Georgia State University. "Service Dogs May Reduce Suicidal Impulses, Stress among Veterans." Medical Xpress, 17 July 2018. medicalxpress.com/news/2018-07-dogs -suicidal-impulses-stress-veterans.html.

Gross, Natalie. "Do Service Dogs Really Help with PTSD? A New Study Has Answers." *Reboot Camp*, 19 March 2018. rebootcamp.militarytimes.com/news/transi tion/2018/03/16/do-service-dogs-really-help-with-ptsd-a-new-study-has-answers/.

Houtert, Emmy A. E. Van, et al. "The Study of Service Dogs for Veterans with Post-Traumatic Stress Disorder: A Scoping Literature Review." *European Journal of Psychotraumatology* 9, supplement 3 (13 August 2018), doi:10.1080/20008198.2018.1 503523.

"How Common Is PTSD in Adults?" National Center for PTSD. Accessed 30 September 2018. www.ptsd.va.gov/understand/common/common_adults.asp.

Huckaby, Megan. "Study Shows Service Dogs Are Associated with Lower PTSD Symptoms among War Veterans." Purdue University, 8 February 2018. www.purdue.edu /newsroom/releases/2018/Q1/study-shows-service-dogs-are-associated-with-lower -ptsd-symptoms-among-war-veterans-.html.

Interviews with Steve Gagnon; Danielle Cockerham and Cece McConnell, Paws4People; several men and women incarcerated in West Virginia Division of Corrections and Rehabilitation prisons; a Marine veteran visiting the prison for canine selection; Wil Nobles; and Judy McDonald, Little Angels Service Dogs.

National Center for PTSD. Accessed March 2017. www.ptsd.va.gov/.

Nickel, Abbey. "Research Shows How Service Dogs Can Help Veterans with PTSD." Purdue University, 5 November 2018. www.purdue.edu/newsroom/releases/2018 /Q4/research-shows-how-service-dogs-can-help-veterans-with-ptsd.html.

O'Haire, Marguerite E., and Kerri E. Rodriguez. "Preliminary Efficacy of Service Dogs as a Complementary Treatment for Posttraumatic Stress Disorder in Military Members and Veterans." *Journal of Consulting and Clinical Psychology* 86, no. 2 (February 2018): 179–188, doi:10.1037/ccp0000267.

"PTSD: A Growing Epidemic." *NIH MedlinePlus* 4, no. 1 (Winter 2009). medlineplus .gov/magazine/issues/winter09/articles/winter09pg10-14.html.

"PTSD Statistics." PTSD United. Accessed 30 September 2018. www.ptsdunited.org /ptsd-statistics-2/.

Ramchand, Rajeev, et al. "Disparate Prevalence Estimates of PTSD among Service

Members Who Served in Iraq and Afghanistan: Possible Explanations." *Journal of Traumatic Stress* 23, no. 1 (February 2010): 59–68, doi:10.1002/jts.20486.

Robe, Mike, dir. *Within These Walls*, 2001. Lifetime Television.

Todd, Zazie. "Do Service Dogs Help Military Veterans with PTSD?" *Psychology Today*, 19 June 2018. www.psychologytoday.com/us/blog/fellow-creatures/201806/do-service-dogs-help-military-veterans-ptsd.

Yarborough, Bobbi Jo H., et al. "Benefits and Challenges of Using Service Dogs for Veterans with Posttraumatic Stress Disorder." *Psychiatric Rehabilitation Journal* 41, no. 2 (June 2018): 118–124, doi:10.1037/prj0000294.

CHAPTER 10: STAND BY ME

Blake, Eric S., and David A. Zelinsky. *Hurricane Harvey*. National Weather Service, 9 May 2018. www.nhc.noaa.gov/data/tcr/AL092017_Harvey.pdf.

Brooks, Helen Louise, et al. "The Power of Support from Companion Animals for People Living with Mental Health Problems: A Systematic Review and Narrative Synthesis of the Evidence." *BMC Psychiatry* 18, no. 1 (5 February 2018), doi:10.1186/s12888-018-1613-2.

Courthouse Dogs Foundation. Accessed 28 September 2018. courthousedogs.org/.

Ebert, Roger. Review of *Irreversible*. RogerEbert.com, 14 March 2003. www.rogerebert.com/reviews/irreversible-2003.

Hafner, Josh. "The Judge in the Larry Nassar Trial: Incredible Quotes to Victims and Their Abuser." *USA Today*, 24 January 2018. www.usatoday.com/story/news/nation-now/2018/01/24/judge-larry-nassar-trial-incredible-quotes-victims-and-their-abuser/1061691001/.

"How California's Most Destructive Wildfire Spread, Hour by Hour." *New York Times*, 21 October 2017. www.nytimes.com/interactive/2017/10/21/us/california-fire-damage-map.html.

Interviews with Ashley Vance, counselor, Small Talk Children's Assessment Center; Dan Cojanu, founder, Canine Advocacy Program; Celeste Walsen, DVM, executive director, Courthouse Dogs Foundation; Kelley Kostin, 52nd District Court judge, Oakland County, Michigan; Joan Hoerner; Jim Kelaher, MD; Pam Bertz, regional director, Pacific Southwest Region, Hope Animal-Assisted Crisis Response; Kathy Felix, volunteer, Hope Animal-Assisted Crisis Response; several fire victims at the Local Assistance Center, Santa Rosa, California.

Kindelan, Katie. "Meet Preston, the Therapy Dog Comforting Larry Nassar's Victims." ABC News, 22 January 2018. abcnews.go.com/US/meet-preston-therapy-dog-comforting-larry-nassars-victims/story?id=52522137.

"Kyle Stephens the First Victim to Address Larry Nassar at Sentencing." YouTube video, 3:19, published by MLive, 16 January 2018. https://youtu.be/Vkuj0IaeH3s.

"Larry Nassar Victims Speak Out Ahead of Sentencing | NBC News." YouTube video, 3:37:42, published by NBC News, 19 January 2018. https://youtu.be/2WUEmrBG6Zc.

Lass-Hennemann, Johanna, et al. "Therapy Dogs as a Crisis Intervention After Traumatic Events? An Experimental Study." *Frontiers in Psychology* 9 (15 October 2018), doi:10.3389/fpsyg.2018.01627.

Lundqvist, Martina, et al. "Patient Benefit of Dog-Assisted Interventions in Health Care: A Systematic Review." *BMC Complementary and Alternative Medicine* 17, no. 1 (10 July 2017), doi:10.1186/s12906-017-1844-7.

"Most Destructive California Wildfires in History: Camp Fire Tops the List." ABC7 News, 25 November 2018. abc7news.com/camp-fire-is-californias-most-destructive-wildfire/2516857/.

Preston's Guide to Court: A Fun and Informative Activity Book (Lansing, MI: Small Talk Children's Assessment Center, 2017).

"Remembering the Victims of the North Bay Fires." *Santa Rosa Press Democrat*, 27 December 2017. www.pressdemocrat.com/news/7808264-181/remembering-the -victims-of-the.

"Top 20 Most Destructive California Wildfires." Cal Fire, 8 February 2019. www.fire .ca.gov/communications/downloads/fact_sheets/Top20_Destruction.pdf.

EPILOGUE: BEDSIDE MANNER REDEFINED

Allela, Loïs, et al. "Ebola Virus Antibody Prevalence in Dogs and Human Risk." *Emerging Infectious Diseases* 11, no. 3 (March 2005): 385–390, doi:10.3201/eid1103.040981.

Angle, Craig, et al. "Canine Detection of the Volatilome: A Review of Implications for Pathogen and Disease Detection." *Frontiers in Veterinary Science* 3 (24 June 2016), doi:10.3389/fvets.2016.00047.

Blackwell, Michael. "Can You Really Get Ebola from Your Dog? (Op-Ed)." *LiveScience*, 1 November 2014. www.livescience.com/48574-can-you-get-ebola-from-your-dog .html.

Byrne, Ceara, et al. "Predicting the Suitability of Service Animals Using Instrumented Dog Toys." *Proceedings of the ACM on Interactive, Mobile, Wearable and Ubiquitous Technologies* 1, no. 4 (December 2017): 1–20, doi:10.1145/3161184.

Centers for Disease Control and Prevention. "Ebola (Ebola Virus Disease)." 22 May 2018. www.cdc.gov/vhf/ebola/transmission/index.html.

Gibbens, Sarah. "Can Old Dogs Learn New Tricks? New 'Brain Games' May Help Them Stay Young." *National Geographic*, 8 February 2018. news.nationalgeographic.com /2018/02/dog-cognitive-brain-games-touchscreen-lab-video-spd/.

Interviews with Melody Jackson, PhD, director, Animal-Computer Interaction Lab, Georgia Institute of Technology, and director, FIDO project; Thad Starner, PhD, wearable computing pioneer, founder and director, Contextual Computing Group, College of Computing, Georgia Tech; Claire Guest, cofounder and CEO, Medical Detection Dogs; Clara Mancini, PhD, founder and head, Animal-Computer Interaction (ACI) and Pervasive Interaction labs, Open University (UK); Craig Angle, PhD, codirector, Canine Performance Sciences, College of Veterinary Medicine, Auburn University; Patrick Hilverink, Royal Dutch Guide Dog Foundation; and Andreas Mershin, PhD, research scientist and director, Label Free Research Group, Massachusetts Institute of Technology.

Jackson, Melody M., et al. "FIDO—Facilitating Interactions for Dogs with Occupations: Wearable Communication Interfaces for Working Dogs." *Personal and Ubiquitous Computing* 19, no. 1 (January 2015): 155–173, doi:10.1007/s00779-014-0817-9.

Johnston-Wilder, Olivia, et al. "Sensing the Shape of Canine Responses to Cancer." *Proceedings of the 12th International Conference on Advances in Computer Entertainment Technology* (16–19 November 2015), doi:10.1145/2832932.2837017.

Mancini, Clara, et al. "Re-Centering Multispecies Practices." *Proceedings of the 33rd Annual ACM Conference on Human Factors in Computing Systems* (18–23 April 2015): 2673–2682, doi:10.1145/2702123.2702562.

Müller, Corsin A., et al. "Dogs Can Discriminate Emotional Expressions of Human Faces." *Current Biology* 25, no. 5 (March 2015): 601–605, doi:10.1016/j.cub.2014.12.055.

Robinson, Charlotte, et al. "Designing an Emergency Communication System for Human and Assistance Dog Partnerships." *Proceedings of the 2015 ACM International Joint Conference on Pervasive and Ubiquitous Computing* (7–11 September 2015): 337–347, doi:10.1145/2750858.2805849.

"Can Wearable Computing for Dogs Keep Humans Safer? | Melody Moore Jackson |

TEDxPeachtree." YouTube video, 18:26, published by TEDx Talks, 19 November 2014. https://youtu.be/aMuVpnUElMg.

Valentin, Giancarlo, et al. "Wearable Alert System for Mobility-Assistance Service Dogs." *Journal on Technology & Persons with Disabilities* 3 (2015): 184–203. scholarworks .csun.edu/bitstream/handle/10211.3/151196/JTPD-2015-p184.pdf.

Wallis, Lisa J., et al. "Utilising Dog-Computer Interactions to Provide Mental Stimulation in Dogs Especially during Ageing." *Proceedings of the Fourth International Conference on Animal-Computer Interaction* (21–23 November 2017), doi:10.1145 /3152130.3152146.

ACKNOWLEDGMENTS

I'd like to introduce you to a robot in Budapest. His name is Ethon, and he is being created in a university laboratory to behave more like a dog than a human. Ethon doesn't look like a dog or a human. At this stage of his development he looks a little more like a souped-up standing lawn mower.

If all goes as hoped, Ethon will soon be able to "listen" to someone and respond to simple requests. While he won't speak with words, he'll "talk" with subtle doglike body language and cute bio sounds. (Think R2-D2, only more birdlike.) Ethon's progeny may one day work in nursing homes and other senior care facilities. They'll be like therapy dogs but more autonomous, and available every day, maybe even around the clock.

Ethon shares his* laboratory with a robot dog, who was also built there. Life seemed to be going well for the robot dog, but then came the sad day when a real dog lifted his leg on him. The whiz sizzled his circuits, and now he sits in the laboratory, essentially dead.

If this book could have had more pages, you would have read about Ethon and the fried robot dog earlier in the book. I had written about them in a chapter that included the renowned researchers

---

*I realize Ethon is neither male nor female, but I could not call him "it." Since his name is close to Ethan, I've always thought of Ethon as male.

at the Family Dog Project, part of the ethology department at Eöt-vös Loránd University (ELTE). Ádám Miklósi, PhD, considered by many the father of canine cognition research, welcomed me into the fold for a few chilly November days in 2017, when I visited to learn more about how dogs think and sense the world—important information when it comes to future doctor dogs.

But because even the book you have in your hands now is significantly longer than my publisher had expected, something had to get cut. Actually, many stories—some fully written, some just drafted—ended up in book heaven. They were no less worthy than the others. The people in them are spectacularly interesting, and the dogs are skilled and devoted.

What follows is a list of the people who took time out of their busy lives to meet with me, tell their stories, and let me see their dogs at work, but who didn't make it into the main part of the book. I thank you all so much for the gift of your time. I will never forget your stories, and I may even find other places to tell some of them.

Besides Dr. Miklósi, others I met with in Budapest included Kálmán Czeibert, DVM; Enikö Kubinyi, PhD; Péter Pongrácz, PhD; Attila Andics, PhD; Márta Gácsi, PhD; Claudia Fugazza, PhD; Beáta Korcsok; Bence Ferdinandy, PhD; Tamás Faragó, PhD; and Levente Raj, PhD. Your work fascinates me, and it was a privilege to be able to see it in person, against the backdrop of the beautiful blue Danube.

Also a big part of the chopped chapter was neuroscientist Gregory Berns, PhD, and his Dog Project, at Emory University in Atlanta. I spent an afternoon there watching dogs happily walk into a loud MRI machine and lie down so researchers could get a better view of their brains while the dogs looked at various objects presented to them. Dr. Berns, it was a lot of fun, even if your peanut butter sandwich caused Mark Spivak to have to vacate the premises for a while.

Biological anthropologist and comparative psychologist Evan MacLean, PhD, runs the Canine Cognition Center at the University of Arizona. He's doing research into, among other things, whether dogs and their people experience an increase in oxytocin—often called the love or cuddle hormone, but much more complex—when they're with each other. I spent part of a day with him and his colleagues, and his adorable black Lab, Sisu.*

We decided to see if I had an oxytocin increase after hanging out on my own with Sisu. I gave saliva and urine samples before and after. Dr. MacLean also obtained saliva samples from Sisu. The results (which are not part of his study) were mixed, but apparently I liked spending time with Sisu better than she liked being petted and made googly talk to by a stranger. Dr. MacLean, thanks for humoring me! I look forward to following your research.

Brenda Kennedy, DVM, and the rest of the people I interviewed at Canine Companions for Independence in Santa Rosa, California, were gracious, informative, and generous with their time. CCI provides gorgeously trained assistance dogs free of charge. Originally I'd planned to include mobility assistance dogs in the book, but in the end, they were also a casualty of space constraints.

Derek Herrera was a MARSOC (US Marine Corps Forces Special Operations Command) captain who was shot in the spine by enemy fire while leading his team on patrol in the Helmand Province, Afghanistan, in 2012. Even though the ambush paralyzed him from the chest down, and one of his lungs had collapsed, he somehow continued to lead his Marines until the attackers were suppressed.

Derek received, among many awards, a Bronze Star for his heroism. He has accomplished so many seemingly impossible feats since his injury, and he is an inspiration to many people, including me. He has a service dog, Shaggy, who helps him with some mobility tasks, but mostly keeps him company. Derek, I'm so sorry I didn't get to tell your story in *Doctor Dogs*, but you deserve an entire book of your own. I hope you will find time to write it.

---

*Quiz time! If you read my book *Top Dog*, do you remember the meaning of the Finnish word *sisu*?

Shaggy had been a shelter dog and was rescued and trained by Mike Lorraine, of the CAMO foundation in South Florida. CAMO trains service dogs for disabled veterans at no cost to the vets. Mike also trained the dog of Matt Kleemann, a former Navy diver who was paralyzed from the chest down after a car accident. Matt and his dog, Charlie Brown, are a phenomenal team who now work with Mike. Matt and Mike, I enjoyed my time there, and thanks to you, I can now add to my résumé that I have trained chickens to peck at blue poker chips.

And now from Florida to Alaska. April Gettys founded Midnight Sun Service Dogs after going through some hellish times in her life. These days the Anchorage-area organization specializes in service dogs for veterans and active-duty military. April and her crew of volunteers have even trained a chocolate Lab named TOML (That Others May Live) to help mitigate PTSD and combat stress, anxiety, and depression for members of Alaska's Air National Guard's 212th Rescue Squadron. As I write this, TOML is back from his second deployment and apparently knocked it out of the ballpark again.

When I thought I was going to be writing about service dog law in this book, I contacted a few people for interviews, including Chris Diefenthaler, operations manager for Assistance Dogs International. Thanks for your help, Chris. Even though I didn't write about it in the book, our talks helped inform me on this important topic.

Once upon a time, Kim Denton had a dedicated diabetic-alert dog named Hatcher. I met them and was touched by the way Hatcher was always gently looking after Kim. Horribly, Hatcher was subsequently attacked on two occasions by random dogs, and this sweet, sensitive guy no longer felt comfortable or secure outside Kim's home or office. He stopped alerting in public.

Kim made the selfless decision to give him up to a boy who needed a diabetic-alert dog in his home only. She said it was like giving up a child. It took a while for Dogs4Diabetics to match her with another dog, but they did a great job, and her handsome new dog, Troy, has become a top-notch medical alert dog and best friend. (Hatcher is happy in his home and loves his boy, and his boy and family love him right back.) Kim, I hope to meet Troy in person soon!

I can feel my editor giving me the "wrap it up with this part of the acknowledgments" cue from afar (this happens after four books together), so I'm going to quickly mention the last four big stories that didn't make it into the book: Onyx and his amazing young woman, Bailey Bish, of Tucson; the Winokur family of the Atlanta area and their hard-working dog, Quinn (Donnie, thank you for spending all that time with me; you are a gem, and your book, *Chancer,* is lovely); the Martins family of Atlanta, with their adorable "dynamic duo" of Alex and Blue; and Tara Bedford, of Chipping Norton, England, and her dear dog, Willow.

I usually thank almost everyone who appears in my books by name in the acknowledgments. They deserve to be called out individually. But I'm not going to be able to do that this time, because 1) there are so many more people in this book than my others; and 2) I just mentioned most of the people whose stories didn't make it, and that took up valuable book real estate.

Instead, I'm going to do it this way: If you are in this book, I greatly appreciate that you took the time to talk to me, share your stories, and welcome me into your lives and homes and laboratories. You are special to me, and I enjoyed each and every one of you, and I hope we will keep in touch.

I'm especially grateful to Claire Guest of Medical Detection Dogs and Cindy Otto of the Penn Vet Working Dog Center for letting me spend days watching amazing dogs and trainers at work. And to Masao Miyashita, *arigato gozaimashita* for your kindness and generosity of spirit in helping me navigate my complex but greatly enjoyable trip to Japan. I feel that I have not only gained three stellar colleagues but three friends as well.

Speaking of Japan, I want to thank Keimi Miura for her role in helping arrange interviews with some of the good people of

Kaneyama. And a big thank-you to Mayor Hiroshi Suzuki and other town leaders for welcoming me so warmly. Kaneyama calls my name, so I hope we will all meet again.

I would also like to thank Tomoko Otake, an excellent, longtime reporter at the *Japan Times*, for her assistance in helping me locate a source for the book when it was proving impossible to do so in English. This opened doors that enriched the story.

Back in August 2017, I attended the Canine Science Conference, at Arizona State University. The conference—the first of its kind in the United States—was a gargantuan undertaking for coordinator Clive Wynne, whom you briefly met in the introduction.

Ta-Hsuan Ong, PhD, of MIT Lincoln Laboratory, gave a presentation called "Supporting Explosive-Detection Canine Training with the Help of a Real-Time Trace Vapor Detection Mass Spectrometer." Right up my alley. He and I talked afterward, and we kept in touch about mass spectrometry and dogs. He introduced me to Matthew Staymates, PhD, who ended up mailing me the dog nose you encountered in the very first sentence of this book.

So thank you, Dr. Ong. Without this, I would probably still be figuring out how to begin the book.

And Jeff and Jess, without you to watch Gus during some of my interminably long writing days, I'd still be on Chapter 1. As I type this, he is waiting at the door for you to pick him up.

Patty Stansfield Tarbox and Jack O'Mara, your encouragement of my pursuing writing or journalism way back when I was a kid in Maine was instrumental in my career choice. And Glenn Tremblay, you helped stoke my fascination with science, which came in handy in this book. Teachers deserve so much thanks for the work they do but rarely get it. So thank you! (And if this book tanks, you can say, "Who is that crazy lady? I never taught her!")

This is my fourth book with Dutton executive editor Stephen Morrow. Stephen, as always, it has been an incredible journey and a joy to work with you—even as you wielded the ax to parts of the book. Your intelligence, enthusiasm, and eye and ear for stories helped me maintain a steady course on our most challenging book yet. I also appreciated Stephen's fantastic editorial assistants, Maddy Newquist and Hannah Feeney, who helped keep us both on track.

Also terrific to have on Team *Doctor Dogs* were ace copy editor Mary Beth Constant, book jacket designer extraordinaire Steve Meditz, and friend and fellow writer Erin Van Rheenen, who helped me locate the delightfully colorful Dr. Hywel Williams when I was too busy traveling for research to do so. As always I am grateful for my wonderful agents, Carol Mann and Deirdre Mullane.

And then there's Sam Barry, who has worked in the world of books for much of his career. After I completed the bulk of my travels and interviews, I brought Sam on as a sort of editorial consultant because the amount of material felt overwhelming. I needed someone who would hold me accountable on a regular basis—someone local I could meet with over coffee, who could help me hash out ideas and see the forest for the trees. Sam, thank you. Your humor and keen editorial sense took me from deer-in-the-headlights to horse-cantering-in-the-meadow. Or something like that.

I extend a big, heartfelt thank-you to friends and family for once again patiently waiting for me as I took the deepest plunge yet into a book. I'll call out just a smattering here:

Tammi Goldstein, for your friendship and support, and for joining me on my taiko journey just when I needed to hit something hard and have fun doing it. (I'm sorry Dr. Benji didn't make it into the book. Wait—he just did!) And San Francisco Taiko Dojo, thanks for welcoming me aboard the taiko train with open, bachi-wielding arms and calloused hands. Tuesday City rocks! (No diggity!)

Catherine Oenbrink, for being my great buddy since we met in scuba class in our twenties. And for making me mostly work instead of mostly play when I visited you in Florida this year and was met with an unexpected *Doctor Dogs* deadline. You earned that frozen yogurt.

Scott Eyman and Lynn Kalber, for being there.

Heike Eilers, Colleen Wentworth, Jacquie Steiner, Ann Dages, Sean M., Sally Deneen, and Liz Genolio, because it takes a village.

Naomi Fujimori Castro, for your help getting my vocabulary and cultural skills tuned up for my visit to Japan and for introducing me to the "joys" of natto.

Christina Ketchum Georgiou, because who else would take me on a Danube dinner cruise in Budapest to get my equilibrium back after I watched a deceased dog's brain taken out of her head? Where will our next adventure take us?

David Rosenfelt, for your dry wit and drier wisdom, and because you write something like a thousand books a year and make it look easy.

Gus's "dad," Craig Hanson, for doggedly reading the manuscript as the clock ticked.

My fun-loving Italian relatives who put me up during my travels to Italy: in Cassino, Franca DeMagistris and family, including my delightful *nipote*, Anna Laura; and in Rome, cousin Valeria Mancone, and her mom, sister, other cousins, and her adorable daughter, Nicole, with whom it is fun to brush teeth.

My shipmates at US Coast Guard Auxiliary flotilla 1-2, Station Golden Gate, for being so understanding about my going semi-AWOL during my travels and the most intensive writing months. *Semper Gumby!*

And finally, to Gus, and all the other dogs in this book. I would thank you all by name, but since most of you can't read, that would be pointless. But you are amazing, special creatures, and I am lucky to have you in this book and in my life.

INDEX